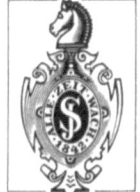

F. Wachsmann G. Drexler

Graphs and Tables for Use in Radiology
Kurven und Tabellen für die Radiologie
Graphiques et Tables pour la Radiologie
Gráficas y Tablas para Radiología

With the collaboration of – Unter Mitarbeit von

Avec la collaboration de – Con la colaboración de

K. Bunzl M. Busch H. Czempiel J. David M. Gossrau
G. Grünauer R. G. Jaeger H. L. Keller H. Oeser W. Panzer
H. Paretzke K. R. Trott L. Widenmann

Second completely revised and enlarged edition
Zweite, völlig neu bearbeitete und erweiterte Auflage
Deuxième édition revisée et completée
Segunda edición totalmente revisada y aumentada

Springer-Verlag Berlin Heidelberg New York 1976

Professor Dr.-Ing. Felix Wachsmann

Dr.-Ing. Günter Drexler

Institut für Strahlenschutz
Gesellschaft für Strahlen- und Umweltforschung mbH,
8042 Neuherberg bei München

Titel der ersten Auflage: Kurven und Tabellen für die Strahlentherapie
© S. Hirzel Verlag, Stuttgart 1957

ISBN-13: 978-3-642-67898-1   e-ISBN-13: 978-3-642-67896-7
DOI: 10.1007/978-3-642-67896-7

Library of Congress Cataloging in Publication Data. Wachsmann, Felix, 1904-. Graphs and tables for use in radiology = Kurven und Tabellen für die Radiologie. First ed. (c 1957) published under title: Kurven und Tabellen für die Strahlentherapie. Text in English, French, German, and Spanish. Bibliography: p. Includes index. 1. Radiology, Medical-Tables. I. Drexler, Günter, 1935-, joint author. II. Title. III. Title: Kurven und Tabellen für die Radiologie. R895.W3 1976 616.07'57'0212 76-14437

© by Springer-Verlag Berlin Heidelberg 1976
Softcover reprint of the hardcover 2nd edition 1976

The authors wish to thank:
Die Verfasser danken:
Les auteurs remercient:
Los autores agradecen a:

For valuable suggestions and for the translation of the texts into
English, French, and Spanish
Für wertvolle Anregungen und die Übersetzung der Texte ins Englische,
Französische und Spanische
Pour leurs précieuses suggestions et pour leurs traductions en ang-
lais, français et espagnol
Por sus valiosas sugestiones y la traducción de los textos al Inglés,
Francés y Espagnol

        M. Cohen, Montreal; Mrs. E. Lanzl, Chicago
        Mme A. Dutreix, Paris
        R.D. Perches, Mexico City; M.D. Reboiras, Madrid;

for the typing of the text, the drawings, and the photographic work,
für das Schreiben des Textes, das Zeichnen der Graphiken und die Er-
ledigung der Fotoarbeiten
pour la dactylographie du texte, les dessins, et le travail photogra-
phique,
por la escritura del texto, diagramas, y el trabajo de fotografiado,

        K. Semmelmann, I. Zink, I. Schellmann;

for making possible the work performed at the Gesellschaft für Strah-
len- und Umweltforschung mbH Munich, the scientific director
für die Ermöglichung der Arbeiten bei der Gesellschaft für Strahlen-
und Umweltforschung mbH München ihrem Wissenschaftlichen Geschäftsfüh-
rer,
pour avoir rendu possible le travail effectué au Gesellschaft für
Strahlen- und Umweltforschung mbH Munich, son directeur scientifique
por hacer posible le realización del trabajo en la Gesellschaft für
Strahlen- und Umweltforschung mbH Munich a su director scientifico

        R. Wittenzellner;

for the publication of the book, and for its responsiveness to our
wishes, the
für die Herausgabe und das verständnisvolle Eingehen auf unsere Wünsche dem
pour la publication et pour la compréhension de nos désirs
por la publicación, y comprensión de a nuestros deseos

        Springer-Verlag, Heidelberg

Foreword

The first edition of this book was published more than 15 years ago and created considerable interest among radiotherapists and medical physicists. The present new edition takes into consideration the latest scientific developments. It is a completely revised version and the information included has been considerably expanded. The presentation of the material in different languages and in the form of adjacent tables and diagrams is of particular value because it enables the reader to choose the presentation he prefers.

Whereas the data in the first edition were mainly related to radiotherapy, the new edition also includes information on nuclear medicine, X-ray diagnosis, radiation protection, and biomedical findings.

I hope that this book will be of value to a wide range of readers throughout the world and I am convinced that its use in daily work will contribute considerably to the badly needed improvement in the medical applications of ionizing radiation.

Professor Dr. W. Seelentag
Chief Medical Officer, Radiation Medicine
World Health Organization, Geneva

Vorwort

Die vor mehr als 15 Jahren erschienene 1. Auflage des vorliegenden Buches hatte bei Strahentherapeuten und medizinischen Physikern großen Anklang gefunden. Die vorliegende Neuauflage wurde auf den neuesten Stand des Wissens gebracht, völlig neu bearbeitet und im Informationsgehalt wesentlich erweitert. Der besondere Wert des Buches liegt wiederum in der Mehrsprachigkeit und der parallelen Darstellung in Kurven und Tabellen, welche dem Leser erlauben, die ihm zusagende Darstellungsform zu benutzen.

Zu den in der 1. Auflage enthaltenen Kurven und Tabellen, die vorzugsweise auf die Strahlentherapie ausgerichtet waren, sind Abschnitte über Nuklearmedizin, Röntgendiagnostik und den Strahlenschutz hinzugekommen, sowie schließlich ein Abschnitt mit Zahlenangaben über allgemeine biologisch-medizinische Erkenntnisse.

Ich wünsche dem Buch eine gute Aufnahme in der ganzen Welt und bin davon überzeugt, daß sein Gebrauch in der täglichen Arbeit wesentlich zur dringend erforderlichen Verbesserung der medizinischen Strahlenanwendungen beitragen wird.

Professor Dr. W. Seelentag
Leiter der Abteilung Strahlenmedizin der
Weltgesundheitsorganisation, Genf

Publiées pour la première fois il y a une quinzaine d'années, les
"Courbes et Tables de Radiothérapie" ont suscité un très grand inté-
rêt parmi les radiothérapeutes et les radiophysiciens. Depuis, les
connaissances scientifiques ont beaucoup progressé, rendant nécessaire une mise à jour. Le présent volume contient donc une version
complètement remaniée et complétée du texte précédent. La somme d'informations qui y figure est plus vaste que dans la première édition,
et on retrouve dans la présente version un des grands avantages de
la première, c'est-à-dire la présentation en plusieurs langues et
des tables et courbes côte à côte, ce qui permet au lecteur de choi-
sir la présentation qui lui convient le mieux.

Alors que la première édition était essentiellement consacrée à la
radiothérapie, la nouvelle contient également des chapitres sur la
médecine nucléaire, le radiodiagnostic et la radioprotection, ainsi
que sur des données biomédicales générales.

J'espère que ce livre pourra être utile à une très large gamme d'
utilisateurs dans le monde et je suis convaincu qu'il contribuera,
dans la pratique quotidienne, à l'amélioration tant souhaitable des
applications médicales des rayonnements ionisants.

Professeur Dr. W. Seelentag
Médecin Chef, Section de Médecine radiologique
Organisation Mondiale de la Santé, Genève

La primera edición del presente libro, aparecida hace más de 15
años, ha encontrado gran aceptación entre los radioterapeutas y fí-
sico-médicos. La presente edición ha sido puesta al día al nivel de
los conocimientos actuales, totalmente refundida y sensiblemente
aumentada en el contenido de sus materias. Por otro lado, el libro
posee un valor especial al estar presentado en varios idiomas y
ofrecer paralelamente representaciones gráficas y tablas que permiten al lector elegir la forma que más le convenga.

Además de las curvas y tablas de la 1ª edición, principalmente
orientadas a la radioterapia, se incluye en esta, información sobre
medicina nuclear, diagnóstico por rayos X y protección radioactiva,
asi como una sección al final dedicada a datos numéricos sobre conocimientos generales de biomedicina.

Deseo que el libro alcance una buena acogida en todo el mundo y
estoy convencido de que su manejo en el trabajo diario contribuirá
apreciablemente a la urgente y necesaria mejora de las aplicaciones
médicas de la radiación.

Profesor Dr. W. Seelentag
Director del Departamento de Medicina radiologica
de la Organización Mundial de la Salud, Ginebra

Table of contents

Detailed tables of contents can be found at the beginning of each section on the pages listed below:

Inhaltsverzeichnis

Die aufgegliederten Inhaltsverzeichnisse befinden sich am Anfang der einzelnen Abschnitte auf den nachstehend genannten Seiten:

Table des matières

Les tables des matières détaillées se trouvent au commencement de
chaque chapitre sur les pages suivantes:

Tabla de materias

Las tablas de materias detalladas se encuentran en el comienzo de
cada capítulo en las páginas que se indican:

Table of contents - Inhaltsverzeichnis
Table des matières - Tabla de materias

1.1 Editors' Comments

In this book, the numerical data needed by the radiologist and radiation physicist are given in the form of graphs and tables:

Graphic representations were chosen when it was important primarily to show the relationship between variables. Graphs have the additional advantages of providing information rapidly and of making available any desired intermediate values.

Tables, on the other hand, provide specific values with greater speed and reliability, and often with greater precision than graphs. For many topics in which not only a representation by curves, but also the easy availability of particular numbers was important, graphs and tables were placed side by side.

The accuracy of the tables was chosen to correspond to practical needs. We avoided the use of uncertain decimal places which would give the impression of pseudoaccuracy. In particular cases where it was impossible to give precise values, we used the designation "average or approximate values". If numbers cited in the literature were not in agreement, a critical selection of the most probable values according to our present knowledge was made. Special attention was paid to making the values given in the various graphs and tables compatible to facilitate comparison. Uncertain values were indicated in the graphs by dotted lines and in the tables, by parentheses.

The material was chosen in such a way that the data needed in daily practice are as complete as possible. Due to the limitations of the length of the book, however, this goal could not be attained perfectly. In addition, we included some material in which general relationships can be recognized qualitatively, and which may be of interest to those users of the graphs and tables who need information on related subjects.

The literature cited under the individual subjects is by no means complete. Instead, particularly those reports and textbooks were selected from which additional information can be obtained. Unfortunately it was impossible to have English-American, German, French, and Spanish literature represented equally.

The texts for the graphs and tables are given in four languages. The resulting space limitations forced us to use brief formulations; we hope that these are always clear. In exceptional cases, especially in some tables, only English, or Latin for medical terms, was used when this seemed possible without creating linguistic problems.

Some difficulties arose, for example, the marking of decimal fractions by periods or commas or, in the English text, the use of British or American spelling; we consistently used the British form. If we have not succeeded in satisfying all demands, we ask the reader's forbearance.

The Editors

1.1 Bemerkungen der Herausgeber

Das vom Radiologen und Strahlenphysiker benötigte Zahlenmaterial ist
im vorliegenden Buch in Kurven und Tabellen wiedergegeben:

Graphische Darstellungen wurden dort gewählt, wo es vor allem darauf
ankam, den Verlauf von Zusammenhängen zu zeigen. Diese bieten darüber
hinaus den Vorteil einer schnellen Information und daß aus ihnen be-
liebige Zwischenwerte abgelesen werden können.

Tabellen dagegen lassen Einzelwerte schneller, sicherer und oft ge-
nauer ablesen als Kurven. Bei vielen Themen, bei denen es sowohl auf
die Darstellung des Verlaufes als auch auf die bequeme Ablesbarkeit
von Einzelwerten ankam, wurden Kurven und Tabellen nebeneinander ge-
stellt.

Die Genauigkeit der angegebenen Werte ist so gewählt, daß sie prak-
tischen Bedürfnissen entspricht. Es wurde vermieden, durch Angabe
nicht gesicherter Dezimalstellen eine Pseudogenauigkeit vorzutäuschen.
Bei einzelnen Darstellungen, bei denen genaue Werte anzugeben unmög-
lich ist, wurde dies durch den Vermerk "Richtwerte" gekennzeichnet.
Wenn in der Literatur voneinander abweichende Werte genannt sind,
wurden die nach unserem heutigen Wissen wahrscheinlichsten kritisch
ausgewählt bzw. Mittelwerte gebildet. Es wurde besonders darauf ge-
achtet, daß die in den verschiedenen Kurven und Tabellen genannten
Werte miteinander vergleichbar sind. Unsichere Werte wurden in den
graphischen Darstellungen durch gestrichelte Linien und in den Tabellen dadurch gekennzeichnet, daß die Zahlenwerte in Klammern gesetzt
wurden.

Die Auswahl des Stoffes erfolgte so, daß die in der täglichen Praxis
benötigten Angaben möglichst vollständig aufgenommen wurden. Mit
Rücksicht auf den Umfang des Buches ließ sich dieses Ziel leider nicht
vollständig erreichen. Darüber hinaus wurden aber auch einige Darstellungen gebracht, die allgemeine Zusammenhänge qualitativ erkennen
lassen und für die Benutzer der Kurven und Tabellen von Interesse sein
mögen, um sich über Randgebiete zu informieren.

Die bei den einzelnen Themen angegebene Literatur ist keineswegs vollständig! Es wurden vielmehr bevorzugt nur solche Arbeiten und Lehr-
bücher zitiert, aus denen weitere Informationen entnommen werden können. Dabei konnte die deutsche, englisch-amerikanische, französische
und spanische Literatur leider nicht gleichmäßig berücksichtigt werden.

Die Kurven und Tabellen sind grundsätzlich viersprachig beschriftet.
Der hierdurch bedingte Platzbedarf hat zu knappen Formulierungen ge-
zwungen, die hoffentlich immer verständlich sind. Nur in Ausnahmefäl-
len, d.h. besonders in einigen Tabellen, wurde dort, wo dies möglich
erschien, ohne sprachliche Schwierigkeiten aufkommen zu lassen, nur
englisch bzw. bei medizinischen Ausdrücken lateinisch beschriftet.

Schwierigkeiten ergaben sich auch z.B. bezüglich der Kennzeichnung
von Dezimalbrüchen durch Punkt oder Komma oder im Englischen bezüglich der englischen oder amerikanischen Schreibweise; wir wählten ein-
heitlich die englische. Wenn wir dabei nicht alle Wünsche erfüllt haben, bitten wir um Nachsicht.

                                                    Die Verfasser

1.1 Commentaires des editeurs

Dans ce livre, les valeurs numériques nécessaires aux radiologistes et aux radiophysiciens sont données sous la forme de graphiques et de tables:

La représentation graphique a été choisie chaque fois qu'il a paru surtout important de montrer les relations entre variables. Les graphiques présentent en outre l'avantage de fournir rapidement les informations et de faciliter la détermination pour des valeurs intermédiaires des variables.

Les tables, d'autre part, fournissent des valeurs en des points spécifiques, plus rapidement, de façon plus fiable et souvent avec une plus grande précision que les graphiques. Dans de nombreux cas, pour lesquels la représentation graphique, mais également la disponibilité de valeurs numériques est importante, les graphiques et les tables ont été placés l'un à côté de l'autre.

La précision des valeurs a été choisie en fonction des besoins pratiques. Nous avons évité d'utiliser des décimales qui donneraient une impression de pseudoprécision. Dans les cas particuliers où il est impossible de donner des valeurs précises, nous avons utilisé l'expression "valeurs moyennes" ou "valeurs approchées". Lorsque les valeurs citées dans la littérature ne sont pas en accord, une sélection critique des valeurs les plus probables suivant l'état actuel de nos connaissances, a été effectuée. On s'est assuré tout spécialement de la compatibilité des valeurs données dans les différents tableaux et graphiques afin de faciliter les comparaisons. Les valeurs qui ne sont pas très sûres sont indiquées dans les graphiques par des lignes pointillées et dans les tables par des parenthèses.

Le choix a été fait de façon à ce que les données nécessaires dans la pratique quotidienne soient aussi complètes que possible. Cependant, du fait de la limite imposée à la taille de ce livre, ce but n'a pu être atteint parfaitement. En outre, nous avons ajouté quelques données montrant les relations générales qualitatives et pouvant être utiles aux lecteurs qui recherchent des informations sur des sujets en rapport avec ceux traités dans les tables et les graphiques.

Les références bibliographiques citées ne sont en aucune façon complètes. Au contraire on a choisi seulement les rapports et les livres dans lesquels des informations supplémentaires pouvaient être trouvées. Malheureusement il a été impossible de représenter également les littératures française, anglaise, américaine, allemande et espagnole.

Les textes accompagnant les graphiques et les tables sont donnés en quatre langues. En conséquence, l'espace a été très limité et nous avons été obligés d'utiliser des expressions très simples. Dans quelques cas exceptionnels, spécialement dans certaines tables, seul l' Anglais ou le Latin a été utilisé. Nous espérons qu'elles sont néanmoins toujours claires. Nous avons rencontré quelques difficultés: par exemple, la séparation des fractions décimales par des points ou des virgules, ou encore, le choix entre les orthographes britanniques ou américaines; nous avons toujours choisi la forme britannique. Nous demandons l'indulgence du lecteur si nous n'avons pas réussi à satisfaire à toutes des demandes.

Les Editeurs

1.1 Notas de los editores

El presente libro ofrece en curvas y tablas, los datos numéricos que necesitan el radiólogo y el radio-físico.

Las representeciones gráficas se eligieron cuando se consideró apropiado poner de manifiesto la dependencia continua entre variables. Estas ofrecen, además de la ventaja de una rápida información, la posibilidad de lectura de valores intermedios.

Las tablas, por el contrario, permiten leer valores particulares de forma más rápida, segura y exacta que en las curvas. En muchos temas, en los cuales hubo que atender tanto a la representación gráfica como a la lectura cómoda de una magnitud, se ofrecen las curvas y tablas unas al lado de las otras.

La exactitud de los valores se ha elegido de forma que corresponda a las necesidades prácticas. Se ha querido evitar el hacer creer en una pseudoexactitud dando cifras decimales que no son seguras. En casos particulares, en los que es imposible dar valores exactos, se indicaron estos mediante la notación "valores estimativos". En el caso de valores que se encuentran en la literatura y se desvian entre si, se eligieron con criterio crítico los más probables, de acuerdo con nuestros conocimientos actuales, o se estimaron los valores medios. Se ha puesto especial cuidado en que los valores indicados en diferentes curvas y tablas sean comparables entre si. Los valores inseguros se indicaron en la representaciones gráficas mediante líneas articuladas y en las tablas poniendolos entre paréntesis.

En la elección de la temática se tuvo en cuenta que estuvieran recogidos de forma lo más completa posible los datos necesarios en la práctica diaria. Este fin, por desgracia, no se ha podido alcanzar totalmente en consideración a la extensión del libro. Además se incluyen algunas gráficas en las que se recogen relaciones generales cualitativas y que son de interés para el manejo de las curvas y tablas, para informarse sobre cuestiones adicionales.

La literatura indicada para cada tema particular no es de ninguna forma exhaustiva! Se prefirió mucho antes citar solamente aquellos trabajos y tratados, que puedan proporcionar informaciones más amplias.

Las curvas y tablas llevan una leyenda en cuatro idiomas; por ello, las disponibilidades de espacio nos han obligado a formulaciones abreviadas que esperamos resulten siempre comprensivas. Unicamente en casos escepcionales, concretamente en algunas tablas, se escribió solo inglés, o latin en expresiones médicas, pero unicamente en aquellos casos en que ha sido posible sin crear dificultades de comprensibilidad.

Dificultades han surgido también por ejemplo en lo referente a la utilización del punto o la coma en los números decimales o en las formas de expresión inglesas o americanas; nosotros hemos elegido siempre las inglesas. Si con ello no hemos satisfecho todas las exigencias, rogamos indulgencia para

los autores

15

1.2   Abbreviations and symbols

1.2	Decimal fraction: "1 unit, 2 tenths"; instead of the notation used in Germany and France: 1,2
x	multiplication sign (e.g., "2 x 3 = 6"); in equations also · (e.g., "2·3 = 6")
=	equals
~	similar to (approximately equal)
≈	approximately (nearly or practically equal) (the two penultimate symbols, respectively placed after "V" the abbreviation for the unit of voltage, e.g., "kV=, kV~, or
≋	kV≋", mean direct-current voltage, alternating-current voltage, or threephase alternating current)
>	greater than ... (e.g., "8>5")
<	less than ... (e.g., "5<8")
	decimal fractions and multiples: a, f, p, n, µ, m, c, k, M, G, T, P, E (10^{-18}...10^{18}); for details, see page 41
ℓ	liter (unit of volume)
m	meter (SI unit of length)
g	gram (unit of mass; SI unit kg)
s	second (SI unit of time)
min	minute (unit of time)
h	hour (hora - unit of time)
d	day (dies - unit of time)
a	year (annum - unit of time)
T	time (tempus - general)
$T_{1/2}$	half-life (time in which half of a radioactive substance decays); also HL
τ	lifetime (= time in which a radioactive substance has decayed to 1/e, i.e. to about 37% of the initial value)
A	ampere (SI unit of electrical current)
V	volt (unit of electric potential)
C	coulomb (SI unit of electric charge)
W	watt (SI unit of power)
J	joule (SI unit of energy)
mAs	milliampere-second (quantity used for radiographic exposures)
R	röntgen (unit of exposure)
rad	rad (radiation absorbed dose = unit of absorbed dose)
Gy	gray (SI unit of absorbed dose)
rem	rem (radiation equivalent man = equivalent dose)
Ci	curie (unit of radioactivity, = $3.71 \cdot 10^{10}$ decays/s)
Bq	becquerel (SI unit of radioactivity; = 1 decay/s)
RBE	relative biologic effectiveness
q	quality factor (= RBE for radiation protection, for values see p.44)

e	1. elementary electric charge (see page 40) and 2. basis of the natural logarithm (e = 2.718282)
eV	electron volt (unit of energy, 1 J = $6.2435 \cdot 10^{18}$ eV)
LET	linear energy transfer (energy discharged by a particle during its passage through matter per unit path length)
°C	degree centigrad (unit of temperature referred to the freezing point of water)
°F	degrees Fahrenheit (unit of temperature referred to -32°C)
K	kelvin (formerly degrees Kelvin) unit of temperature referred to the absolute zero point -273°C
α	alpha (symbol for alpha particles or alpha radiation)
β	beta (symbol for beta particles or beta radiation)
γ	gamma (symbol for gamma particles or gamma radiation)
n	neutron (particles or radiation)
p	proton (particles or radiation)
e^-, e^+	electron resp. positron (particles or radiation)
d	deuteron (particles or radiation)
Γ	gamma (specific gamma-ray constant, $\frac{R \cdot m^2}{h \cdot Ci}$, see page 150)
η	eta (symbol for degree of effectiveness)
ρ	rho (symbol for the density of a substance)
λ	lambda (symbol for the wavelength of radiation)
FSD	focus-skin (surface)-distance
SD	source distance
SSD	source-skin-(surface)-distance
HVL	half-value layer (measure of the energy of a radiation)
HVD	half-value depth in tissue
MPC	maximum permissible concentration
D	dose (general)
$\bar{D}$	(time) average of the dose ($\bar{X}$ general = time average of a quantity)
$\dot{D}$	dose rate ($\dot{X}$ general = time-related quantity)
D_0	dose which kills 1 - 1/e (= 63%) of irradiated individuals
LD_{50}	lethal dose 50, i.e., dose by which 50% of irradiated individuals are killed
^3_1H	hydrogen (or other chemical elements, as on page 24 and 27) with the atomic number 1 written as subscript before the symbol and the mass number 3 as superscript before the symbol
SI	International System of Units
ICRU	International Commission on Radiation Units and Measurements
ICRP	International Commission on Radiological Protection
ISO	International Standard Organisation
DIN	German Standard Institute (Deutsches Institut für Normung)

1.2 Abkürzungen und Formelzeichen

1.2 Dezimalbruch: 1 Ganzes, 2 Zehntel (anstelle der in der deutschen und französischen benutzen Schreibweise: 1,2)

x Zeichen für Multiplikation (z.B. 2 x 3 = 6); in Formeln auch: · (z.B. 2·3 = 6)

= gleich

∿ ähnlich (ungefähr gleich)

≋ angenähert (nahezu oder praktisch) gleich (diese drei Symbole hinter dem Kurzzeichen für die Einheit der Spannung V (z.B. kV=, kV∿ oder kV≋) bedeuten Gleichspannung, Wechselspannung oder Drehstrom)

> größer als ... (z.B. 8>5)

< kleiner als ... (z.B. 5<8)

Dezimale Brüche und Vielfache a, f, p, n, μ, m, c, k, M, G, T, P, E ($10^{-18}...10^{18}$), siehe Seite 41

ℓ Liter (Einheit des Volumens)

m Meter (SI-Längeneinheit)

g Gramm (Masseneinheit; SI-Einheit kg)

s Sekunde (SI-Zeiteinheit)

min Minute (Zeiteinheit)

h Stunde (hora - Zeiteinheit)

d Tag (dies - Zeiteinheit)

a Jahr (annum - Zeiteinheit)

T Zeit (tempus - allgemein)

$T_{1/2}$ Halbwertzeit (Zeit, in der die Hälfte eines radioaktiven Stoffes zerfallen ist) auch HWZ

τ mittlere Lebensdauer (= Zeit, in der ein radioaktiver Stoff auf 1/e, d.h. rund 37 % des Ausganswertes, zerfallen ist)

A Ampere (SI-Einheit der elektrischen Stromstärke)

V Volt (Einheit der elektrischen Spannung)

W Watt (SI-Einheit der Leistung)

J Joule (SI-Einheit der Energie)

mAs Milli-Ampere-Sekunden Produkt (zur Kennzeichnung der für die Belichtung von Röntgenaufnahmen benutzten Größe)

R Röntgen (Einheit der Ionendosis)

rad Rad (radiation absorbed dose - Einheit der Energiedosis; in Deutschland Abkürzung auch rd)

Gy Gray (Si-Einheit der Energiedosis)

rem rem (radiation equivalent man - Äquivalentdosis)

Ci Curie (Einheit der Radioaktivität = $3{,}71 \cdot 10^{10}$ Zerfälle/s)

Bq Becquerel (SI-Einheit der Radioaktivität in Zerfällen/s)

RBW Relative Biologische Wirksamkeit (englisch RBE)

q Qualitätsfaktor (= RBW für Strahlenschutzzwecke abgerundet festgelegte Werte siehe Seite 44)

C	Coulomb (SI-Einheit der elektrischen Ladung)
e	1. elektrische Elementarladung (siehe Seite 40) und 2. Basis des natürlichen Logarithmensystems (e = 2,718282)
eV	Elektronenvolt (Einheit der Energie, 1 J = $6,2435 \cdot 10^{18}$ eV)
LET	Linear Energy Transfer (Energie, die ein Teilchen beim Durchgang durch Materie je Weglänge abgibt), deutsch auch LEÜ
°C	Grad Celsius (auf den Gefrierpunkt des Wassers bezogene Einheit der Temperatur)
°F	Grad Fahrenheit (auf -32°C bezogene Einheit der Temperatur, siehe Seite 42)
K	Kelvin (auf den absoluten Nullpunkt -273°C bezogene SI-Einheit der Temperatur °C, °F und K, siehe Seite 42)
α	Alpha (Symbol für Alpha-Teilchen oder Alpha-Strahlung)
β	Beta (Symbol für Beta-Teilchen oder Beta-Strahlung)
γ	Gamma (Symbol für Gamma-Quanten oder Gamma-Strahlung)
e^-, e^+	Elektron bzw. Positron (Teilchen oder Strahlung)
p	Proton (Teilchen oder Strahlung)
d	Deuteron (Teilchen oder Strahlung)
n	Neutron (Teilchen oder Strahlung)
Γ	Gamma (spezifische Gamma-Strahlenkonstante in $\frac{R \cdot m^2}{h \cdot Ci}$, s.Seite 150)
η	Eta (Symbol für Wirkungsgrad)
ρ	Rho (Symbol für die Dichte eines Stoffes)
λ	Lamda (Symbol für die Wellenlänge einer Strahlung)
FA	Fokusabstand (englisch FD, SD) bzw. QA = Quellenabstand
FHA	Fokus-Haut-Abstand (englisch FSD)
HWSD	Halbwertschichtdicke (Maß für die Härte einer Strahlung; englisch HVL)
GHWT	Gewebehalbwerttiefe (englisch HVD)
MZK	maximal zulässige Konzentration (englisch MPC)
D	Dosis (allgemein)
$\bar{D}$	(zeitlicher) Mittelwert der Dosis ($\bar{X}$ allgemein zeitlicher Mittelwert)
$\dot{D}$	Dosisleistung ($\dot{X}$ allgemein auf die Zeit bezogene Größe)
D_0	Dosis, die 1 - 1/e (= 63%) der bestrahlten Individuen abtötet
LD_{50}	Letal Dosis 50, d.h. Dosis, durch die 50 % der bestrahlten Individuen abgetötet werden
^3_1H	Wasserstoff (bzw. andere chemische Elemente)mit der Ordnungszahl 1 vor dem Symbol tiefgestellt und der Massenzahl 3 vor dem Symbol hochgestellt, siehe Seite 24 und 27
SI	Internationales Einheitensystem
ICRU	International Commission on Radiation Units and Measurements
ICRP	International Commission on Radiological Protection
ISO	International Standard Organisation
DIN	Deutsches Institut für Normung

1.2   Abréviations et symboles

1.2	fraction décimale: 1 unité, 2 dixièmes (au lieu de la notation française ou allemande 1,2)
x	signe de multiplication (par ex. 2 x 3 = 6); en formule aussi· (par ex. 2·3 = 6)
=	égale
$\sim$	semblable à (à peu près égal)
$\approx$	valeur approchée (presque égal ou pratiquement égal) (les deux derniers symboles, ainsi que le symbole$\approx$, placés après "V" l'abréviation pour l'unité de tension (par ex. kV=,
$\approx$	kV$\sim$, ou kV$\approx$), signifient tension constante, tension alternative ou tension alternative triphasée)
>	plus grand que... (par ex. 8>5)
<	plus petit que... (par ex. 5<8)
	multiples et sous-multiples a, f, p, n, µ, m, c, k, M, G, T, P, E (10^{-18}...10^{18}) pour plus de détails, voir page 41
ℓ	litre (unité de volume)
m	mètre (unité SI de longueur)
g	gramme (unité de masse; SI unité kg)
s	seconde (unité SI de temps)
min	minute (unité de temps)
h	heure (unité de temps)
d	jour (dies - unité de temps)
a	année (annum - unité de temps)
T	temps (tempus - en général)
$T_{1/2}$	période demi vie, PDV (temps au bout duquel la moitié des atomes radioactifs se sont désintégrés)
τ	durée de vie (= temps au bout duquel une substance radioactiv a décru à 1/e = $\sim$37% de la valeur initiale)
A	Ampère (unité SI de courant électrique)
V	Volt (unité de potentiel électrique)
C	Coulomb (unité SI de charge électrique)
W	Watt (unité SI de puissance)
J	Joule (unité SI d'énergie)
mAs	milliampère seconde (quantité utilisée pour les radiographies)
R	röntgen (unité d'exposition)
rad	rad (radiation absorbed dose = unité de dose absorbée)
rem	rem (radiation equivalent man = dose équivalente)
Gy	gray (unité SI de dose absorbée)
Ci	Curie (ancienne unité de radioactivité = $3.71 \cdot 10^{10}$ désinté- grations/s)
Bq	Becquerel (unité SI de radioactivité = 1 désintégration/s)
EBR	efficacité biologique relative (anglais: RBE)

q	facteur de qualité (= EBR dans le domaine de la radioprotection; pour les valeurs approchées admises, voir page 44)
e	1. charge électrique élémentaire (voir page 40) et 2. base des logarithmes naturels (e = 2.718282)
eV	electron-volt (unité d'énergie. 1 J = $6.2435 \cdot 10^{18}$ eV)
TEL	transfert d'énergie linéique (anglais LET)
°C	degré centigrade (unité de température)
°F	degrés Fahrenheit (unité de température rapportée à -32°C)
K	Kelvin (auparavant degrés Kelvin) unité de température rapportée au zéro absolu (-273°C); °C, °F et K voir page 42
α	alpha (symbole pour particules ou rayonnement α)
β	beta (symbole pour particules ou rayonnement β)
γ	gamma (symbole pour particules ou rayonnement γ)
n	neutron (symbole pour particules ou rayonnement)
p	proton (symbole pour particules ou rayonnement)
d	deuteron (symbole pour particules ou rayonnement)
e^-, e^+	symboles pour les electrons et les positrons
Γ	gamma (constante de débit d'exposition; voir page 150)
η	eta (symbole pour le degré d'efficacité)
ρ	rho (symbole pour la densité d'une substance)
λ	lambda (symbole pour la longueur d'onde d'un rayonnement)
DFP	distance foyer-peau resp. DS distance de la source
CDA	couche de demi-atténuation (mesure de la qualité d'un rayonnement)
PDA	profondeur demi absorption tissulaire
CMA	concentration maximale admissible
D	dose (en général)
$\bar{D}$	dose moyenne (par rapport au temps) (en général $\bar{X}$ = moyenne d'une quantité X par rapport au temps)
$\dot{D}$	débit de dose (en général $\dot{X}$ = quantité X rapportée à l'unité de temps)
D_0	dose tuant 1 - 1/e (= 63%) d'individus irradiés
DL_{50}	dose létale 50, c'est-à-dire dose tuant 50% des individus irradiés
$^3_1 H$	hydrogène (ou autre élément chimique décrit page 24) le nombre atomique 1 est écrit en bas et en avant du symbole et le nombre de masse 3 est écrit en haut en avant du symbole
SI	système international d'unites
ICRU	Commission internationale sur les unités radiologique (CIUR)
ICRP	Commission internationale sur la protection contre les radiations (CIPR)
ISO	Organisation internationale de normalisation
DIN	Institut allemand de normalisation (Deutsches Institut für Normung)

1.2   Abreviaturas y símbolos

1.2   número decimal: 1 unidad, 2 decena (en lugar de la forma usual de escritura alemana y francesa: 1,2)

x   símbolo de multiplicación (p. ej. 2 x 3 = 6); en las fórmulas también: · (p. ej. 2·3 = 6)

=   igual a

∿   semejante (aproximadamente igual a)

≈   muy cerca de (casi o practicamente) igual; (estos tres símbolos después de las unidades de tensión V (p. ej. kV=, kV∿ o kV≋) indican corriente continua, alterna o trifásica respectivamente)

>   mayor que ... (p. ej. 8>5)

<   menor que ... (p. ej. 5<8)

        números decimales y exponenciales a, f, p, n, µ, m, c, k, M, G, T, P, E (10^{-18}...10^{18}), vease página 41

ℓ   litro (unidad de volumen)

m   metro (unidad de longitud en el SI)

g   gramo (unidad de masa; unidad en el SI kg)

s   segundo (unidad de tiempo en el SI)

min   minuto (unidad de tiempo)

h   hora (unidad de tiempo)

d   día (unidad de tiempo)

a   año (unidad de tiempo)

T   tiempo (en general)

$T_{1/2}$ período de vida media (tiempo en el cual se disgrega la mitad de una sustancia radiactiva) también PVM

τ   vida media (= tiempo en el cual una sustancia radiactiva se disgrega hasta $1/e$, de su valor inicial)

A   amperio (unidad de intensidad de corriente eléctrica en el SI)

V   voltio (unidad tensión eléctrica)

W   watio (unidad de potencia en el SI)

J   julio (unidad de energía en el SI)

mAs   producto de miliamperios por segundo (para denominar la magnitud utilizada en la impresión de radiografias)

R   röntgen (unidad de dosis iónica o exposición)

rad   Rad (dosis absorbida - unidad de dosis de energía)

Gy   Gray (unidad de dosis de energía en el SI)

rem   rem (radiación equivalente en el hombre - dosis equivalente)

Ci   Curie (unidad de radioactividad = $3,71 \cdot 10^{10}$ desintegraciones/s)

Bq   Becquerel (unidad de radioactividad del SI en desintegraciones/s)

EBR   efectividad biológica relativa (en inglés RBE)

q   factor de calidad (= EBR valores fijos redondeados para el radioprotección, vease página 44)

C   Coulomb (unidad de carga eléctrica en el SI)

e	1. carga eléctrica elemental (vease pág. 40) y 2. base del sistema de logaritmos natural (e = 2,718282)
eV	electrónvoltio (unidad de energía, 1 J = $6,2435 \cdot 10^{18}$ eV)
TLE	transmisión lineal de energía (energía que cede una partícula al pasar a través de un determinada porción de materia; ingles RBE)
°C	grado Celsius (unidad de temperatura referida al punto de congelación del agua)
°F	grado Fahrenheit (unidad de temperatura referida a -32 °C, vease pág. 42)
K	Kelvin (unidad de temperatura en el SI referida al punto del cero absoluto -273 °C, °C, °F y K vease pág. 42)
α	alfa (símbolo para las partículas o rayos alfa)
β	beta (símbolo para las partículas o rayos beta)
γ	gamma (símbolo para los cuantos o rayos gamma)
e^-, e^+	electrón o positrón (partículas o radiación)
p	protón (partículas o radiación)
d	deuterón (partículas o radiación)
n	neutrón (partículas o radiación)
Γ	gamma (constante de radiación gamma específica en $\frac{R \cdot m^2}{h \cdot Ci}$, v.p.150)
η	eta (símbolo del grado de eficacia)
ρ	ro (símbolo de la densidad de una sustancia)
λ	lambda (símbolo de la longitud de onda de una radiación)
DF	distancia focal o distancia fuente (inglés FD)
DFP	distancia foco- o sea fuente-piel (inglés FSD o sea SSD)
CHR	capa hemirreductora (medida de la dureza de una radiación, inglés HVL)
PHR	Profundidad hemi-reductora (tejido)
CMP	concentración máxima permisible (inglés MPC)
D	dosis (en general)
$\bar{D}$	valor medio de la dosis (temporal) ($\bar{X}$ valor medio temporal en general)
$\dot{D}$	intensidad de la dosis (X en general magnitud referida al tiempo)
D_0	dosis, el 1 - 1/e (= 63 %) de individuos radiados muertos
LD	dosis letal 50, es decir, la dosis mediante la cual se morirían el 50 % de los individuos irradiados
^3_1H	hidrógeno (u otro elemento químico) con el número atómico 1 como subíndice antes del símbolo y número másico 3 como super-indice antes del símbolo, vease páginas 24 y 27
SI	Sistema de Unidades Internacional
ICRP	Comisión Internacional de Radioprotección
ICRU	Comisión Internacional de Unidades de Radiación
ISO	Organización Internacional de Normalización
DIN	Instituto Alemán de Normalización

	I	II	III	IV	V
1	${}^{1}_{1}$H Hydrogen Wasserstoff Hydrogène Hidrógeno				
2	${}^{7}_{3}$Li Lithium Lithium Lithium Litio	${}^{9}_{4}$Be Beryllium Beryllium Béryllium Berilio	${}^{11}_{5}$B Boron Bor Bore Boro	${}^{12}_{6}$C Carbon Kohlenstoff Carbone Carbono	${}^{14}_{7}$N Nitrogen Stickstoff Azote Nitrógeno
3	${}^{23}_{11}$Na Sodium Natrium Sodium Sodio	${}^{24}_{12}$Mg Magnesium Magnesium Magnésium Magnesio	${}^{27}_{13}$Al Aluminium Aluminium Aluminium Aluminio	${}^{28}_{14}$Si Silicon Silizium Silicium Silicio	${}^{31}_{15}$P Phosphorus Phosphor Phosphore Fósforo
4	${}^{39}_{19}$K β Potassium Kalium Potassium Potasio ${}^{63}_{29}$Cu Copper Kupfer Cuivre Cobre	${}^{40}_{20}$Ca Calcium Kalzium Calcium Calcio ${}^{64}_{30}$Zn Zinc Zink Zinc Cinc	${}^{45}_{21}$Sc Scandium Skandium Scandium Escandio ${}^{69}_{31}$Ga Gallium Gallium Gallium Galio	${}^{48}_{22}$Ti Titanium Titan Titane Titanio ${}^{74}_{32}$Ge Germanium Germanium Germanium Germanio	${}^{51}_{23}$V Vanadium Vanadium Vanadium Vanadio ${}^{75}_{33}$As Arsenic Arsen Arsenic Arsénico
5	${}^{85}_{37}$Rb β Rubidium Rubidium Rubidium Rubidio ${}^{107}_{47}$Ag Silver Silber Argent Plata	${}^{88}_{38}$Sr Strontium Strontium Strontium Estroncio ${}^{114}_{48}$Cd Cadmium Kadmium Cadmium Cadmium	${}^{89}_{39}$Y Yttrium Yttrium Yttrium Itrio ${}^{115}_{49}$In β Indium Indium Indium Indio	${}^{90}_{40}$Zr Zirconium Zirkon Zirconium Circonio ${}^{120}_{50}$Sn Tin Zinn Étain Estano	${}^{93}_{41}$Nb Niobium Niob Niobium Niobio ${}^{121}_{51}$Sb Antimony Antimon Antimoine Antimonio
6	${}^{133}_{55}$Cs Cesium Zäsium Césium Cesio ${}^{197}_{79}$Au Gold Gold Or Oro	${}^{138}_{56}$Ba Barium Barium Barium Bario ${}^{202}_{80}$Hg Mercury Quecksilber Mercure Mercurio	57–71 Rare earths Seltene Erden Terres rares Tierras raras ${}^{205}_{81}$Tl Thallium Thallium Thallium Talio	${}^{180}_{72}$Hf Hafnium Hafnium Hafnium Hafnio ${}^{208}_{82}$Pb Lead Blei Plomb Plomo	${}^{181}_{73}$Ta Tantalum Tantal Tantale Tántalo ${}^{209}_{83}$Bi Bismuth Wismut Bismuth Bismuto
7	${}^{223}_{87}$Fr (α) Francium Francium Francium Francio	${}^{226}_{88}$Ra α Radium Radium Radium Radio	${}^{227}_{89}$Ac β Actinium Aktinium Actinium Actinio	${}^{232}_{90}$Th α Thorium Thorium Thorium Torio	${}^{231}_{91}$Pa α Protactinium Protaktinium Protactinium Protactinio

Système périodique des éléments - Tabla periódica de los elementos

VI	VII	VIII			O
					$^{4}_{2}He$ Helium Helium Hélium Helio
$^{16}_{8}O$ Oxygen Sauerstoff Oxygène Oxígeno	$^{19}_{9}F$ Fluorine Fluor Fluor Flúor				$^{20}_{10}Ne$ Neon Neon Néon Neón
$^{32}_{16}S$ Sulphur Schwefel Soufre Azufre	$^{35}_{17}Cl$ Chlorine Chlor Chlore Cloro				$^{40}_{18}Ar$ Argon Argon Argon Argón
$^{52}_{24}Cr$ Chromium Chrom Chrome Cromo	$^{55}_{25}Mn$ Manganese Mangan Manganèse Manganeso	$^{56}_{26}Fe$ Iron Eisen Fer Hierro	$^{59}_{27}Co$ Cobalt Kobalt Cobalt Cobalto	$^{58}_{28}Ni$ Nickel Nickel Nickel Níquel	
$^{80}_{34}Se$ Selenium Selen Sélénium Selenio	$^{79}_{35}Br$ Bromine Brom Brome Bromo				$^{84}_{36}Kr$ Krypton Krypton Krypton Criptón
$^{98}_{42}Mo$ Molybdenum Molybdän Molybdène Molibdeno	$^{99}_{43}Tc(\beta)$ Technetium Technetium Technécium Tecnecio	$^{102}_{44}Ru$ Ruthenium Ruthenium Ruthénium Rutenio	$^{103}_{45}Rh$ Rhodium Rhodium Rhodium Rodio	$^{106}_{46}Pd$ Palladium Palladium Palladium Paladio	
$^{130}_{52}Te$ Tellurium Tellur Tellurium Teluro	$^{127}_{53}I/^{127}_{53}J$ Iodine Jod Iode Iodo				$^{132}_{54}X$ Xenon Xenon Xénon Xenón
$^{184}_{74}W$ Wolfram Wolfram Tungstène Wolframo	$^{187}_{75}Re\ \beta$ Rhenium Rhenium Rhénium Renio	$^{192}_{76}Is$ Osmium Osmium Osmium Osmio	$^{193}_{77}Ir$ Iridium Iridium Iridium Iridio	$^{195}_{78}Pt$ Platinum Platin Platine Platino	
$^{210}_{84}Po\ \alpha$ Polonium Polonium Polonium Polonio	$^{211}_{85}At(\alpha)$ Astatine Astatin Astate Astatio				$^{222}_{86}Rn\ \alpha$ Radon Radon Radon Radón
$^{238}_{92}U\ \alpha$ Uranium Uran Uranium Uranio	$_{93}...$ Transuranic elements Transurane Transuraniens Transuránicos				

	$^{139}_{57}$La γ Lanthanum Lanthan Lanthane Lantano	$^{140}_{58}$Ce Cerium Zer Cérium Cerio	$^{141}_{59}$Pr Praseodymium Praseodym Praséodyme Praseodimio	$^{144}_{60}$Nd Neodymium Neodym Néodymium Neodimio
Rare earths (57 - 71) Seltene Erden	$^{147}_{61}$Pm(β) Promethium Prometheum Prométhéum Promedio	$^{152}_{62}$Sm α Samarium Samarium Samarium Samario	$^{153}_{63}$Eu Europium Europium Europium Europio	$^{158}_{64}$Gd Gadolinium Gadolinium Gadolinium Gadolinio
Terres rares Tierras raras	$^{159}_{65}$Tb Terbium Terbium Terbium Terbio	$^{164}_{66}$Dy Dysprosium Dysprosium Dysprosium Disprosio	$^{165}_{67}$Ho Holmium Holmium Holmium Holmio	$^{166}_{68}$Er Erbium Erbium Erbium Erbio
	$^{169}_{69}$Tm Thulium Thulium Thulium Tulio	$^{174}_{70}$Yb Ytterbium Ytterbium Ytterbium Iterbio	$^{175}_{71}$Cp β Lutecium Lutetium Lutécium Lutecio	

	$^{237}_{93}$Np(β) Neptunium Neptunio	$^{239}_{94}$Pu(α) Plutonium Plutonio	$^{241}_{95}$Am(α) Americium Americo
	$_{96}$Cm(α) Curium Curio	$_{97}$Bk(α) Berkelium Bercelio	$_{98}$Cf(α) Californium Californio
Transuranic elements (93 ...) Transurane Transuraniens Transurânicos	$_{99}$Es Einsteinium Einsteinio	$_{100}$Fm Fermium Fermio	$_{101}$Md Mendelevium Mendelevio
	$_{102}$No Nobelium Nobelio	$_{103}$Lr Lawrencium Lawrencio	$_{104}$Ku Kurchatovium Kurchatovio
	$_{105}$Ha Hahnium	$_{106}$	

Note - Bemerkung - Remarque - Nota:

The index left of each symbol on the lower bottom is the atomic number and that on the upper the mass number of the most frequent isotope. α, β, γ indicate the type of radiation of natural and (α), (β), (γ) that of artificially produced radioactive elements.

Der Index links vom Symbol unten gibt die Ordnungszahl, der oben die Massenzahl des häufigsten Isotops an; α, β, γ ist die Art der ausgesandten Strahlung natürlicher, (α), (β), (γ) künstlich erzeugter Radionuklide.

L'index à gauche en bas du symbole est le numéro atomique, en naut le nombre de masse de l'isotope naturel le plus fréquent, α, β, γ indiquent le type de rayonnement d'un radioélément naturel et (α), (β), (γ) celui d'un radioélément artificiel.

El índice izquierdo inferior del símbolo es el número atómico, el superior el número másico del isótopo más fréquente. α, β y γ indican el tipo de radiación de los elementos naturales y (α), (β) y (γ) la de los elementos artificiales.

Lit.: 1. LANDOLT-BÖRNSTEIN: I. 5. Berlin: Springer 1952
2. WANG, Y.: Handbook, Cleveland: Chemical Rubber Co. 1969

1.4 The chemical elements and their most important properties
Die chemischen Elemente und ihre wichtigsten Eigenschaften
Les éléments chimiques et leurs principales propriétés
Los elementos químicos y sus propiedades más importantes

1. Symbol - Symbol - Symbole - Símbolo
2. Atomic number - Ordnungszahl - Numéro atomique - Número atómico
3. Atomic weight - Atomgewicht - Poids atomique - Peso atómico
4. Mass number and composition in % of isotopes - Massenzahl und %-Anteil der Isotope - Nombre de masses et pourcentage des isotopes - Número másico y porcentaje de los isótopos
5. Mean energy of K photons - Mittlere Energie der K Photonen - Energie moyenne des photons K - Energía media de fotones K:keV
6. Mean energy of L photons - Mittlere Energie der L Photonen - Energie moyenne des photons L - Energía media de fotones L:keV

1	2	3	4			5	6
H	1	1.008	1 99.985	2 0.015		(0.013)	-
He	2	4.003	3 10^{-4}	4 100		(0.025)	-
Li	3	6.939	6 7.42	7 92.58		0.054	-
Be	4	9.012	9 100			0.109	-
B	5	10.811	10 19.78	11 80.22		0.184	-
C	6	12.010	12 98.89	13 1.11		0.279	-
N	7	14.007	14 99.63	15 0.37		0.393	-
O	8	16.000	16 99.76	17 0.04	18 0.20	0.524	-
F	9	18.998	19 100			0.675	-
Ne	10	20.183	20 90.92	21 0.26	22 8.82	0.849	0.018
Na	11	22.990	23 100			1.04	0.031
Mg	12	24.312	24 78.70	25 10.13	26 11.17	1.25	0.048
Al	13	26.982	27 100			1.49	0.069
Si	14	28.086	28 92.21	29 4.70	30 3.09	1.74	0.136
P	15	30.974	31 100			2.02	0.169

Lit.: 1. LANDOLT-BÖRNSTEIN: Zahlenwerte und Funktionen, I, 5 Berlin: Springer 1952
2. STORM, E., ISRAEL, H.J.: L.A.-3753 UC-34 Physics 1967
3. WANG, Y.: Handbook of Radioactive Nuclides, Cleveland 1969

1	2	3	4				5	6
S	16	32.064	32 95.0	33 0.76	34 4.22	36 0.014	2.32	0.205
Cl	17	35.453	35 75.53	37 24.47			2.64	0.243
Ar	18	39.948	36 0.34	38 0.06	40 99.60		2.98	0.286
K	19	39.102	39 93.1	40 0.01	41 6.9		3.34	0.262
Ca	20	40.08	40 96.97 46 0.003	42 0.64 48 0.18	43 0.14	44 2.06	3.72	0.385
Sc	21	44.956	45 100				4.12	0.438
Ti	22	47.90	46 7.93 50 5·.34	47 7.28	48 73.94	49 5.51	4.55	0.495
V	23	50.942	50 0.24	51 99.76			5.00	0.555
Cr	24	51.996	50 4.31	52 83.76	53 9.55	54 2.38	5.47	0.582
Mn	25	54.938	55 100				5.96	0.646
Fe	26	55.847	54 5.82	56 91.66	57 2.19	58 0.33	6.47	0.714
Co	27	58.933	59 100				7.00	0.785
Ni	28	58.71	58 67.84	60 26.23	61 1.19	62 3.66	7.56	0.859
Cu	29	63.546	63 63.09	65 30.91			8.14	0.937
Zn	30	65.37	64 48.89 70 0.62	66 27.81	67 4.11	68 18.57	8.74	1.02
Ga	31	69.72	69 60.4	71 39.6			9.37	1.11
Ge	32	72.59	70 20.52 76 7.76	72 27.43	73 7.76	74 36.54	10.01	1.21
As	33	74.92	75 100				10.69	1.30

1	2	3	4				5	6
Se	34	78.96	74 0.87	76 9.02	77 7.58	78 23.52	11.38	1.40
			80 49.82	82 9.19				
Br	35	79.90	79 50.54	81 49.46			12.09	1.50
Kr	36	83.80	78 0.35	80 2.27	82 11.56	83 11.55	12.84	1.61
			84 56.90	86 17.37				
Rb	37	85.47	85 72.15	87 27.85			13.60	1.72
Sr	38	87.62	84 0.56	86 9.86	87 7.02	88 82.55	14.39	1.84
Y	39	88.905	89 100				15.20	1.96
Zr	40	91.22	90 51.46	91 11.23	92 17.11	94 17.40	16.04	2.08
			96 2.80					
Nb	41	92.906	93 100				16.90	2.21
Mo	42	95.94	92 15.84	94 9.04	95 15.7	96 16.53	17.78	2.34
			97 9.46	98 23.78	100 9.63			
Tc	43	(99)					18.69	2.48
Ru	44	101.07	96 5.51	98 1.87	99 12.72	100 12.62	19.63	2.65
			101 17.07	102 31.61	104 18.60			
Rh	45	102.91	103 100				20.59	2.80
Pd	46	106.4	102 0.96	104 10.97	105 22.23	106 27.33	21.58	2.95
			108 26.71	110 11.81				
Ag	47	107.87	107 51.82	109 48.18			22.59	3.11
Cd	48	112.40	106 1.22	108 0.88	110 12.39	111 12.72	23.63	3.27
			112 24.07	113 12.26	114 28.86	116 7.58		
In	49	114.82	113 4.28	115 95.72			24.75	3.44

1	2	3	4				5	6
Sn	50	118.69	112 0.96	114 0.66	115 0.35	116 14.30	25.84	3.61
			117 7.61	118 24.03	119 8.58	120 32.85		
			122 4.72	124 5.94				
Sb	51	121.75	121 57.25	123 42.75			26.96	3.78
Te	52	127.60	120 0.09	122 2.46	123 0.87	124 4.61	28.12	3.96
			125 6.99	126 18.71	128 31.79	130 34.48		
I	53	126.90	127 100				29.29	4.14
Xe	54	131.30	124 0.10	126 0.09	128 1.92	129 26.4	30.49	4.33
			130 4.08	131 21.18	132 26.89	134 10.44		
			136 8.87					
Cs	55	132.91	133 100				31.72	4.52
Ba	56	137.34	130 0.10	132 0.10	134 2.42	135 6.59	32.99	4.72
			136 7.81	137 11.30	138 71.66			
La	57	138.91	138 0.09	139 99.91			34.27	4.93
Ce	58	140.12	136 0.19	138 0.25	140 88.48	142 11.07	35.59	5.14
Pr	59	140.91	141 100				36.94	5.35
Nd	60	144.24	142 27.11	143 12.17	144 23.85	145 8.30	38.31	5.56
			146 17.22	148 5.73	150 5.62			
Pm	61	(147)					39.72	5.79
Sm	62	150.35	144 3.09	147 14.97	148 11.24	149 13.83	41.16	6.02
			150 7.44	152 26.72	154 22.71			
Eu	63	151.96	151 47.82	153 52.18			42.63	6.25
Gd	64	157.25	152 0.20	154 2.15	155 14.73	156 20.47	44.13	6.49
			157 15.6	158 24.9	160 22.0			

1	2	3	4				5	6
Tb	65	158.92	159 100				45.66	6.73
Dy	66	162.50	156 0.05	158 0.09	160 2.29	161 18.88	47.23	6.99
			162 25.53	163 24.97	164 28.18			
Ho	67	164.93	165 100				48.82	7.23
Er	68	167.26	162 0.14	164 1.56	166 33.41	167 22.94	50.45	7.49
			168 27.07	170 14.88				
Tm	69	168.93	169 100				52.11	7.75
Yb	70	173.04	168 0.13	170 3.03	171 14.27	172 21.77	53.80	8.02
			173 16.08	174 31.92	176 12.80			
Lu	71	174.97	175 97.4	176 2.6			55.53	8.30
Hf	72	178.49	174 0.18	176 5.20	177 18.50	178 27.14	57.30	8.58
			179 13.75	180 35.24				
Ta	73	180.95	180 0.01	181 99.99			59.10	8.86
W	74	183.85	180 0.14	182 26.40	185 14.40	184 30.64	60.94	9.17
			186 28.41					
Re	75	186.2	185 37.07	187 62.93			62.81	9.47
Os	76	190.2	184 0.02	186 1.59	187 1.64	188 13.3	64.72	9.77
			189 16.1	190 26.4	192 41.0			
Ir	77	192.2	191 37.3	193 62.7			66.67	10.08
Pt	78	195.0	190 0.01	192 0.78	194 32.9	195 33.8	68.65	10.40
			196 25.3	198 7.2				
Au	79	196.97	197 100				70.68	10.72
Hg	80	200.59	196 0.15	198 10.12	199 17.04	200 23.25	72.75	11.04
			201 13.18	202 29.54	204 6.72			

1	2	3	4				5	6
Tl	81	204.37	203 29.5	205 70.5			74.85	11.37
Pb	82	207.19	204 1.54	206 22.62	207 22.62	208 53.22	77.00	11.72
Bi	83	208.98	209 100				79.19	12.07
Po	84	(210)	radioactive				81.43	12.42
At	85		radioactive				83.70	12.78
Rn	86	(222)	radioactive				86.02	13.15
Fr	87		radioactive				88.40	13.52
Ra	88	(226)	radioactive				90.81	13.90
Ac	89	(227)	radioactive				93.28	14.29
Th	90	232.04	232 100 radioactive				95.79	14.69
Pa	91	(231)	231 100 radioactive				98.35	15.10
U	92	238.03	234 0.01	235 0.72	238 radioactive 99.27		100.96	15.51
Np	93	(237)	radioactive				103.63	15.93
Pu	94	(242)	radioactive				106.35	16.08
Am	95	(241)	radioactive				109.14	16.80
Cm	96	(242)	radioactive				111.98	17.25
Bk	97	243	radioactive				114.89	17.71
Cf	98	244	radioactive				117.86	18.18
Es	99	−	radioactive				120.92	18.65
Fm	100	−	radioactive				124.05	19.14
Md	101	−	radioactive					
No	102	−	radioactive					
Lr	103	−	radioactive					
Ku	104	−	radioactive					
Ha	105	−	radioactive					
?	106	−	radioactive					

1.5 Most important elementary particles
Wichtigste Elementarteilchen
Principales particules élémentaires
Partículas elementales mas importantes

Group Art Groupe Grupo	Name Name Nom Nombre	Symbol Symbol Symbole Simbolo	Restmass Ruhemasse Masse au repos Masa en reposo		Charge Ladung Charge Carga	Energy Energie Énergie Energia	HL *) HWZ PDV PVM
			m_o kg$\cdot 10^{-27}$	m_o/m_{eo} -		$E=m_o c_o^2$ MeV	s$\cdot 10^{-9}$
Leptons Leptonen Leptons Leptones	Photon	γ	0	0	0	0	∞
	Neutrino	ν	0	0	0	0	∞
	Electron	e^-, β^-	0.00091	1	-1	0.511	∞
	Positron	e^+, β^+	0.00091	1	+1	0.511	∞
	Muon	μ^-	0.1884	206.78	-1	105.66	1525
Mesons Mesonen Mésons Mesones	Pion	π^0	0.2407	264.2	0	135.0	$6\cdot 10^{-8}$
	π-Meson	π^+, π^-	0.2489	273.2	+1-1	139.6	18
	K-Meson	K^+	0.8805	966.6	+1	493.8	0.06
	K^0-Meson	K^0	0.8874	974.2	0	497.9	$6\cdot 10^{-2}$
Nucleons Nucleonen Nucléons Nucleones	Proton	p^+	1.6725	1836.1	+1	938.26	∞
	Neutron	n	1.6748	1838.6	0	939.55	700 s
	Deuteron	d	3.3443	-	+1	1875.5	∞
	Triton	t	5.0070	-	+1	2808.8	12.3 a
	α-particle	α	6.644	-	+2	3727.2	∞

*) HL = Half-live
   HWZ = Halbwertzeit
   PDV = Période demi vie
   PVM = Período de vida media

Lit.: 1. COHEN, E.R., DUMOND I.W.M.: Rev.Mod.Phys. **37**, 537 (1965)
      2. EBERT, H.: Physikalisches Taschenbuch, Braunschweig: Vieweg 1967
      3. KOHLRAUSCH, F.: Praktische Physik, Bd. I - III, Stuttgart: Teubner 1968
      4. JAEGER, G., HÜBNER, H.: Dosimetrie und Strahlenschutz, Stuttgart: Thieme 1974

1.6   Range of electrons, protons, deuterons and α particles
Reichweite von Elektronen, Protonen, Deuteronen und α-Teilchen
Parcours des électrons, protons, deutérons et des particules α
Alcance de los electrones, protones, deuterones y particulas α

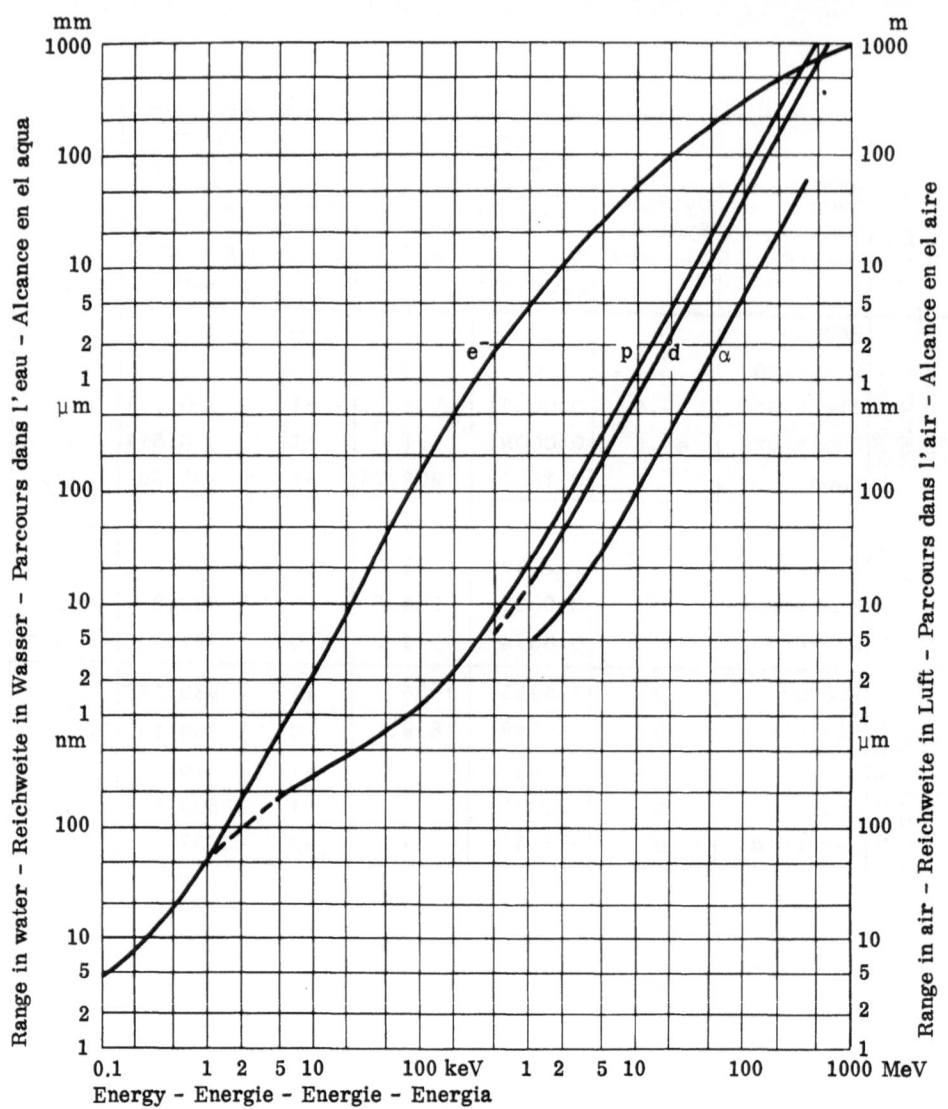

Energy - Energie - Energie - Energia

e⁻ : Electrons - Elektronen - Electrons - Electrones
p : Protons - Protonen - Protons - Protones
d : Deuterons - Deuteronen - Deutérons - Deuterones
α : α Particles - α-Teilchen - Particules α - Particulas α

Lit.: 1. LEA, D.E.: Actions of radiations on living cells, Cambridge:
University Press 1946
2. ROSSI, B.: High energy particles, N.Y., Prentice-Hall 1952
3. HEISENBERG, W.: Kosmische Strahlen, Berlin: Springer 1953
4. ICRU Report 16, Washington 1970

Energy Energie Energie Energía E	Range - Reichweite - Parcours - Alcance in - in - dans - en:				H₂O	Air Luft Air Aire
	e⁻	p	d	α		
0.1 keV	4.5	-	-	-		
0.2	8.0	-	-	-		
0.5	18	-	-	-		
1	53	(56)	-	-		
2 •	170	(95)	-	-	nm	μm
5	760	180	-	-		
10	2.5	280	-	-		
20	8.3	420	-	-		
50	42	750	-	-		
100	140	1.25	-	-		
200	500	2.4	-	-		
500	1.7	8.2	(6.0)	-		
1 MeV	4.3	22	16	4.5		
2	10	80	45	9.4	μm	mm
5	25	340	200	14		
10	55	1.2	750	105		
20	96	4.3	2.4	305		
50	190	19	12	1.7		
100	300	77	43	6.0		
200	480	250	150	22	mm	m
500	770	(1100)	730	(90)		
1000	1000	(3200)	(2300)	-		

The range of the particles in air is approximately 1000 times greater than that in water because the density of air is approximately 1/1000 that of water.

Die Reichweite der Teilchen in Luft ist wegen der gegenüber Wasser etwa 1000 mal geringeren Dichte rund 1000 mal größer als die in Wasser.

Le parcours des particules dans l'air est à peu près 1000 fois plus grand que dans l'eau puisque la densité de l'air est à peu près 1/1000 de celle de l'eau.

El alcance de las partículas en el aire es aproximadamente 1000 veces major que el correspondiente en agua, puesto que la densidad del aire es aproximadamente 1000 veces menor que la del agua.

1.7 Densities ρ of different materials
Dichte ρ verschiedener Stoffe
Densité ρ de différents matériaux
Densidad ρ de diferentes materiales

At - bei - à - a 20 - 25° C (1.013 bar = 760 mm Hg)

Elements - Elemente - Éléments - Elementos

Metals - Metalle - Métaux - Metales						Others - Andere - Autres - Otros		Gases-Gase Gaz-Gases	
Sym-bol	ρ (g/cm³)	Sym-bol	ρ (g/cm³)	Sym-bol	ρ (g/cm³)	Sym-bol	ρ (g/cm³)	Sym-bol	ρ (g/ℓ)
Li	0.53	Ni	8.90	Es	1.87	B	~3.35	H	0.09
Be	1.85	Cu	8.96	Ba	3.5	C	1.8-2.3	He	0.18
Na	0.97	Zn	7.13	Ta	16.65	P	1.8-2.7	N	1.25
Mg	1.74	Ga	5.90	W	19.3	S	1.9-2.1	O	1.43
Al	2.70	Ge	5.32	Os	22.57	Br	3.12	Ne	0.90
Si	2.33	Se	~4.5	Ir	22.42	Sb	6.22	Br	7.59
K	0.86	Sr	2.54	Pt	21.45	I/J	4.93	Ar	1.78
Ca	1.55	Y	4.47	Au	19.32			Kr	3.73
Ti	5.54	Mo	10.22	Hg	13.55			I/J	11.27
V	6.11	Pd	12.02	Tl	11.85			X	5.89
Cr	7.19	Ag	10.50	Pb	11.35	Air - Luft - Air - Aire			
Mn	~7.3	Cd	8.65	Bi	9.75	760 mm Hg (= 1.013 bar)			
Fe	7.87	Sn$_{gr}$	5.75	Th	11.72	0° C			1.293
Co	8.9	Sn$_w$	7.31	U	18.95	20° C			1.205

Composite materials - Zusammengesetzte Stoffe - Materiaux divers - Sustancias compuestas	ρ g/cm³
Foam plastic-Schaumstoff-Plastique expansé-Espumas artific.	0.03-0.05
Cork - Kork - Liège - Corcho	0.22-0.26
Balsa wood - Balsa Holz - Balsa - Madera balsa	0.11-0.14
Soft wood - Weichholz - Bois tendres - Madera blanda	0.4 -0.8
Hard wood - Hartholz - Bois durs - Madera dura	0.7 -1.3
Plastics - Kunststoff - Plastique - Plásticos	0.9 -1.8
Sand,gravel - Sand,Kies - Sable,gravier - Arena,grava	1.6 -1.9
Brick massive-Ziegel massiv-Brique pleine-Ladrillo comp.	1.4 -2.2
Brick hollow-Ziegel hohl-Brique creuse-Ladrillo hueco	1.0 -1.4
Concrete, normal - Beton norm. - Béton norm. - Hormigón	1.5 -2.4
Concrete, heavy-Beton schwer-Béton lourd-Hormigón pesado	3.0 -6.0
Concrete foam-Schaumbeton-Béton expansé-Hormigón espumado	0.45-0.60
Paraffine - Paraffin - Paraffine - Parafina	0.87-0.91
Glass - Glas - Verre - Vidrio	2.4 -2.8
Flint glass-Bleiqals-Verre au plomb-Vidrio de plomo	3.3 -6.2
Soil (dry)-Erde (trocken)-Terre (sèche)-Tierra (seca)	1.3 -2.0

Liquids - Flüssigkeiten - Liquides - Líquidos	ρ g/cm³
Alcohol - Alkohol - Alcool - Alcohol	0.79-0.81
Ether - Äther - Ether - Eter	0.74
Glycerin - Glycerin - Glycérine - Glicerina	1.26
Gasoline - Benzin - Essence - Gasolina	0.66-0.69
Mineral oil - Erdöl - Huile minérale - Petróleo	0.81-0.85
Water - Wasser - Eau - Agua	1.00

Lit.: 1. WEAST, R.C.: Handbook of Chemistry and Physics, Cleveland, Ohio: CRC-Press 1974 - 1975
2. JAEGER, R., HÜBNER, W.: Dosimetrie und Strahlenschutz, Stuttgart: Thieme 1974

1.8   Linear energy transfer (LET) and specific ionization density
       (ID) for different radiations in water (soft tissue)

       Lineare Energieübertragung (LEÜ) und spezifische Ionisations-
       dichte (ID) verschiedener Strahlungen in Wasser (Weichgewebe)

       Transfert d'énergie linéique (TEL) et densité d'ionisations
       linéique (DI) pour differents rayonnements dans l'eau

       Transferencia lineal de energía (TLE) y densidad de ioniza-
       tion específica (DI) en el agua, para differentes radiaciones

LET: energy transferred by a ionizing particle to matter along its
path in keV/μm. *)

LEÜ: von einem ionisierenden Teilchen in Materie entlang seiner Bahn
abgegebene Energie in keV/μm. *)

TEL: énergie transferée au milieu par la particule ionisante le long
de sa trajectoire exprimé en keV/μm. *)

TLE: energía transferida al medio por una partícula ionizada a lo
largo de su trayectoria, expresada en keV/μm. *)

ID: specific ionization density of ionizing particles in matter expressed in pairs/μm.

ID: spezifische Ionisationsdichte ionisierender Teilchen in Materie
ausgedrückt in Paaren/μm.

DI: densité linéique d'ionisation des particules ionisantes dans le
milieu, exprimée en paires d'ions/μm.

DI: Densidad de ionización específica de las partículas ionizadas
en el medio, expresada en pares ionicos/μm.

Terms used in graph and table - In der graphischen Darstellung und
in der Tabelle benützte Begriffe - Termes utilisées dans les
graphiques et les tables - Conceptos utilizados en el grafica y tabla

1. LET and ID of primary electrons of specific energy
   LEÜ und ID von Primärelektronen bestimmter Energie
   TEL et DI des électrons primaires d'énergie donnée
   TLE y DI de electrones primarios de energía determinada

2. LET and ID of electrons, including ionisation due to secondary
   electrons
   LEÜ und ID von Elektronen einschließlich der Ionisation durch
   Sekundärelektronen
   TEL et DI des électrons, y compris les ionisations dûes aux
   électrons secondaires
   TLE y DI des electrones incluyendo la ionización debida a elec-
   trones secundarios

3. LET and mean ID of electrons, integrated over the entire path
   length
   LEÜ und mittlere ID von Elektronen integriert über die gesamte
   Bahnlänge
   TEL et DI moyens des électrons intégrés sur la totalité de la
   trajectoire
   TLE y DI media de electrones, integrada sobre la longitud total
   de la trayectoria

*) For definitions see - Definitionen siehe - Pour les definitions voir - Para las
   definiciones ver: ICRU Report No. 19, Washington D.C. 1971

4. LET and mean ID of electrons released by X-rays
   LEÜ und mittlere ID von durch Röntgenstrahlung ausgelösten Elek-
   tronen
   TEL et DI moyens des électrons mis en mouvement par les rayons X
   TLE y DI media de los electrones provocados por rayos X

5. LET and ID of protons of specific energy
   LET und ID von Protonen bestimmter Energie
   TEL et DI des protons d'énergie donnée
   TLE y DI de protones de una energía determinada

6. LET and ID of deuterons of specific energy
   LEÜ und ID von Deuteronen bestimmter Energie
   TEL et DI des deuterons d'énergie donnée
   TLE y DI de deuterones de una energía determinada

7. LET and ID of alpha-particles of specific energy
   LEÜ und ID von Alphateilchen bestimmter Energie
   TEL et DI des particules alpha d'énergie donnée
   TLE y DI de partículas alfa de una energía determinada

8. $\bar{E}$ mean energy of electrons released by monoenergetic X-rays
   $\bar{E}$ mittlere Energie der von monoenergetischer Röntgenstrahlung
   ausgelösten Elektronen
   $\bar{E}$ Energie moyenne des électrons mis en mouvement par les rayons X
   monoénergétiques
   $\bar{E}$ energía media de los electrones provocados por rayos X mono-
   energéticos

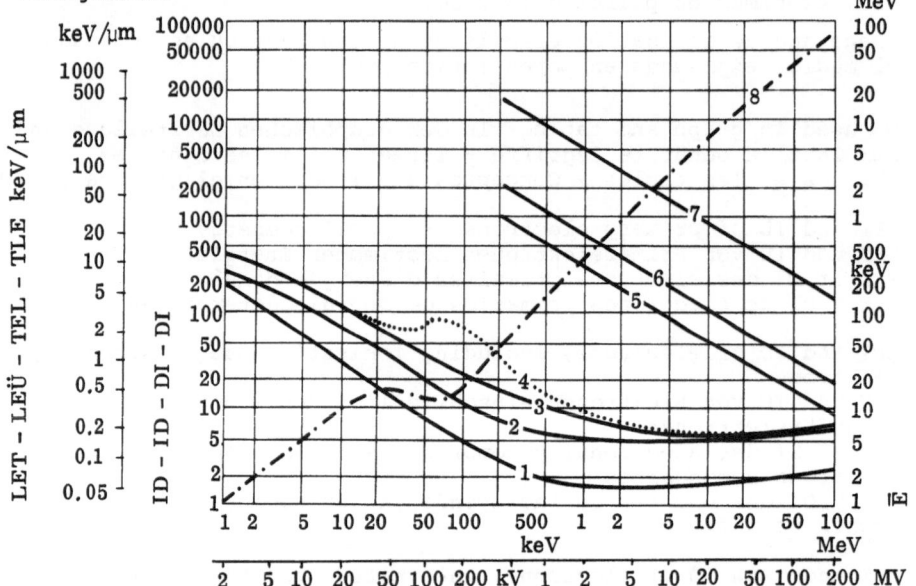

Energy of monoenergetic radiations - Energie der monoenergetischen
Strahlungen - Energie des rayonnements monoénergétiques - Energía
de las radiaciones monoenergeticas

Tube voltage for normal X-radiation - Röhrenspannung von Normal-
röntgenstrahlung - Tension normale du tube de rayons X - Voltaje del
tubo par rayos X normales (see page - siehe Seite - voir page -
ver página 70)

LET, ID, and E at various particle energies E
LEÜ, ID und E bei verschiedener Teilchenenergie E — keV/µm
TEL, DI et E pour différentes énergies des particules — n/µm
TLE, DI y E para diferentes energías de las partículas

	E *)	1 **)	2	3	4	5	6	7	8
LET - LEÜ - TEL - TLE: keV/µm	keV								
	1	6.2	8.4	13	13	-	-	-	1 keV
	2	4.9	6.2	9.6	9.6	-	-	-	2 keV
	5	1.95	3.9	5.9	5.9	-	-	-	5 keV
	10	0.96	2.3	3.9	3.9	-	-	-	10 keV
	20	0.55	1.3	2.2	2.6	-	-	-	15 keV
	50	0.26	0.65	1.2	2.6	-	-	-	13 keV
	100	0.16	0.39	0.72	2.3	-	-	-	16 keV
	200	0.11	0.28	0.55	1.15	32	72	485	45 keV
	500	0.065	0.18	0.39	0.49	17	36	260	140 keV
	MeV								
	1	0.060	0.19	0.31	0.32	9.8	21	160	350 keV
	2	0.055	0.18	0.24	0.26	6.2	11.7	95	950 keV
	5	0.060	0.18	0.21	0.23	3.1	6.2	49	3 MeV
	10	0.065	0.19	0.21	0.23	1.95	3.7	29	7 MeV
	20	0.068	0.20	0.22	0.22	1.14	2.3	18	15 MeV
	50	0.080	0.21	0.23	0.23	0.58	1.10	9.2	36 MeV
	100	0.094	0.24	0.26	0.26	0.32	0.65	4.9	70 MeV
ID - ID - DI - DI: n/µm ***)	keV								
	1	190	260	400	400	-	-	-	1 keV
	2	150	190	290	290	-	-	-	2 keV
	5	60	120	180	180	-	-	-	5 keV
	10	30	70	120	120	-	-	-	10 keV
	20	17	42	66	70	-	-	-	15 keV
	50	8.0	20	35	70	-	-	-	13 keV
	100	5.0	12	22	65	-	-	-	16 keV
	200	3.2	8.5	17	38	1000	2200	15000	45 keV
	500	2.0	5.6	12	15	530	1100	8000	140 keV
	MeV								
	1	1.8	5.7	9.5	10	300	650	4900	350 keV
	2	1.8	5.7	7.5	8.0	190	360	2900	950 keV
	5	1.8	5.7	6.5	7.0	95	190	1500	3 MeV
	10	2.0	5.8	6.5	7.0	60	115	900	7 MeV
	20	2.1	5.9	6.6	6.6	35	70	520	15 MeV
	50	2.5	6.5	7.2	7.2	18	34	280	36 MeV
	100	2.9	7.5	8.0	8.0	10	20	150	70 MeV

*) E = Energy of the radiation - Strahlenenergie - Energie de la radiation - Energía de los rayos

**) 1 - 8 See pages - Siehe Seiten - Voir pages - Ver páginas 37-38

***) n = Paires - Paare - Paires - Pares

Lit.: 1. GENTNER, W., MAIER-LEIBNITZ, H., BOTHE, W.: Atlas typischer Nebelkammerbilder, Berlin: Springer 1940
2. LEA, D.E.: Actions of Radiation on Living Cells, Cambridge 1946
3. CORMACK, C.V., JOHNS, H.E.: Brit.J.Radiol. 25, 369 (1952)
4. - 5.: WACHSMANN, F.: Strahlenther.86,440(1952); 89,128(1952)
6. ROSSI, B.: High energy particles, New York:Prentice-Hall (1952)
7. BURCH, P.R.J.: Brit.J.Radiol. 30, 524 (1957)

1.9   Physical units, constants and formulas
       Physikalische Einheiten, Konstanten und Formeln
       Unités, constantes et formules physiques
       Unidades, constantes y fórmulas físicas

1. SI basic units - SI-Grundeinheiten - Unités fondamentales SI -
   Unidades básicas SI

Meter	Meter	Mètre	Metro	m
Kilogram	Kilogramm	Kilogramme	Kilogramo	kg
Second	Sekunde	Seconde	Segundo	s
Ampere	Ampere	Ampère	Ampere	A
Kelvin	Kelvin	Kelvin	Kelvin	K
Candela	Candela	Candela	Candela	cd
Mole	Mol	Mole	Mole	mol

2. Units of force, pressure, energy, and power - Einheiten von
   Kraft, Druck, Energie und Leistung - Unités de force, de pression,
   d'énergie et de puissance - Unidades de fuerza, presión, energía
   y potencia

Newton	1 N	=	$1 \ kg \cdot m/s^2$
Dyne	1 dyn	=	$1 \ g \cdot cm/s^2$
Torr	1 Torr	=	$1 \ mm \ Hg = 1.333224 \cdot 10^2 \ N/m^2$
Pascal	1 Pa	=	$1 \ N/m^2$
Joule	1 J	=	$1 \ W \cdot s = 10^7 \ erg = 6.2435 \cdot 10^{18} eV$
Calorie	1 cal	=	$4.186047 \ J$
Watt	1 W	=	$1 \ N \cdot m/s = 10^7 \ erg/s$
Bar	1 bar	=	$10^5 \ N/m^2 = 10^6 \ dyn/cm$

3. Physical constants - Physikalische Konstanten - Constantes
   physiques - Constantes físicas

Velocity of light
Lichtgeschwindigkeit
Vitesse de la lumière $c \quad = \quad 2.997925 \cdot 10^8 \ m/s$
Velocidad de la luz

Electron charge
Elektrische Elementarladung
Charge de l'électron $e \quad = \quad 1.60210 \cdot 10^{-19} \ C$
Carga electrónica

Planck's constant $h \quad = \quad 6.6256 \cdot 10^{-34} \ J \cdot s$

Boltzmann's constant $k \quad = \quad 1.38054 \cdot 10^{-23} \ J/K$

Avogadro's number $N_A \quad = \quad 6.02252 \cdot 10^{-23}/mol$

Loschmidt's constant $N_{L_2} \quad = \quad 2.6871 \cdot 10^{-19}/cm^3$

Mass-energy equivalent (= 1 kg)
Massenenergieäquivalent (= 1 kg)
Energie équivalente à une $mc^2 \quad = \quad 8.98755 \cdot 10^{16} \ J$
masse de 1 kg
Energía equivalente de 1 kg
de masa

Dielectric constant
Dielektrische Konstante
Constante diélectrique $\varepsilon_o \quad = \quad 8.85419 \cdot 10^{-12} A \cdot s/V \cdot m$
Constante dieléctrica

4. Decimal multiples and fractions - Dezimale Vielfache und Teile -
   Multiples et sousmultiples décimaux - Múltiplos y submúltiplos
   decimales

deca	da	10^1		deci	d	10^{-1}
hecto	h	10^2		centi	c	10^{-2}
kilo	k	10^3		milli	m	10^{-3}
mega	M	10^6		micro	μ	10^{-6}
giga	G	10^9		nano	n	10^{-9}
tera	T	10^{12}		pico	p	10^{-12}
peta	P	10^{15}		femto	f	10^{-15}
exa	E	10^{18}		atto	a	10^{-18}

5. Electric and magnetic units - Elektrische und magnetische Einheiten - Unités d'électricité et de magnétisme - Unidades eléctricas
   y magnéticas

Ampere	1 A	=	1 C/s
Volt	1 V	=	1 W/A
Coulomb	1 C	=	1 A·S
Ohm	1 Ω	=	1 V/A
Farad	1 F	=	1 A·s/V
Henry	1 H	=	1 V·s/A
Weber	1 Wb	=	1 V·s
Oerstedt	1 Oe	=	$10^3/4\pi \cdot A/m$
Gauss	1 G	=	$10^{-4} Wb/m^2$
Electrostatic unit	1 esu	=	$3.3356 \cdot 10^{-10}$ C

6. Mathematical formulas - Mathematische Formeln - Formules mathé-
   matiques - Fórmulas matemáticas

   Error analysis - Fehlerrechnung - Analyse d'erreurs - Análisis de
   error

   Arithmetic mean - Arithmetisches Mittel - Valeur moyenne -
   Media aritmética

$$\bar{x} = \frac{1}{n} (x_1 + x_2 + \ldots + x_i + \ldots + x_n) = \frac{1}{n} \sum_{i=1}^{n} x_1$$

   Mean-square error - Mittlerer quadratischer Fehler - Variance -
   Error cuadratico-medio

$$s = \frac{1}{n-1} \sum_{i=1}^{n} (x_i - \bar{x})^2$$

   Standard deviation - Standardabweichung - Ecart type - Desviación
   standard

$$s_{\bar{x}} = \frac{s}{\sqrt{n}} \sqrt{\frac{1}{n(n-1)} \sum_{i=1}^{n} (x_i - \bar{x})^2}$$

7. Photon energies and wave lengths (λ) - Photonenenergien und Wellenlängen (λ) - Energie et longueurs d'onde (λ) des photons - Energías de los fotónes y longitudes de onda (λ)

Values rounded off - Zahlenwerte abgerundet - Valeurs arrondies - Valores redondeados

Photon energy - Photonenenergie Energie des photons Energía de los fotones			λ	Type of radiation Art der Strahlung Type de rayonnement Tipo de radiación
E	Joule	cal	nm	
1 eV	$1.6 \cdot 10^{-19}$	$3.82 \cdot 10^{-20}$	$1.24 \cdot 10^3$	Infrared-Infrarot
5 eV	$8.0 \cdot 10^{-19}$	$1.91 \cdot 10^{-19}$	$2.48 \cdot 10^2$	Visible light
10 eV	$1.6 \cdot 10^{-18}$	$3.82 \cdot 10^{-19}$	$1.24 \cdot 10^2$	Ultraviolet (UV)
50 eV	$8.0 \cdot 10^{-18}$	$1.91 \cdot 10^{-19}$	$2.48 \cdot 10^1$	
100 eV	$1.6 \cdot 10^{-17}$	$3.82 \cdot 10^{-18}$	$1.24 \cdot 10^1$	
500 eV	$8.0 \cdot 10^{-17}$	$1.91 \cdot 10^{-18}$	2.48	
1 keV	$1.6 \cdot 10^{-16}$	$3.82 \cdot 10^{-17}$	1.24	
5 keV	$8.0 \cdot 10^{-16}$	$1.91 \cdot 10^{-17}$	$2.48 \cdot 10^{-1}$	X- and γ-rays X- und γ-Strahlung Rayons X et γ Rayos X y γ
10 keV	$1.6 \cdot 10^{-15}$	$3.82 \cdot 10^{-17}$	$1.24 \cdot 10^{-1}$	
50 keV	$8.0 \cdot 10^{-15}$	$1.91 \cdot 10^{-17}$	$2.48 \cdot 10^{-2}$	
100 keV	$1.6 \cdot 10^{-14}$	$3.82 \cdot 10^{-17}$	$1.24 \cdot 10^{-2}$	"
500 keV	$8.0 \cdot 10^{-14}$	$1.91 \cdot 10^{-17}$	$2.48 \cdot 10^{-3}$	"
1 MeV	$1.6 \cdot 10^{-13}$	$3.82 \cdot 10^{-17}$	$1.24 \cdot 10^{-3}$	"
5 MeV	$8.0 \cdot 10^{-13}$	$1.91 \cdot 10^{-17}$	$2.48 \cdot 10^{-4}$	"
10 MeV	$1.6 \cdot 10^{-12}$	$3.82 \cdot 10^{-17}$	$1.24 \cdot 10^{-4}$	"
50 MeV	$8.0 \cdot 10^{-12}$	$1.91 \cdot 10^{-17}$	$2.48 \cdot 10^{-5}$	"
100 MeV	$1.6 \cdot 10^{-11}$	$3.82 \cdot 10^{-17}$	$1.24 \cdot 10^{-5}$	"

8. Temperature - Temperatur - Température - Temperatura

Kelvin   K $1 \text{ K} = -273.16\ ^\circ\text{C} = -459.72\ ^\circ\text{F}$

$^\circ$Celsius $^\circ$C $x\ ^\circ\text{C} = (y\ ^\circ\text{F}-32)/1.8 = x + 273.16 \text{ K}$

$^\circ$Fahrenheit $^\circ$F $y\ ^\circ\text{F} = x\ ^\circ\text{C} \cdot 1.8 + 32 = x \cdot 1.8 + 241 \text{ K}$

Equivalent temperatures - Äquivalente Temperaturen - Températures équivalentes - Temperaturas equivalentes

$^\circ$C	$^\circ$F	$^\circ$C	$^\circ$F	$^\circ$C	$^\circ$F	$^\circ$C	$^\circ$F
-100	-148	-35	-31	$\mp$ 0	+32	+40	+104
-90	-130	-30	-22	$\mp$ 5	+41	+45	+113
-80	-112	-25	-13	+10	+50	+50	+122
-70	-94	-20	-4	+15	+59	+60	+140
-60	-76	-15	+5	+20	+68	+70	+158
-50	-58	-10	+14	+25	+77	+80	+176
-45	-49	-5	+23	+30	+86	+90	+194
-40	-40	$\pm$0	+32	+35	+95	+100	+212

Table of contents - Inhaltsverzeichnis
Table des matières - Tabla de materias

2.1 Radiological quantities and units
Radiologische Größen und Einheiten
Grandeurs et unités radiologiques
Cantidades y unidades radiológicas

2.1.1 Quantities - Größen - Grandeurs - Cantidades

Quantity Größe Grandeur Cantidad	Defining equation Definitionsgleichung Equation de definition Ecuación que las define
Activity Aktivität Activité Actividad	$A = \dfrac{dN}{dt}$	Number of disintegrations dN/ time interval dt Anzahl von Zerfällen dN/Zeitinter- vall dt Nombre de désintégrations dN/ intervalle de temps dt Número de desintegraciones dN/ intervalo del tiempo dt
Absorbed dose Energiedosis Dose absorbée Dosis absorbida	$D = \dfrac{dW_D}{dm}$	Absorbed energy dW_D/mass dm Absorbierte Energie dW_D/Masse dm Energie absorbée dW_D/masse dm Energía absorbida dW_D/masa dm
Absorbed dose rate Energiedosisleistung Débit de dose absorbée Indice de dosis absorbida	$\dot{D} = \dfrac{dD}{dt}$	Absorbed dose dD/time interval dt Energiedosis dD/Zeitintervall dt Dose absorbée dD/intervalle de temps dt Dosis absorbida dD/intervalo del tiempo dt
Exposure (Standard-)Ionendosis Exposition Exposición	$X = \dfrac{dQ}{dm_L}$	Induced charge dQ/mass dm_L of air Erzeugte Ladung dQ/Luftmasse dm_L Charge produite dQ/masse dm_L d'air Carga producide dQ/masa dm_L de aire
Exposure rate Ionendosisleistung Débit d'exposition Indice de exposición	$\dot{X} = \dfrac{dX}{dt}$	Exposure dX/time interval dt Ionendosis dX/Zeitintervall dt Exposition dX/intervalle de temps dt Exposición dX/intervalo del tiempo dt
Dose equivalent Äquivalentdosis Dose équivalente Dosis equivalente	$H = Q \cdot N \cdot D$ $D_q = q \cdot D$	Quality factor q x absorbed dose D Bewertungsfaktor q x Energiedosis D Facteur de qualité q x dose absorbée D Factor de calidad q x dosis absorbida D

Quality factors of different radiations
for radiation protection purposes:
Bewertungsfaktoren verschiedener Strahlen-
arten für Strahlenschutzzwecke:
Facteurs de qualité de différents rayonnements en vue de la radioprotection:
Factores de calidad de diferentes radiaciones para protección radiológica:

	q
β, γ, röntgen =	1
n =	3 - 10
α, p =	10

2.1.2 Units - Einheiten - Unités - Unidades

Quantity Größe Grandeur Cantidad	SI unit SI Einheit Unité SI SI unidad	Special name Besonderer Name Nom special Nombre especial (Symbol)	Non-SI unit Bisherige Einheit Unité hors système SI Unidad fuera de sistema SI
Activity Aktivität Activité Actividad	s^{-1}	becquerel (Bq)	curie (Ci) 1 Ci = $3.7 \cdot 10^{10} s^{-1}$
Absorbed dose Energiedosis Dose absorbée Dosis absorbida	$J \cdot kg^{-1}$	gray (Gy)	rad (rad) 1 rad = $0.01\ J \cdot kg^{-1}$
Absorbed dose rate Energiedosisleistung Débit de dose absorbée Indice de dosis absorbida	$W \cdot kg^{-1} =$ $J \cdot kg^{-1} s^{-1}$	gray/s $(Gy \cdot s^{-1})$	rad/s (rad s^{-1}) 1 rad s^{-1} = $0.01\ J \cdot kg^{-1} s^{-1}$
Exposure Ionendosis Exposition Exposición	$C \cdot kg^{-1}$	-	röntgen (R) 1 R = $2.5 \cdot 10^{-1} C \cdot kg^{-1}$
Exposure rate Ionendosisleistung Débit d'exposition Indice de exposición	$A \cdot kg^{-1} =$ $C \cdot kg^{-1} s^{-1}$	-	röntgen/s (R$\cdot s^{-1}$) 1 R$\cdot s^{-1}$ = $2.5 \cdot 10^{-4} A \cdot kg^{-1}$
Dose equivalent Äquivalentdosis Dose equivalente Dosis equivalente	$J \cdot kg^{-1}$	-	rem (rem) 1 rem = $0.01\ J \cdot kg^{-1}$

2.2 Radiological units formerly in use – Früher benützte radiologische Einheiten – Unités radiologiques anciennement utilisées – Unidades radiológicas empleadas anteriormente

Unit – Einheit / Unité – Unidad	Symbol / Symbole	Method – Methode / Methode – Método	Properties-Eigenschaften – Propriétés	Used-Gebraucht- / Utilisées: in	Equivalent rad/unit
Sabouraud-Noiré	Sab	Change of color / Verfärbung / Variation de couleur	High energy dependence / Stark energieabhängig / Forte variation avec l'énergie	Europe 1915-25	~ 200 – 400
Holzknecht	H		"	Europe 1910-30	~ 50 – 200
Kienböck	X	Photographic	"	Germany 1920-30	~ 15 – 40
Fürstenau	F	Change of resistance	"	Germany 1920-30	~ 3 – 10
Solomon	R (French)	Ionization	Low	France 1925-35	0.4 – 1.2
Röntgen	R (German)	"	Wenig / Faible / Baja	World since 1930	≈ 1.00
Röntgen	r (internat.)	"		World since 1930	0.88-0.96
Röntgen equivalent physical	rep	"	Also valid for α,β... / Auch gültig für	USA since 1955	≈ 1.00
Neutron	n	"	Valid for neutrons	USA since 1960	~ 1
Erythema dose	ED	Skin reaction / Hautreaktion	Inexact, but energy-independent	World since 1900	~ 600
Skin standard dose	HED (German)	Reaction cutanée / Reacción de la piel	Ungenau, aber energieunabhängig	Germany 1920-35	~ 800

Radioactivity – Radioaktivität – Radioactivité – Radioactividad

Unit – Einheit / Unité – Unidad	Symbol / Symbole	Method – Methode / Methode – Método	Properties-Eigenschaften – Propriétés
Rutherford	rd	Disintegrations	1 rd = 10^6/s
Stat	St	Ionization	1 St = amount of Rn 222 to produce $3.33\cdot10^{-10}$ A in air
mCi destroyed	mcd	"	1 mcd = 133 mgh with Rn 222
mg element h	mgeh/cm	"	1 mgeh/cm ≈ 6.5 rad
Eman		Disintegr./l	1 Eman = 0.275 ME (only Rn 222)
Mache	ME	"	1 ME = 3.64 Eman

Lit.: 1. ADLER, E.: Strahlenther. 5, 465 (1914) – 2. FÜRSTENAU, R.: Leitfaden, Stuttgart: Enke 1921
3. BEHNKEN, H., JAEGER, R.: Z.f.techn.Phys.7,563(1926) – 4. KÜSTNER, H.:Strahlenther.26,120(1927)
5. GREBE, L.: Strahlenther. 27, 358 (1928) – 6. HOLTHUSEN, H.:Grundlagen.., Leipzig:Thieme 1933
7. JAEGER, R., HÜBNER, W.: Dosimetrie u. Strahlenschutz, Stuttgart: Thieme 1974

2.3 Chemical composition and number of electrons/g of some materials and human tissues
Chemische Zusammensetzung und Elektronenzahl/g einiger Materialien und menschlicher Gewebe
Composition chimique et nombre d'électrons/g de quelques matériaux et des tissus humains
Composición química y número de electrones/g de algunas sustancias y tejidos humanos

Material / Material / Matière / Material	ρ g/cm³	Proportion (weight) – Gewichtsanteile – Pourcentage (poids) – Porción en peso – Element – Élément – Elemento %									N_e $\frac{10^{23}}{g}$	1.	2.	3.
		H	C	N	O	Mg	P	Ar	Ca	Ti				
Air – Luft	$1.293\cdot10^{-3}$			76	23			1			3.01	0.499	3.67	223
H₂O	1	11			89						3.34	0.555	3.66	227
Graphite	2.25		100								3.01	0.500	3.00	108
Paraffin	0.88	15	85								3.45	0.573	2.70	92
Mix D	0.99	13	78		3	4				1	3.40	0.565	2.98	196
(CH₂)n	0.92	14	86								3.44	0.570	2.71	92.5
(C₈H₈)n	1.06	8	92								3.24	0.538	2.84	99.6
Perspex	1.18	8	60		32						3.25	0.539	3.16	147
Muscle–Muskel–Muscles–Musculos	1.05	10	12	4	73	0.4	0.2		0.01		3.31	0.549	3.60	230
Fat–Fett–Graisse–Grasa	0.92	12	77		11						3.36	0.558	2.87	111
Bone–Knochen–Os–Huesos	1.50	6	28	3	41	0.2	7		15		3.19	0.530	4.63	874

1. $(Z/A)_{eff}$ For Compton process and slowing down of electrons
Für Comptonprozeß und Elektronenbremsung
Pour l'effet Compton et le ralentissement des électrons
Para el proceso Compton y retención de electrones

2. $(Z^2/A)_{eff}$ For pair production and scattering of electrons
Für Paarbildung und Elektronenstreuung
Pour la production de paires et la diffusion des électrons
Para la formación de par y dispersión de electrones

3. $(Z^4/A)_{eff}$ For photoelectric effect – Für photoelektrischen Prozess
Pour l'effet photoélectrique – Para efecto fotoeléctrico

Z = Atomic number
Ordnungszahl
Nombre atomique
Número atómico

A = Atomic weight
Atomgewicht
Masse atomique
Peso atómico

N_e = Number of electrons/g
Zahl der Elektronen/g
Nombre d'électrons/g
Número de electrones/g

Lit.: 1. ATTIX, F.H., TOCHILIN, E.: Radiation Dosimetry, New York, London: Academic-Press 1969
      2. JAEGER, R.G., HÜBNER, W.: Dosimetrie und Strahlenschutz, Stuttgart: Thieme 1974

2.4 Correction of the air density for ionization chambers
Korrektur der Luftdichte für Ionisationskammern
Corrections pour la densité de l'air pour chambres d'ionisation
Correcciones por densidad de aire en cámaras de ionización

The dose X_1, measured at air density ρ, (temperature t, pressure p) by means of an unsealed chamber which has been calibrated at ρ_0 (t_0, p_0) has to be corrected to yield the true value of X:

Die Dosis X_1, welche bei Luftdichte ρ (Temperatur t, Luftdruck p) mit einer nicht luftdichten Kammer gemessen wird, welche bei einer Luftdichte ρ_0 (t_0, p_0) calibriert wurde, muß korrigiert werden, um den wahren Wert X zu erhalten:

La dose X_1 mesurée avec une densité de l'air ρ (température t, pression p) au moyen d'une chambre non scellée étalonnée avec une densité de l'air ρ_0 (t_0, p_0) doit être corrigée pour obtenir la valeur vraie X:

Para obtener el verdadero valor de una dosis X, cuando la dosis X_1, ha sido medida por medio de una cámara no sellada a una densidad del aire ρ (temperatura t, presión p), calibrada a una densidad del aire ρ_0 (t_0, p_0), se debe corregir la lectura por medio de la siguiente fórmula:

$$X = X_1 \cdot \frac{\rho_0}{\rho} \qquad \rho = \frac{1.293}{1 + 0.00366\ t} \cdot \frac{p}{760} \ (mg/cm^3)$$

$$t\ (^{\circ}C) \qquad\qquad p\ (Torr)$$

Pressure Druck Pression Présion	Air density – Luftdichte – Densité de l'air – Densidad del aire								mg/cm³
	Temperature – Temperatur – Température – Temperatura °C								
Torr / mbar	0	5	10	15	20	25	30	35	40
640 / 853	1.089	1.069	1.050	1.032	1.015	0.997	0.981	0.965	0.950
650 / 866	1.106	1.086	1.067	1.048	1.030	1.013	0.996	0.980	0.965
660 / 880	1.123	1.103	1.083	1.064	1.046	1.029	1.012	0.995	0.979
670 / 893	1.140	1.119	1.100	1.081	1.062	1.044	1.027	1.010	0.994
680 / 906	1.157	1.136	1.116	1.097	1.078	1.060	1.042	1.025	1.009
690 / 920	1.174	1.153	1.132	1.113	1.094	1.075	1.058	1.041	1.024
700 / 933	1.191	1.170	1.149	1.129	1.110	1.091	1.073	1.056	1.039
710 / 946	1.208	1.186	1.165	1.145	1.125	1.107	1.088	1.071	1.054
720 / 960	1.225	1.203	1.182	1.161	1.141	1.122	1.104	1.086	1.068
730 / 973	1.242	1.220	1.198	1.177	1.157	1.138	1.119	1.101	1.083
740 / 986	1.259	1.236	1.214	1.193	1.173	1.153	1.134	1.116	1.098
750 / 1000	1.276	1.253	1.231	1.210	1.189	1.169	1.150	1.131	1.113
760 / 1013	1.293	1.270	1.247	1.226	1.205	1.185	1.165	1.146	1.128
770 / 1026	1.310	1.286	1.264	1.242	1.221	1.200	1.180	1.161	1.143
780 / 1040	1.327	1.303	1.280	1.258	1.236	1.216	1.196	1.176	1.157
790 / 1053	1.344	1.320	1.297	1.274	1.252	1.231	1.211	1.191	1.172
800 / 1066	1.361	1.337	1.313	1.290	1.268	1.247	1.226	1.206	1.187
810 / 1080	1.378	1.353	1.329	1.306	1.284	1.262	1.242	1.221	1.202
820 / 1093	1.395	1.370	1.346	1.322	1.300	1.278	1.257	1.237	1.217

1 Torr = 1.33 mbar   1 mbar = 0.75 Torr
$^{\circ}C$ = K-273   K = $^{\circ}C$+273
$^{\circ}C$ = 5/9 · ($^{\circ}F$-32) $^{\circ}F$ = 9/5 · ($^{\circ}C$+32)

2.5 Energy- and photon fluence per röntgen
Energie- und Photonenfluenz pro Röntgen
Fluence en énergie et en nombre de photons par röntgen
Flujo de energía y de fotones por röntgen

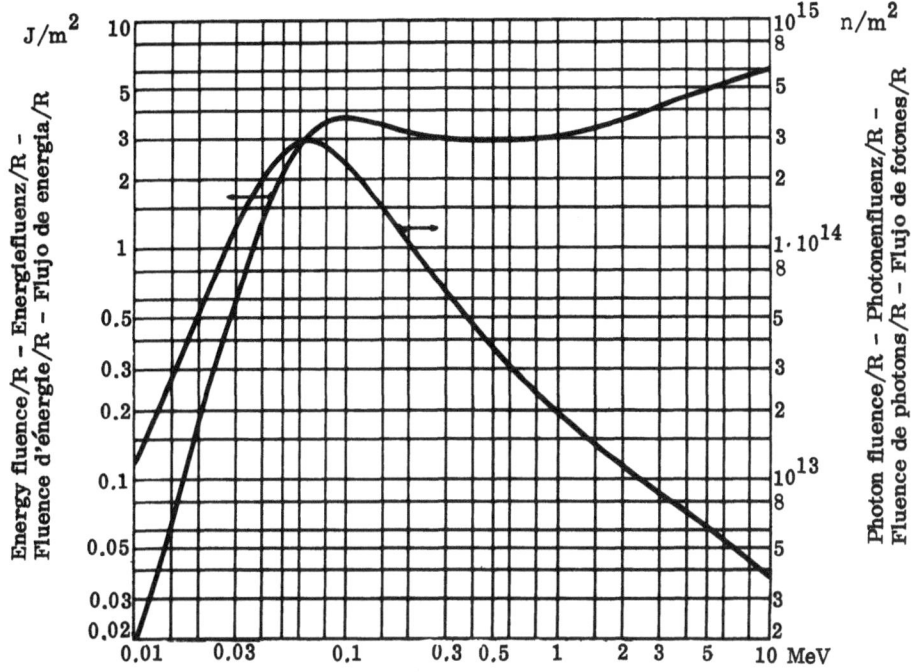

Energy - Energie - Energie - Energia

Photon energy Photonenenergie Energie des photons Energía de los fotones MeV	Fluence per röntgen - Fluenz pro Röntgen Fluence par röntgen - Flujo por röntgen	
	Energy Energie J/m² Énergie Energía	Number of photons Photonenzahl Nombre de photons n/m² Número de fotones
0.01	0.019	$1.18 \cdot 10^{13}$
0.02	0.170	5.31
0.04	1.301	20.30
0.06	2.849	29.70
0.08	3.576	27.90
0.10	3.714	23.20
0.20	3.243	10.10
0.40	2.946	4.60
0.66	2.956	2.79
0.80	3.007	2.35
1.00	3.126	1.95
1.25	3.267	1.63
2.0	3.714	1.16
4.0	4.672	0.73
8.0	5.717	0.447
10.0	5.993	0.375

2.6   Conversion of exposure to absorbed dose
              Umrechnung von Ionendosis in Energiedosis
              Conversion de l'exposition en dose absorbée
              Conversión de exposición en dosis energía

2.6.1   X- and gamma rays - Röntgen- und Gammastrahlung -
            Rayonnements X et gamma - Rayos X y gamma

2.6.1.1   Water - Wasser - Eau - Agua

Conversion factor - Umrechnungsfaktoren - Facteurs de conversion - Factores de conversión F_γ (rad/R)			
Radiation quality - Strahlenqualität - Qualité du rayonnement - Calidad de la radiación			
Monochromatic Monochromatisch Monochromatique Monocromática	"Normal radiation" *) "Normalstrahlung" "Rayonnement normal" "Radiación normal"	HVL - HWSD CDA - CHR	F_γ
E_0			rad/R
16 keV	32 kV	0.5 mm Al	0.89
21.5 keV	43 kV	1.0 mm Al	0.88
26.5 keV	53 kV	2.0 mm Al	0.87
35 keV	70 kV	4.0 mm Al	0.87
42.5 keV	85 kV	6.0 mm Al	0.88
50 keV	100 kV	8.0 mm Al	0.89
62.5 keV	125 kV	0.5 mm Cu	0.89
80 keV	160 kV	1.0 mm Cu	0.91
95 keV	190 kV	2.0 mm Cu	0.93
130 keV	260 kV	3.0 mm Cu	0.95
150 keV	300 kV	4.0 mm Cu	0.96
Cs 137	(Cs 137)	Cs 137	0.95
1 MeV	2 MV	-	0.95
Co 60	(Co 60)	Co 60	0.95
2 MeV	4 MV	-	0.94
3 MeV	6 MV	-	0.93
4 MeV	8 MV	-	0.93
5 MeV	10 MV	-	0.92
6 MeV	12 MV	-	0.91
7.5 MeV	15 MV	-	0.90
10 MeV	20 MV	-	0.90
12.5 MeV	25 MV	-	0.89
15 MeV	30 MV	-	0.88
17.5 MeV	35 MV	-	0.88

*) Definition "normal radiation" see page 70
   Definition "Normalstrahlung" siehe Seite 70
   Définition "rayonnement normal" voir page 70
   Definición "radiación normal" véase página 70

Lit.: 1. ICRU Report 23, Washington 1973

2.6.1.2 **Ratio of mass absorption coefficients, tissue/air**
Verhältnis der Massenabsorptionskoeffizienten Gewebe/Luft
Rapport des coefficients d'absorption massique tissu/air
Relación del coeficiente de absorción masico tejido/aire

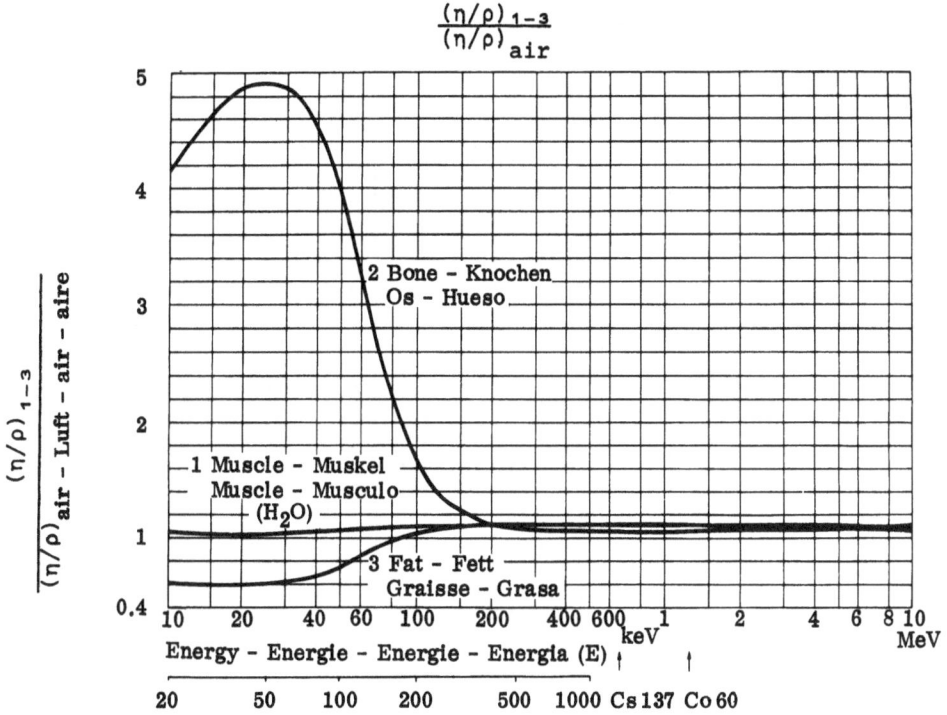

$$\frac{(\eta/\rho)_{1-3}}{(\eta/\rho)_{air}}$$

Energy - Energie - Energie - Energia (E)

Tube voltage - Röhrenspannung - Tension d'alimentation
Voltaje del tubo

E	$\frac{(\eta/\rho)_{1-3}}{(\eta/\rho)_{air}}$			E	$\frac{(\eta/\rho)_{1-3}}{(\eta/\rho)_{air}}$		
keV	1	2	3	MeV	1	2	3
10	1.04	4.17	0.61	0.2	1.11	1.12	1.11
15	1.01	4.59	0.59	0.3	1.11	1.08	1.12
20	1.00	4.81	0.58	0.5	1.11	1.07	1.12
30	1.01	4.86	0.59	Cs 137	1.11	1.06	1.12
40	1.01	4.55	0.64	1	1.11	1.06	1.12
50	1.03	3.97	0.74	Co 60	1.11	1.06	1.12
60	1.05	3.27	0.84	2	1.12	1.06	1.12
80	1.08	2.21	0.98	3	1.11	1.07	1.11
100	1.09	1.65	1.07	5	1.10	1.08	1.09
150	1.11	1.22	1.10	10	1.08	1.10	1.04

Lit.: 1. ATTIX, F.H., ROESCH, W.C.: Radiation Dosimetry, New York: Academic Press 1968
2. JAEGER, R., HÜBNER, W.: Dosimetrie und Strahlenschutz, Stuttgart: Thieme 1974

2.6.1.3 Exemples - Beispiele - Exemples - Ejemplos

Corresponding values - Es entsprechen - Valeurs correspondantes Valores corespondientes in - in - en - en 1 Gy (= 100 rad)						
Radiation HVL Strahlung HWSD Rayonnement CDA Radiación CHR	H$_2$O (Muscle Muskel-Muscle Musculo)		Bone Knochen Os - Hueso		Fat - Fett Graisse Grasa	
	R	C/kg	R	C/kg	R	C/kg
0.1 mm Al	111	$2.86 \cdot 10^{-2}$	28	$0.722 \cdot 10^{-2}$	187	$4.82 \cdot 10^{-2}$
0.5 mm Al	112	$2.89 \cdot 10^{-2}$	24	$0.619 \cdot 10^{-2}$	192	$4.95 \cdot 10^{-2}$
1 mm Al	114	$2.94 \cdot 10^{-2}$	24	$0.619 \cdot 10^{-2}$	196	$5.06 \cdot 10^{-2}$
2 mm Al	115	$2.97 \cdot 10^{-2}$	24	$0.619 \cdot 10^{-2}$	200	$5.16 \cdot 10^{-2}$
4 mm Al	115	$2.97 \cdot 10^{-2}$	24	$0.619 \cdot 10^{-2}$	187	$4.82 \cdot 10^{-2}$
6 mm Al	114	$2.94 \cdot 10^{-2}$	26	$0.671 \cdot 10^{-2}$	172	$4.44 \cdot 10^{-2}$
8 mm Al	112	$2.89 \cdot 10^{-2}$	29	$0.748 \cdot 10^{-2}$	156	$4.02 \cdot 10^{-2}$
0.5 mm Cu	112	$2.89 \cdot 10^{-2}$	38	$0.980 \cdot 10^{-2}$	137	$3.53 \cdot 10^{-2}$
1 mm Cu	110	$2.84 \cdot 10^{-2}$	53	$1.37 \cdot 10^{-2}$	120	$3.10 \cdot 10^{-2}$
2 mm Cu	106	$2.73 \cdot 10^{-2}$	65	$1.68 \cdot 10^{-2}$	110	$2.84 \cdot 10^{-2}$
3 mm Cu	105	$2.71 \cdot 10^{-2}$	83	$2.14 \cdot 10^{-2}$	106	$2.73 \cdot 10^{-2}$
4 mm Cu	104	$2.68 \cdot 10^{-2}$	94	$2.43 \cdot 10^{-2}$	106	$2.73 \cdot 10^{-2}$
Cs 137,1 MV,Co 60	105	$2.71 \cdot 10^{-2}$	110	$2.84 \cdot 10^{-2}$	104	$2.68 \cdot 10^{-2}$
2 MV	105	$2.71 \cdot 10^{-2}$	110	$2.84 \cdot 10^{-2}$	104	$2.68 \cdot 10^{-2}$
4 MV	106	$2.73 \cdot 10^{-2}$	111	$2.86 \cdot 10^{-2}$	106	$2.73 \cdot 10^{-2}$
6 MV	106	$2.73 \cdot 10^{-2}$	111	$2.86 \cdot 10^{-2}$	106	$2.73 \cdot 10^{-2}$
8 MV	108	$2.79 \cdot 10^{-2}$	111	$2.86 \cdot 10^{-2}$	108	$2.79 \cdot 10^{-2}$
10 MV	109	$2.81 \cdot 10^{-2}$	111	$2.86 \cdot 10^{-2}$	110	$2.84 \cdot 10^{-2}$
12 MV	109	$2.81 \cdot 10^{-2}$	110	$2.84 \cdot 10^{-2}$	111	$2.86 \cdot 10^{-2}$
15 MV	110	$2.84 \cdot 10^{-2}$	110	$2.84 \cdot 10^{-2}$	112	$2.89 \cdot 10^{-2}$
20 MV	111	$2.86 \cdot 10^{-2}$	109	$2.81 \cdot 10^{-2}$	116	$2.99 \cdot 10^{-2}$

Corresponding values - Es entsprechen - Valeurs correspondantes Valores corespondientes 100 R (= $2.58 \cdot 10^{-2}$ C/kg)						
Radiation HVL Strahlung HWSD Rayonnement CDA Radiación CHR	H O (Muscle Muskel-Muscle Musculo)		Bone Knochen Os - Hueso		Fat - Fett Graisse Grasa	
	rad	Gy	rad	Gy	rad	Gy
0.1 mm Al	90	0.90	361	3.61	53	0.53
0.5 mm Al	89	0.89	409	4.09	52	0.52
1 mm Al	88	0.88	424	4.24	51	0.51
2 mm Al	87	0.87	419	4.19	50	0.50
4 mm Al	87	0.87	409	4.09	53	0.53
6 mm Al	88	0.88	387	3.87	58	0.58
8 mm Al	89	0.89	343	3.43	64	0.64
0.5 mm Cu	89	0.89	266	2.66	73	0.73
1 mm Cu	91	0.91	187	1.87	83	0.83
2 mm Cu	94	0.94	155	1.55	91	0.91
3 mm Cu	95	0.95	120	1.20	94	0.94
4 mm Cu	96	0.96	106	1.06	94	0.94
Cs 137,1 MV,Co 60	95	0.95	91	0.91	96	0.96
2 MV	95	0.95	91	0.91	96	0.96
4 MV	94	0.94	90	0.90	94	0.94
6 MV	94	0.94	90	0.90	94	0.94
8 MV	93	0.93	90	0.90	93	0.93
10 MV	92	0.92	90	0.90	91	0.91
15 MV	91	0.91	91	0.91	89	0.89

2.6.2 Electrons - Elektronen - Electrons - Electrones

2.6.2.1 Water - Wasser - Eau - Agua

Depth / Tiefe / Profondeur / Profundidad cm	Conversion factor - Umrechnungsfaktoren - Facteurs de conversion - Factores de conversión C_e (rad/R) Initial electron energy / Anfangsenergie der Elektronen / Energie initiale des électrons / Energía inicial de los electrones MeV									
	5	10	15	20	25	30	35	40	45	50
1	0.92	0.88	0.84	0.82	0.81	0.80	0.78	0.78	0.77	0.76
2	-	0.89	0.86	0.84	0.82	0.81	0.79	0.79	0.78	0.77
3	-	0.92	0.87	0.85	0.83	0.82	0.80	0.79	0.79	0.78
4	-	0.95	0.89	0.86	0.84	0.82	0.81	0.80	0.79	0.79
5	-	0.96	0.90	0.87	0.85	0.83	0.82	0.81	0.80	0.80
6	-	-	0.93	0.89	0.86	0.84	0.83	0.82	0.81	0.80
7	-	-	0.97	0.90	0.87	0.85	0.83	0.82	0.81	0.80
8	-	-	-	0.94	0.88	0.86	0.84	0.83	0.82	0.81
9	-	-	-	0.96	0.90	0.87	0.85	0.83	0.82	0.81
10	-	-	-	0.93	0.92	0.88	0.86	0.84	0.83	0.82
11	-	-	-	-	0.95	0.89	0.87	0.85	0.83	0.82
12	-	-	-	-	0.94	0.91	0.88	0.86	0.84	0.83
13	-	-	-	-	-	0.93	0.89	0.87	0.85	0.84
14	-	-	-	-	-	0.96	0.91	0.88	0.86	0.84
15	-	-	-	-	-	0.93	0.92	0.89	0.87	0.85
16	-	-	-	-	-	-	0.95	0.90	0.88	0.86
17	-	-	-	-	-	-	0.93	0.92	0.89	0.86
18	-	-	-	-	-	-	-	0.94	0.92	0.88
19	-	-	-	-	-	-	-	-	0.94	0.90
20	-	-	-	-	-	-	-	-	0.94	0.91
21	-	-	-	-	-	-	-	-	0.92	0.92
22	-	-	-	-	-	-	-	-	-	0.95
23	-	-	-	-	-	-	-	-	-	0.92
24	-	-	-	-	-	-	-	-	-	0.92

Lit.: 1. ICRU Report 21, Washington 1972

2.6.2.2 Stopping power ratios (S)
Verhältnis der Massenstoßbremsvermögen (S)
Rapport des pouvoirs d'arrêt massique (S)
Relación de la capacidades de frenado de masa (S)

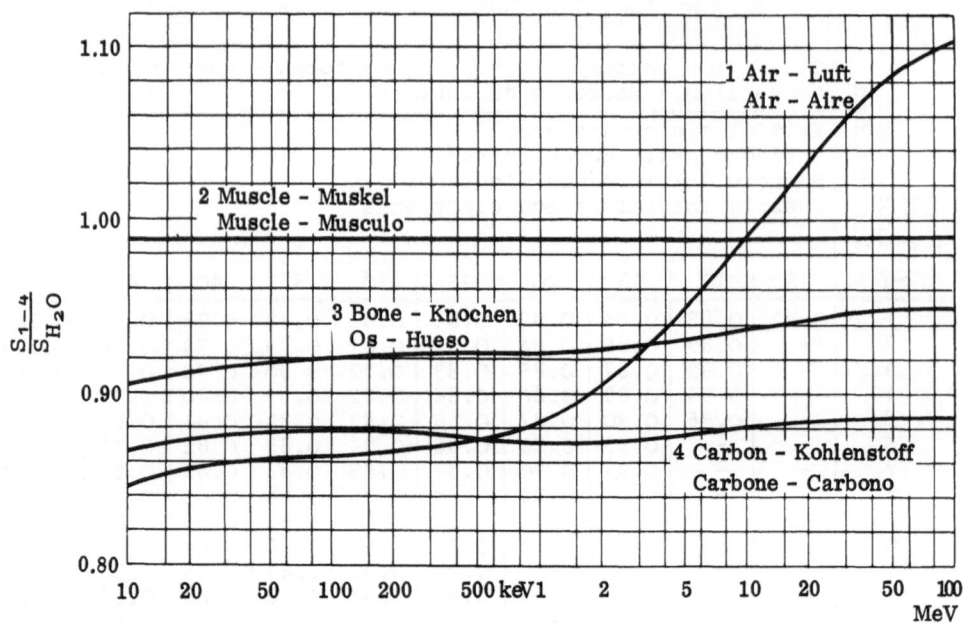

Energy - Energie - Energie - Energía

E	$\frac{S_{1-4}}{S_{H_2O}}$				E	$\frac{S_{1-4}}{S_{H_2O}}$			
keV	1	2	3	4	MeV	1	2	3	4
10	0.85	0.99	0.91	0.87	1	0.88	0.99	0.92	0.87
15	0.85	0.99	0.91	0.87	1.5	0.90	0.99	0.92	0.87
20	0.86	0.99	0.91	0.87	2	0.91	0.99	0.92	0.87
30	0.86	0.99	0.91	0.87	3	0.92	0.99	0.93	0.87
40	0.86	0.99	0.92	0.88	4	0.94	0.99	0.93	0.88
50	0.86	0.99	0.92	0.88	5	0.95	0.99	0.93	0.88
60	0.86	0.99	0.92	0.88	6	0.96	0.99	0.93	0.88
80	0.86	0.99	0.92	0.88	8	0.98	0.99	0.94	0.88
100	0.86	0.99	0.92	0.88	10	0.99	0.99	0.94	0.88
150	0.87	0.99	0.92	0.88	15	1.02	0.99	0.94	0.88
200	0.87	0.99	0.92	0.88	20	1.03	0.99	0.94	0.88
300	0.87	0.99	0.92	0.88	30	1.06	0.99	0.94	0.89
400	0.87	0.99	0.92	0.87	40	1.07	0.99	0.95	0.89
500	0.87	0.99	0.92	0.87	60	1.09	0.99	0.95	0.89
600	0.88	0.99	0.92	0.87	80	1.10	0.99	0.95	0.89
800	0.88	0.99	0.92	0.87	100	1.10	0.99	0.95	0.89

Lit.: 1. ICRP Report 21, Washington 1972

2.7 Change in radiation quality of X-rays with the depth
    Veränderung der Qualität von Röntgenstrahlen in der Tiefe
    Modification de la qualité du rayonnement X avec la profondeur
    Modificación de la calidad de rayos X con la profundidad

2.7.1 1 mm Cu HVL of the incident radiation - HWSD der einfallenden
      Strahlung - CDA du rayonnement incident - CHR de la radiación
      incidente

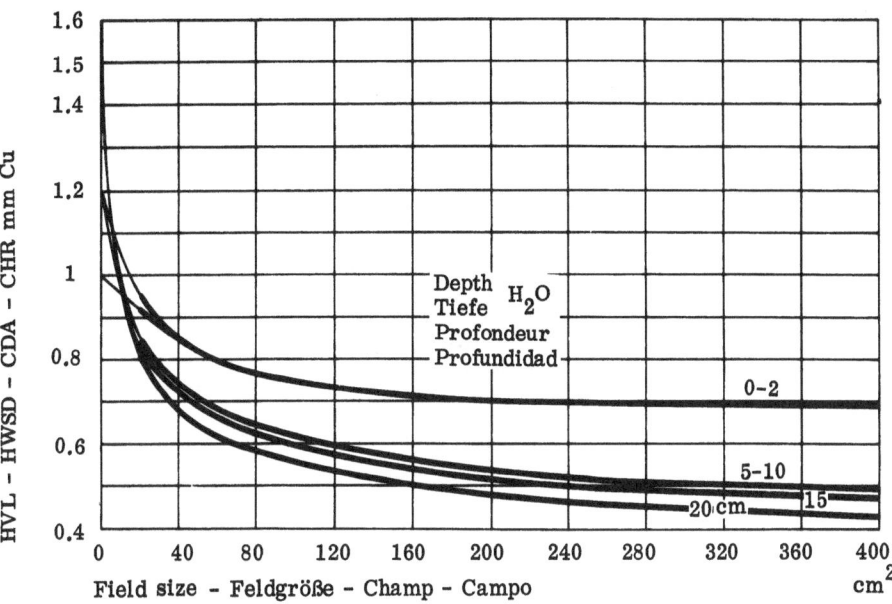

Field size - Feldgröße - Champ - Campo

2.7.2 2 mm Cu

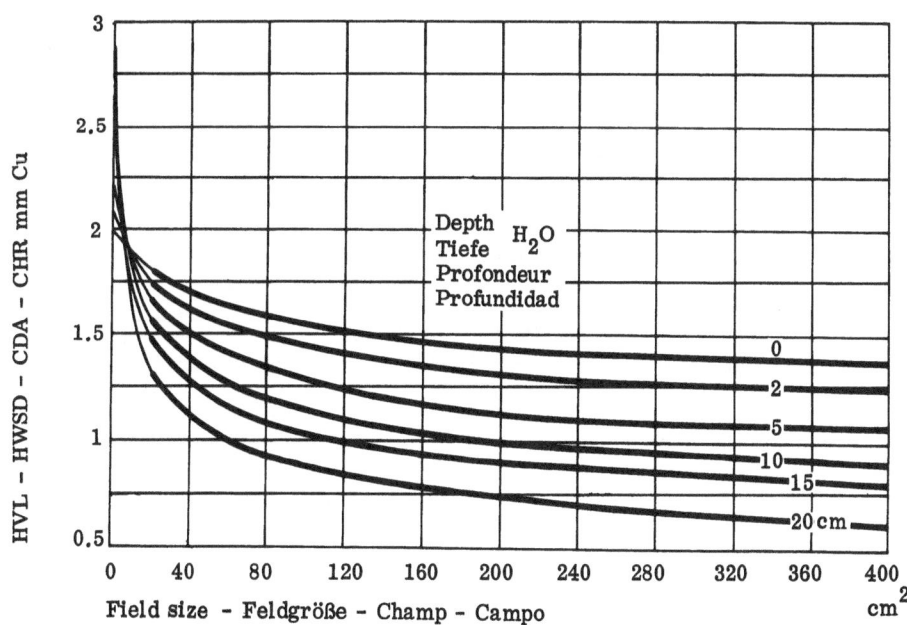

Field size - Feldgröße - Champ - Campo

2.7.3   4 mm Cu

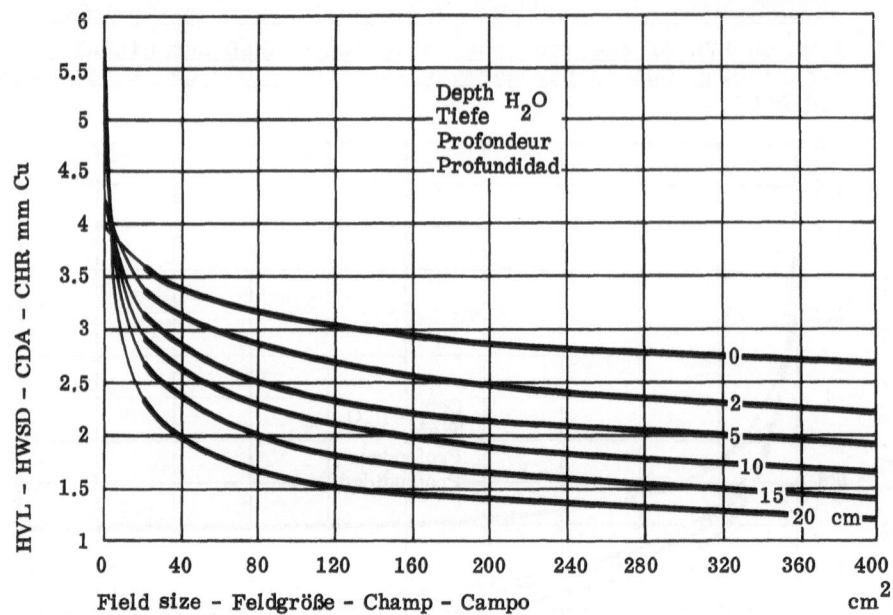

2.7.4   Cs 137

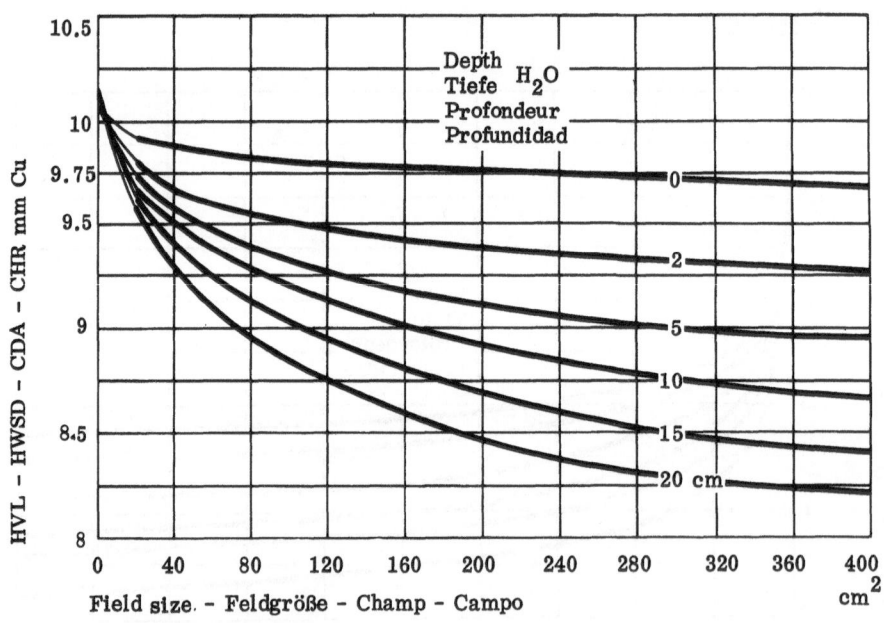

Lit.: 1. LEGARE, J.M., GONCALVES da ROCHA, A.F.: J.Radiol.Electrol. 55, 495 (1974)

2.8 Evaluation of integral dose
Ermittlung der Integraldosis
Evaluation de la dose intégrale
Evaluación de la dosis integral

The integral dose, D_I, is the energy absorbed in the body of the patient and is expressed in g rad. For water-equivalent substances it can be calculated with sufficient accuracy for practical use according to the formula:

$$D_I = D \cdot F \cdot f_i \quad (g\ R \approx g\ rad),$$

where D = dose in R in the centre of the irradiated surface or, for radiations above 1 MeV, at the dose maximum;

F = irradiated area in cm^2 at the surface; and

f_i = integral dose factor, which can be obtained from the graph or from the table next pages.

In moving field therapy, D and F should be expressed in terms of equal SSD.

Die Integraldosis D_I ist die im Körper des Patienten absorbierte Energie und wird in g rad ausgedrückt. Sie kann für wasseräquivalente Körper mit praktisch ausreichender Genauigkeit nach folgender Formel berechnet werden:

$$D_I = D \cdot F \cdot f_i \quad (g\ R \approx g\ rad),$$

wobei D = die Dosis im Zentralstrahl an der Oberfläche bzw. bei Strahlungen über 1 MeV im Dosismaximum in R;

F = die bestrahlte Fläche in cm^2, an der Oberfläche und

f_i = der Integraldosisfaktor ist, der aus der Kurve oder Tabelle (siehe folgende Seiten) entnommen werden kann.

Bei Bewegungsbestrahlung D und F auf einen konstanten FHA beziehen.

La dose intégrale, D_I, est l'énergie absorbée dans le corps du malade et s'exprime en g rad. Pour les corps équivalents à l'eau, elle peut être calculée avec une précision suffisante en pratique, par la formule:

$$D_I = D \cdot F \cdot f_i \quad (g\ R \approx g\ rad)$$

avec D = dose en rad sur l'axe du faisceau à la surface, ou, pour les rayonnements d'énergie supérieure à 1 MeV, à la profondeur du maximum;

F = surface irradiée en cm^2 à la surface

f_i = facteur de dose intégrale relevé sur la courbe ci-jointe ou dans le tableau.

En radiothérapie cinétique D et F doivent être exprimé pour une même DSP.

La dosis integral D_I es la energía absorbida en el cuerpo del paciente y se expresa en g rad. Se puede calcular por cuerpos equivalentes al agua con suficiente exactitud práctica, medianta la siguien fórmula:

$$D_I = D \cdot F \cdot f_i \quad (g\ R \approx g\ rad)$$

donde D = dosis en el rayo central en superficie o, para radiaciones por encima de 1 MeV, en el máximo de dosis en R

F = area irradiada en cm^2 en superficie y

f_i = factor de dosis integral, que se puede sacar de la gráfica o tablas contiguas

En el caso de terapia de movimiento, D y F se referiran al DFP constante.

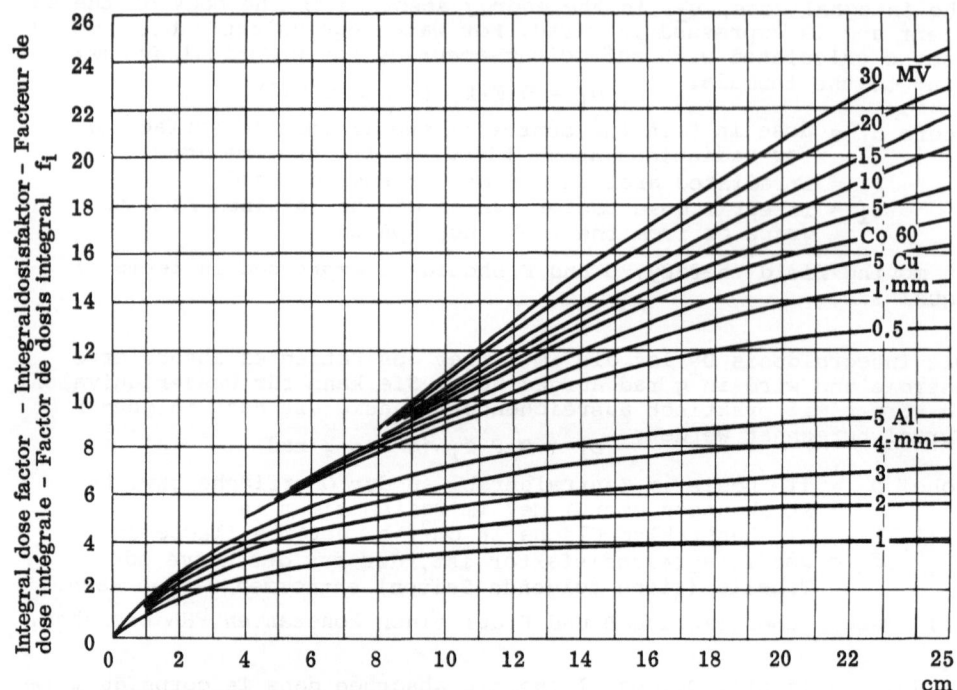

Thickness of the irradiated body (d)
Dicke des bestrahlten Körpers (d)
Epaisseur du corps irradié (d)
Espesor del cuerpo radiado (d)

Lit.: 1. MAYNEORD, W.V.: Brit.J.Radiol. 18, 12 (1945)
      2. WACHSMANN, F.: Strahlentherapie 93, 295 (1954)
      3. WATSON, T.A. et al.: Radiology 62, 165 (1954)
      4. KELLER, H.L.: Fortschr. Röntgenstr. 84, 73 und 85, 333 (1956)
      5. SCHOEN, D.: Strahlentherapie 120, 108/235/335/533 (1963)

d	Integral dose factors - Integraldosisfaktoren - Facteurs de dose intégrale - Factores de la dosis integral f_i							
	Radiation quality - Strahlenqualität - Qualité du rayonnement - Calidad de la radiación							
	HVL - HWSD - CDA - CHR							
	mm Al					mm Cu		
cm	1	2	3	4	5	0.5	1	5
1	1.0	1.15	1.30	1.45	1.6	-	-	-
2	1.7	2.05	2.30	2.55	2.8	-	-	-
3	2.2	2.7	3.1	3.4	3.7	-	-	-
4	2.6	3.2	3.7	4.0	4.4	5.2	-	-
5	2.9	3.6	4.2	4.6	5.0	5.9	6.1	-
6	3.1	3.9	4.5	5.0	5.6	6.5	6.7	7.0
7	3.2	4.1	4.8	5.4	6.0	7.2	7.4	7.6
8	3.3	4.3	5.0	5.8	6.5	7.7	8.0	8.2
9	3.4	4.5	5.3	6.0	6.8	8.2	8.6	9.0
10	3.6	4.7	5.5	6.3	7.2	8.9	9.2	9.6
12	3.8	4.9	5.8	6.8	7.7	9.9	10.4	10.8
14	3.9	5.1	6.1	7.3	8.2	10.8	11.5	12.0
16	4.0	5.2	6.4	7.6	8.6	11.5	12.4	13.1
18	4.0	5.4	6.6	8.0	8.9	12.0	13.2	14.5
20	4.1	5.5	6.8	8.1	9.1	12.5	13.9	15.1
22	4.1	5.6	6.9	8.2	9.2	12.8	14.6	15.7
25	4.2	5.6	7.0	8.3	9.4	13.1	15.0	16.4

d	Integral dose factors - Integraldosisfaktoren - Facteurs de dose intégrale - Factores de la dosis integral f_i					
	Radiation quality - Strahlenqualität - Qualité du rayonnement - Calidad de la radiación MV					
cm	^{60}Co	5	10	15	20	30
8	8.5	8.5	8.6	8.6	8.7	8.8
9	9.2	9.3	9.4	9.6	9.8	10.0
10	9.9	10.1	10.3	10.5	10.9	11.1
11	10.6	10.9	11.2	11.5	11.9	12.1
12	11.3	11.6	11.9	12.3	12.9	13.4
13	12.0	12.4	12.8	13.2	13.9	14.4
14	12.8	13.2	13.6	14.0	14.7	15.4
15	13.4	13.7	14.3	14.7	15.6	16.4
16	14.0	14.5	15.0	15.6	16.5	17.3
17	14.5	15.0	15.5	16.3	17.3	18.2
18	15.0	15.6	16.4	17.3	18.1	19.0
19	15.5	16.3	17.1	17.8	18.9	19.9
20	15.9	16.7	17.5	18.5	19.6	20.8
21	16.2	17.1	18.1	19.0	20.2	21.5
22	16.5	17.5	18.7	19.5	21.0	22.2
23	16.9	18.0	19.3	20.5	21.7	23.0
24	17.2	18.4	19.9	21.2	22.4	24.0
25	17.4	18.8	20.4	21.9	23.0	25.0

2.9 Characteristics of various dosimeters – Eigenschaften verschiedener Dosimeter – Caractéristiques de différents dosimètres – Características de diferentes dosímetros

Suitable for / Geeignet für / Convenables pour / Apropiado para

System	α β γ n Radiations Strahlungen Rayonnements Radiaciónes	1 2 3 4 Dose Dosis Dose Dosis	1 2 3 4 Dose rate Dosisleistung Débit de dose Intensidad	5 6 7 Accumulation Speicherung Intégration Acumulación	1 2 3 Error Fehler Erreur Error	Standard dosimetry	1 2 3 4 Energy dependence Energieabhängigkeit Variation avec l'énergie Dependencia de la energia	2 3 Detector size Detektorgröße Taille détecteur Tamano detector	2 3 4 Expenditure Aufwand Coût Investición
Ionisation	█ █ █ █	█ █	█ █		█ █	●	●	█ █	●
Counter	█ █ █	█ █	█ █ █	●	█ █	●	●	● ●	● ●
Calorimeter	█	●	●	●	●	●	●	●	●
Chemical	█ █ █	●		●	●		●	●	●
Photographic	█ █ █	●		●	●		●	●	●
Radiophotolum.	█ █	●	●	●	●		█	●	●
Thermolumines.	█	●		●	●		█	●	●
Semiconductor	█ █	█	█	●	●	●	█	●	●
Transparency	█		●	●	●		█	●	●
Conductivity				●			●	●	●
Scintillation	█ █ █		█	●	█		█	█	●
Exoelectrons	█	█		●	●		█	●	●

1. Very small/very good – Sehr klein/sehr gut – Très petit/très bon – Muy pequeno/muy bueno
2. Small/good – Klein/gut – Petit/bon – Pequeno/bueno
3. Medium – Mittel/mäßig – Moyen – Medio
4. Large-very large/bad – Groß-sehr groß/schlecht – Grand-très grand/mauvais – Grande-muy grande/mal
5. Impossible – Nicht möglich – Impossible – Imposible
6. Limited possibility – Beschränkt möglich – Limitée – Limitado
7. Quite possible – Gut möglich – Possible – Muy adecuado

Lit.: 1. JAEGER, R.G., HÜBNER, W.: Dosimetrie und Strahlenschutz, Stuttgart: Thieme 1974

2.10 Practical hints for dose measurements

1. The functioning of the dosimeter (leakage and test reading) should be checked regularly. Temperature equilibrium between the chamber and the radioactive check source must be reached, and time for warmup must be allowed. Decrease in activity in the check source since reference date of the calibration protocol must be tanken into account. Tests for sensitivity, done with the check source should consist of several measurements; the relative standard deviation for 10 measurements should not exceed $\pm$ 0.5 %.

2. Measuring chambers should be chosen according to the purpose for which they will be used (energy range and dose range to be measured; directional dependence).

3. The method of measurement and the setup should be chosen correctly: Incident doses "in free air" should be measured without scatter from nearby objects. For low-energy radiations, absorption in air must be taken into account (see page 80); therefore it is recommended that measurements be made at the distance where the object is to be irradiated.

   The surface dose should be measured whith directionally independent chambers on the phantom surface (geometric center of the chamber at zero depth) or should be calculated from the incident dose by multiplication with the backscatter factor (see page 138).

   Reference doses are measured under specified geometric conditions in the phantom. A water phantom is recommended the sides of which are at least 5 cm from the beam edge and the height of which is at least 20 cm.

   Reference depths, according to recommendations by ICRU and DIN (1 - 4):

X- and Gamma Radiation		Electron Beams	
Peak energy	Depth	Incident energy	Depth
10 - 60 keV	0.5 mm	2 - 5 MeV	5 mm
60 - 150 keV	5 mm	5 - 10 MeV	10 mm
150 keV - 3 MeV	50 mm	10 - 20 MeV	20 mm
>3 MeV	100 mm	20 - 50 MeV	30 mm

   Depth doses should be calculated from the measured surface doses or reference doses and from relative depth dose curves (see 86 and beyound. Note: Valid only for substances with water-equivalent absorption!).

   Tumor doses should be measured in the patient ("in vivo") at least occasionally, as a check for the correctness of the dose calculation, e.g., in the oral cavity, vagina, or rectum.

4. Measurements of radiation quality (HVL in mm Al or Cu) should be made in a narrowly collimated beam, with test filters located approximately halfway between the radiation source and the measuring chamber.

5. Correction of measurement results is neccessary if the conditions (energy, direction, field size, air density, etc.) differ from the calibration conditions.
Lit. see page 62

2.10   Praktische Hinweise für die Durchführung von Dosismessungen

1. Die Funktion des Dosimeters (Selbstablauf und Kontrollanzeige) regelmäßig überprüfen. Temperaturgleichgewicht Kammer/radioaktive Kontrollvorrichtung herstellen; Anwärmzeit beachten. Aktivitätsabnahme der Kontrollvorrichtung. Die Kontrolle der Empfindlichkeit mit der Kontrollvorrichtung sollte aus mehreren Einzelmessungen bestehen; die relative Standardabweichung sollte bei 10 Messungen nicht mehr als ± 0,5 % betragen. Prüfprotokoll berücksichtigen!

2. Meßkammern nach Verwendungszweck auswählen; Energie- und Meßbereich, Richtungsabhängigkeit usw. beachten.

3. Meßmethode und -anordnung richtig auswählen: Einfallsdosen "frei in Luft" ohne störende Streukörper messen. Bei weichen Strahlungen Luftabsorption berücksichtigen (siehe Seite 80), d.h. am besten im Bestrahlungsabstand messen.

   Oberflächendosis mit richtungsunabhängigen Meßkammern an der Phantomoberfläche (geometrische Mitte der Kammer in der Tiefe 0) messen oder aus der Einfallsdosis durch Multiplikation mit dem Rückstreufaktor (siehe Seite 132) berechnen.

   Bezugsdosen werden unter definierten geometrischen Bedingungen im Phantom gemessen. Hierzu wird ein Wasserphantom empfohlen, dessen Wände seitlich mindestens 5 cm vom Randstrahl entfernt sind und das eine Tiefe von mindestens 20 cm besitzt.
   Bezugstiefen nach Empfehlungen von ICRU und DIN (1 - 4):

Röntgen- und Gammastrahlung (Grenzenergie)		Elektronenstrahlung (Energie an der Oberfläche)	
10 - 60 keV	0,5 mm	2 - 5 MeV	5 mm
60 - 150 keV	5 mm	5 - 10 MeV	10 mm
150 keV - 3 MeV	50 mm	10 - 20 MeV	20 mm
>3 MeV	100 mm	20 - 50 MeV	30 mm

   Tiefendosen aus den gemessenen Oberflächen- oder Bezugsdosen und Kurven für die relative Tiefendosis (s. S. 86 ff.) berechnen (Achtung: Gilt nur für wasseräquivalent absorbierende Körper!).

   Herddosen wenigstens gelegentlich zur Kontrolle der Richtigkeit der Dosisberechnungen auch am Patienten ("in vivo"), z.B. in der Mundhöhle, im Ösophagus, der Vagina oder im Rectum, gemessen.

4. Messung der Strahlenqualität (HWSD in mm Al oder Cu) im eng ausgeblendeten Strahlenbündel mit Meßfiltern etwa in der Mitte zwischen Strahlenquelle und Meßkammer.

5. Korrektion der Meßergebnisse bei von Kalibrierbedingungen abweichenden Verhältnissen (Energie, Richtung, Feldgröße, Luftdichte usw.).

Lit.: 1.-4. ICRU Report 14 (1969), 17 (1970), 21 (1972), 23 (1973)
     5. MASSEY, J.B.: Manual of Dosimetry in Radiotherapy, IAEA Techn.Rep., Series 110, Vienna (1970)
     6. WACHSMANN, F., KALLERT, S.: Hdb.d.med. Radiologie, Band XVI/1, Heidelberg: Springer 1970
     7. PYCHLAU, P.: IAEA SM 84, 193 (1975)

2.10 Informations pratiques pour la mesure des doses

1 - Le fonctionnement du dosimètre doit être vérifié régulièrement (fuite et tests de lecture). L'équilibre de température entre la chambre et le dispositif radioactif de contrôle doit être établi et un temps de chauffage suffisant doit être assuré. L'activité du dispositif de contrôle doit être corrigée de la décroissance et la validité du protocole de contrôle doit être vérifiée. Pour tester la reproductibilité, plusieurs mesures devraient être effectuées à l'aide du dispositif de contrôle; l'écart type ne devrait pas être supérieur à ± 0,5 % pour 10 mesures successives.

2 - Les chambres devraient être choisies en fonction de la mesure effectuée (domaine d'énergie, domaine de dose, réponse directionnelle, etc.).

3 - La méthode de mesure et le schéma de mise en place devraient être choisis correctement: Les expositions "dans l'air" devraient être mesurées loin de tout diffuseur. Pour les rayonnements de basse énergie, il est nécessaire de tenir compte de l'absorption dans l'air (voir page 80); il est donc recommandé que les mesures soient effectuées à la distance à laquelle l'objet doit être irradié.

La dose à la surface devrait être mesurée avec des chambres sans effet directionnel, à la surface d'un fantôme (le centre géométrique de la chambre étant à la profondeur 0) ou bien elle devrait être calculée à partir de l'exposition dans l'air au moyen du facteur de rétrodiffusion.

Les doses de référence sont mesurées dans des conditions géométriques spécifiées, dans le fantôme. Il est recommandé d'utiliser un fantôme dont les bords soient à au moins 5 cm du bord du faisceau et dont la hauteur soit d'au moins 20 cm.
Les profondeurs de référence suivant les recommandations de l' ICRU (1 - 4) et de DIN sont:

Rayonnements X ou γ		Faisceaux d'électrons	
Energie maximale	Profondeur	Energie primaire	Profondeur
10 - 60 keV	0.5 mm	2 - 5 MeV	5 mm
60 - 150 keV	5 mm	5 - 10 MeV	10 mm
150 keV - 3 MeV	50 mm	10 - 20 MeV	20 mm
>3 MeV	100 mm	20 - 50 MeV	30 mm

Les doses en profondeur devraient être calculés à partir des doses à la surface ou des doses de référence et des rendements en profondeur (voir pages 86 ff). (Note: valables seulement pour les substances équivalentes à l'eau.) Les doses à la tumeur devraient être mesurées dans le malade ("in vivo") au moins occasionnellement, pour vérifier l'exactitude des calculs de dose, par exemple, dans la cavité orale, le vagin, ou le rectum.

4 - Le mesures de qualité du rayonnement (CDA en mm Al ou Cu) devraient être faites dans des conditions de faisceau étroit, très collimaté, et les atténuateurs devraient être placés à peu près à mi-distance entre la source de rayonnement et la chambre d'ionisation.

5 - La correction des résultats des mesures, lorsque c'est nécessaire, doit être faite si les conditions (énergie, direction, champ, densité de l'air, etc.) différent des conditions d'étalonnage.

Lit.: Voir page 62

2.10 Indicaciones prácticas para la realización de medidas dosimétricas

1. Comprobar periodicamente la función del dosímetro (control de aislamiento y medidor de control). Establecer el equilibrio térmico de la cámara/dispositivo de control radioactivo; préstese atención al tiempo de calentamiento. Tengase en cuenta la disminución de actividad del dispositivo de control y la validez del protocolo de prueba. Los controles de sensibilidad con el dispositivo de control deben de realizarse en varias medidas aisladas, la desviación standard relativa no debe ser superior a ± 0,5 % en 10 medidas.

2. Elegir las cámaras de medida de acuerdo con el fin práctico (intervalos de energía y medida, dependencia de la dirección).

3. Elección adecuada del dispositivo y método de medida: medir las dosis de inicidencia "libre en aire" sin cuerpos dispersantes perturbadores. Tengase en cuenta la absorción del aire en el caso de radiaciones blandas (vease pág. 80 o mejor aún medir a la distancia de radiación).

   Medir la dosis superficial con cámara de medida de dirección independiente en la superficie del muneco (centro geométrico de la cámara en profundidad 0) o calcularla multiplicando la dosis de incidencia por el factor de retrodispersión (véase pág. 132).

   La dosis de referencia se medirá en el muneco bajo condiciones geométricas definidas. Para ello se recomienda un muneco de agua, cuyas paredes se encuentren lateralmente del rayo marginal por lo menos 5 cm y que tenga una profundidad mínima de 20 cm. Profundidades de referencia según las recomendaciones de ICRU y DIN (1 - 4).

Rayos X y gamma (energía límite)		Radiación de electrones (energía en la superficie)	
10 - 60 keV	0,5 mm	2 - 5 MeV	5 mm
60 - 150 keV	5 mm	5 - 10 MeV	10 mm
150 keV - 3 MeV	50 mm	10 - 20 MeV	20 mm
>3 MeV	100 mm	20 - 50 MeV	30 mm

   Calcúlese la dosis en profundidad a partir de las dosis superficiales o de referencia medidas y las curvas de dosis en profundidad relativas (vease pág. 86 cont.). (Atención: Solo válido para cuerpo absorbente de equivalente acuoso!)

   Medir la dosis focal también en el paciente ("in vivo") p. ej. en la cavidad bucal, cuello de vagina o recto, al menos de vez en cuando, para controlar la exactitud de las medidas de dosis.

4. Medida de la calidad de la radiación (CHR en mm de Al o Cu) en haz de rayo estrecho atenuado con filtro de medida aproximadamente a la mitad entre la fuente de la radiación y cámara de medida.

5. Corrección de los resultados de medida correspondientes a las desviaciones de las condiciones de calibrado (energía, dirección, magnitud del campo, densidad del aire, etc.).

Lit.: Ver página 62

2.11 <u>What happens during irradiation of matter with 1 R (≈1 rad)?</u>
<u>Was geschieht bei Einstrahlung von 1 R (≈1 rad) in Materie?</u>
<u>Qu'arrive-t-il à un milieu irradié avec 1 R (≈1 rad)?</u>
<u>Que le sucede a la materia cuando se irradia con 1 R (≈1 rad)?</u>

$2.082 \cdot 10^9$ ion pairs/cm³ in air (density 1.293 mg/cm³)

$1.610 \cdot 10^{12}$ ion pairs/cm³ in water

$3.34 \cdot 10^{-10}$ A per 1 R/s in 1 cm³ air

$5.56 \cdot 10^{-12}$ A at 1 R/min in 1 cm³ air

∿84 erg/cm³ water

∿$5 \cdot 10^{-6}$ (= 1/500,000) °C heating of water

∿1800 ion pairs/cell (assumed cell size: 10 x 10 x 10 μm = 1000 μm³)

∿225 ion pairs/cell nucleus (assumed size of cell nucleus: 125 μm³)

∿100 ionisations in a cell during passage of a non-densely
ionising particle (X- or electron radiation), or

∿10,000 ionisations for densely ionising particles (α, p, or n);
in the cell nucleus, ∿50 or 5,000, ionisations respectively.

∿$3.5 \cdot 10^8$ ionisations per second, in a body of 70 kg, due to
exposure to background radiation of 100 mR/year (∿180 ionisations
per cell per year).

$2,082 \cdot 10^9$ Ionenpaare/cm³ in Luft (Dichte 1,293 mg/cm³)

$1,610 \cdot 10^{12}$ Ionenpaare/cm³ in Wasser

$3,34 \cdot 10^{-10}$ A je 1 R/s in 1 cm³ Luft

$5,56 \cdot 10^{-12}$ A bei 1 R/min in 1 cm³ Luft

∿84 erg/cm³ Wasser

∿$5 \cdot 10^{-6}$ (= 1/500.000) °C Erwärmung von Wasser

∿1800 Ionenpaare/Zelle (angenommene Zellgröße: 1000 μm³)

∿225 Ionenpaare/Zellkern (angenommene Größe der Zellkerns: 125 μm³)

∿100 Ionisationen in der Zelle beim Durchgang eines wenig dicht
ionisierenden Teilchens (Röntgen- oder Elektronenstrahlung) bzw.

∿10.000 dgl. bei dicht ionisierenden Teilchen (α, Protonen oder
Neutronen); dgl. im Zellkern ∿50 bzw. 5.000.

∿$3,5 \cdot 10^8$ Ionisationen/s in einem Körper von 70 kg Gewicht durch die
natürliche Strahlenexposition von 100 mR/Jahr (∿180
Ionisationen/Zelle/Jahr).

2,082·10^9 paires d'ions/cm^3 d'air (densité 1,293 mg/cm^3)

1,610·10^{12} paires d'ions/cm^3 d'eau

3,34·10^{-10} A pour 1 R/s dans 1 cm^3 d'air

5,56·10^{-12} A pour 1 R/min dans 1 cm^3 d'air

$\sim$84 erg/cm^3 dans l'eau

$\sim$5·10^{-6} (= 1/500 000) $^{\circ}$C élévation de température de l'eau

$\sim$1800 paires d'ions/cellule (taille moyenne de la cellule:
  10 x 10 x 10 μm = 1000 μm^3)

$\sim$225 paires d'ions/noyau de cellule (taille moyenne du noyau de la
  cellule: 125 μm^3)

$\sim$100 ionisations dans la cellule lors du passage d'un rayonnement
  faiblement ionisant (rayons X ou electrons)

$\sim$10 000 ionisations pour des rayonnements fortement ionisants
  (particules α, protons ou neutrons); $\sim$50 à 5 000 évèments dans
  les noyaux de cellule.

$\sim$3,5·10^8 ionisations/s dans un corps de masse 70 kg pour une exposition à l'irradiation d'origine naturelle de 100 mR/a. ($\sim$180
  ionisations/cellule/a).

2,082·10^9 pares ionicos/cm^3 en aire (densidad 1,293 mg/cm^3)

1,610·10^{12} pares ionicos/cm^3 en agua

3,34·10^{-10} A por cada 1 R/s en 1 cm^3 de aire

5,56·10^{-12} A con 1 R/min en 1 cm^3 de aire

$\sim$84 erg/cm^3 en agua

$\sim$5·10^{-6} (= 1/500 000) $^{\circ}$C de calentamiento del agua

$\sim$1800 pares iónicos/célula (supuesto un tamaño de célula:
  10 x 10 x 10 μm = 1000 μm^3)

$\sim$225 pares iónicos/núcleo celular (supuesto un tamaño de núcleo
  celular: 125 μm^3)

$\sim$100 ionizaciones en la célula por el paso de una partícula poco
  ionizante (rayos X o radiación electrónica) o

$\sim$10.000 asimismo en el caso de partículas fuertemente ionizantes
  (α, protones o neutrones); asimosmo en el núcleo célular

$\sim$50 ó sea 5.000.

$\sim$3,5·10^8 ionizaciones/s en un cuerpo de 70 kg de peso mediante el
  efecto de la radiación natural de 100 mR/año ($\sim$180 ionizaciones/
  célula/año).

Table of contents - Inhaltsverzeichnis
Table des matières - Tabla de materias

3.1   Relationship between tube voltage, filtration and HVL
      Zusammenhang zwischen Röhrenspannung, Filterung und HWSD
      Relations entre tension d'alimentation, filtration et CDA
      Relación entre la voltaje del tubo, filtración y CHR

3.1.1 10 - 150 kV Tube voltage - Röhrenspannung - Tension d'alimen-
       tation - Voltaje del tubo

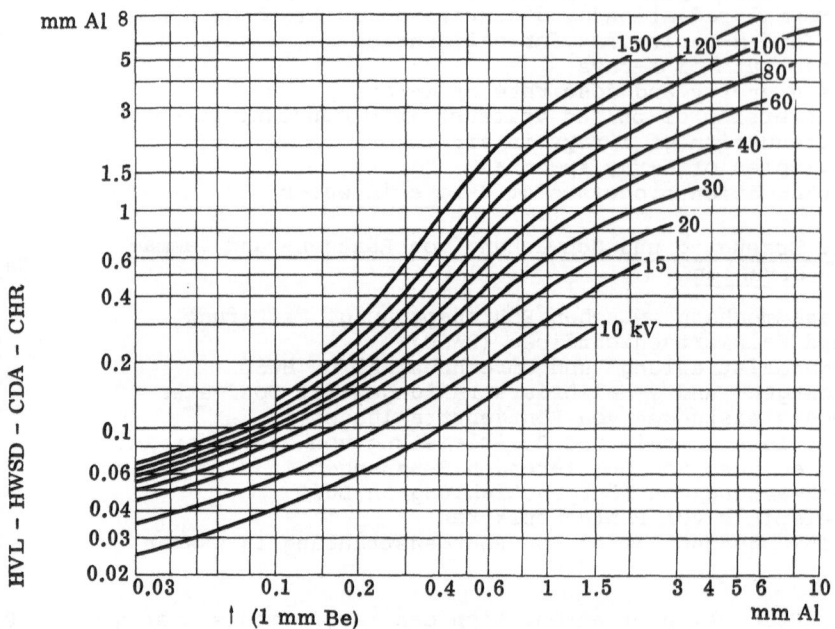

Filtration - Filterung - Filtration - Filtracion

Filtration Filterung Filtration Filtración total	HVL - HWSD - CDA - CHR						mm Al	
	Tube voltage - Röhrenspannung - Tension d'alimentation - Voltaje del tubo							kV
mm Al	10	20	40	60	80	100	120	150
0.03	0.024	0.044	0.054	0.058	0.062	0.066	–	–
0.05	0.030	0.053	0.066	0.071	0.076	0.080	–	–
0.07	0.035	0.061	0.076	0.082	0.088	0.100	–	–
0.1	0.041	0.072	0.095	0.104	0.112	0.124	0.137	–
0.15	0.050	0.092	0.124	0.134	0.15	0.17	0.19	0.23
0.20	0.056	0.110	0.17	0.18	0.20	0.23	0.27	0.31
0.30	0.077	0.15	0.22	0.25	0.30	0.38	0.42	0.57
0.5	0.12	0.24	0.37	0.47	0.60	0.80	0.97	1.35
0.7	0.16	0.33	0.55	0.71	0.94	1.30	1.55	2.15
1.0	0.22	0.45	0.79	1.02	1.30	1.85	2.25	3.05
1.5	0.29	0.60	1.08	1.36	1.97	2.4	3.1	4.3
2.0	–	0.73	1.30	1.7	2.3	3.0	4.0	5.3
3.0	–	0.90	1.7	2.3	3.0	4.0	5.1	7.2
4.0	–	–	2.0	2.6	3.6	4.8	6.1	–
7.0	–	–	–	(3.4)	4.7	6.5	8.2	–
10.0	–	–	–	–	–	7.0	–	–

3.1.2 <u>100 - 1000 kV Tube voltage - Röhrenspannung -</u>
       <u>Tension d'alimentation - Voltaje del tubo</u>

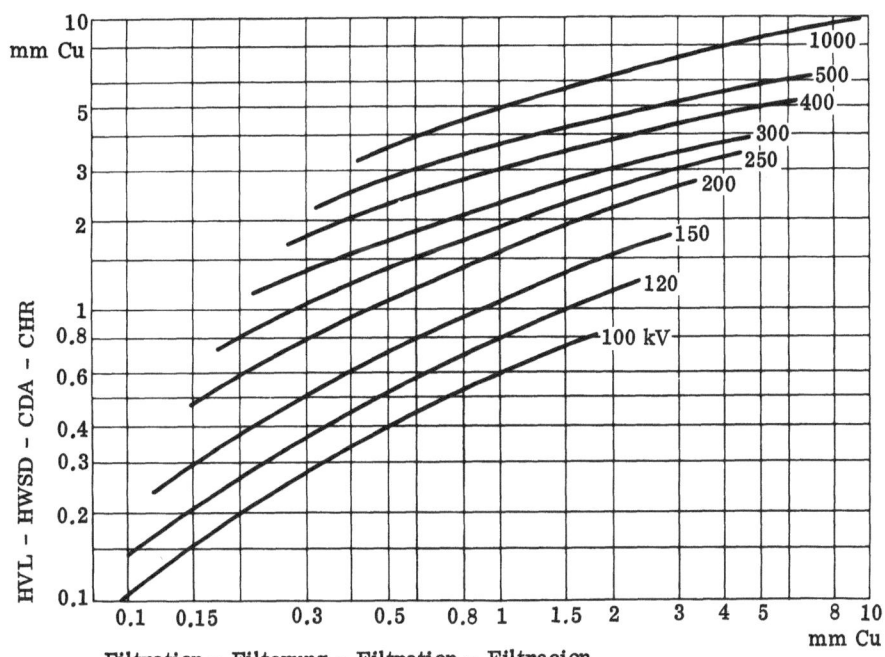

Filtration - Filterung - Filtration - Filtracion

Filtration Filterung Filtration Filtración total	HVL - HWSD - CDA - CHR								mm Cu
	Tube voltage - Röhrenspannung - Tension d'alimentation - Voltaje del tubo								kV
mm Cu	100	120	150	200	250	300	400	500	1000
O.1	0.105	0.145	-	-	-	-	-	-	-
0.15	0.155	0.21	0.295	O.48	-	-	-	-	-
O.2	0.20	0.26	0.38	0.59	0.81	(0.11)	-	-	-
O.3	0.28	0.37	0.51	0.80	1.10	1.40	1.80	(2.1)	
O.4	0.34	0.45	0.61	0.95	1.30	1.55	2.05	2.55	(3.2)
0.5	O.40	0.52	0.72	1.10	1.40	1.70	2.30	2.80	3.7
0.7	0.49	0.62	0.88	1.32	1.65	1.95	2.70	3.25	4.2
1.0	0.60	0.80	1.10	1.60	1.85	2.3	3.0	3.7	5.0
1.5	0.74	1.00	1.36	1.90	2.3	2.7	3.5	4.2	5.7
2.0	0.86	1.20	1.55	2.2	2.6	3.0	3.9	4.6	6.3
3.0	-	-	(1.8)	2.7	3.0	3.5	4.3	5.2	7.2
4.0	-	-	-	-	3.4	3.8	4.8	5.6	8.0
5.0	-	-	-	-	(3.6)	4.0	5.0	5.9	8.4
7.0	-	-	-	-	-	-	(5.3)	6.2	9.3
10.0	-	-	-	-	-	-	-	(6.7)	10.0

Lit.: 1. TROUT, D.E., GAGER, R.M.: Am.J.Radiol. 62, 91 (1949)
      2. - 3. ZIELER, E.: Strahlenther. 93,579 (1954); 100,595 (1956)
      4. HPA Report B, Series No. 7
      5. Authors' measurements - Eigene Messungen - Mesures
         personnelles - Medidas propias

3.2 "Normal radiation" and conversion from Al to Cu HVL
"Normalstrahlung" und Umrechnung von Al in Cu HWSD
"Rayonnement normal" et conversion CDA Al en Cu
"Radiación normal" y conversión CHR Al a Cu

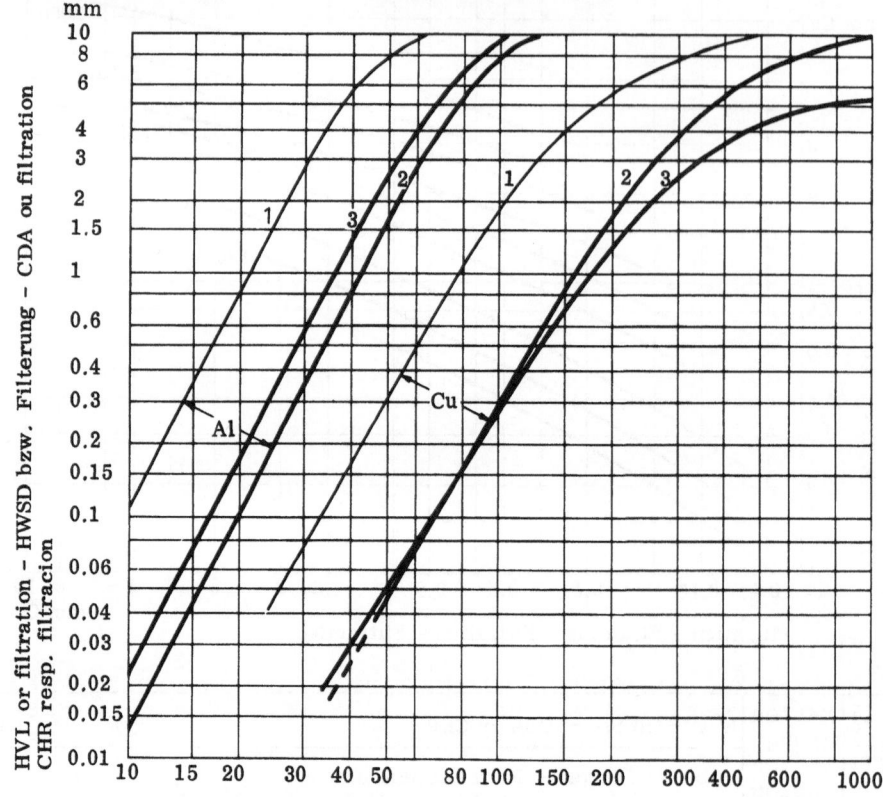

1. Limiting value of the half-value layer (HVL) for monochromatic radiation
   Grenzwert der Halbwertschicht (HWSD), monochromatische Strahlung
   Valeur limite de la couche de demi-atténuation (CDA) pour un rayonnement monochromatique
   Valor límite de la capa hemirreductora (CHR) para una radiación monocromática

2. Half-value layer of the heterogeneous normal radiation
   Halbwertschicht der heterogenen Normalstrahlung
   Couche de demi-attenuation du rayonnement normal hétérogène
   Capa hemirreductora para la radiación normal heterogénea

3. Filtration required to produce "normal radiation"
   Erforderliche Filterung zur Erzeugung von "Normalstrahlung"
   Filtration nécessaire pour la production de "rayonnement normal"
   Filtración necesaria para la obtención de una "radiación normal"

Lit.: 1. WACHSMANN, F.: Strahlenther. 83, 41 (1950)
      2. DIN 6814, Bl. 2, Berlin: Beuth-Verlag 1970

"Normal radiation" - "Normalstrahlung" - "Rayonnement normal" - "Radiación normal" *)							
	HVL-HWSD-CDA-CHR mm Al		Filter Filter Filtre Filtro		HVL-HWSD-CDA-CHR mm Cu		Filter Filter Filtre Filtro
kV	1	2	3	kV	1	2	3
10	0.11	0.013	(0.022)	50	0.30	0.045	(0.05)
15	0.35	0.045	(0.075)	70	0.65	0.11	(0.12)
20	0.83	0.11	0.17	100	1.7	0.30	0.28
25	1.7	0.20	0.33	150	3.8	0.9	0.7
30	2.8	0.35	0.58	200	5.8	1.7	1.2
40	5.8	0.83	1.3	250	7.1	2.8	1.8
50	8.0	1.7	2.4	300	8.0	3.8	2.5
60	10	2.8	4.0	400	9.0	5.8	3.5
70	-	4.0	5.4	500	10	7.1	4.2
80	-	5.3	7.0	600	-	8.0	4.7
90	-	6.7	8.0	800	-	9.0	4.9
100	-	8.0	9.6	1000	-	10	5.1

*) "Normal radiation" means heterogeneous radiation which is filtered in such a way that its HVL is the same as that of homogeneous radiation of half the energy

Unter "Normalstrahlung" versteht man eine heterogene Strahlung, die so gefiltert ist, daß ihre HWSD gleich der einer homogenen Strahlung halber Energie ist

Par "rayonnement normal" on entend un rayonnement filtré de telle sorte que sa CDA soit égale à celle d'un rayonnement homogène ayant la moitié de l'énergie

Se denomina "radiación normal" a la radiación heterogénea que ha sido filtrada en tal forma que su CHR es idéntica a la de la radiación homogénea de la mitad de su energîa

Conversion - Umrechnung - Conversion - Conversión: Al/Cu-Cu/Al **)							
HVL - HWSD - CDA - CHR:							mm
Al	Cu	Al	Cu	Cu	Al	Cu	Al
0.5	(0.016)	3	0.08	0.010	(0.30)	0.1	3.6
0.6	(0.018)	4	0.11	0.015	(0.48)	0.15	5.2
0.7	0.021	5	0.14	0.020	0.66	0.20	6.5
0.8	0.024	6	0.19	0.03	1.00	0.30	8.0
1.0	0.030	7	0.24	0.04	1.35	0.40	9.0
1.5	0.042	8	0.30	0.05	1.8	0.50	9.5
2.0	0.055	9	0.40	0.06	2.2	0.60	(10.5)
2.5	0.68	10	0.55	0.08	3.0	0.70	(11.0)

**) Valid only approximately and only for "normal radiations"
Gilt nur angenähert und nur für "Normalstrahlungen"
Valeur approchée valable seulement pour un "rayonnement normal"
Valor sólo aproximado y únicamente para "radiaciones normales"

3.3   X- and γ radiations for calibration
       Röntgen- und γ-Kalibrierstrahlungen
       Rayonnements X et γ pour l'étalonnage
       Radiaciones X y γ para la calibración

3.3.1 Radiotherapy dosimeters - Therapiedosimeter - Dosimétres
       pour radiothérapie - Dosímetros en radioterapia

3.3.1.1 Bremsstrahlung - Bremsstrahlung - Rayonnement de freinage -
        Radiación de frenaje

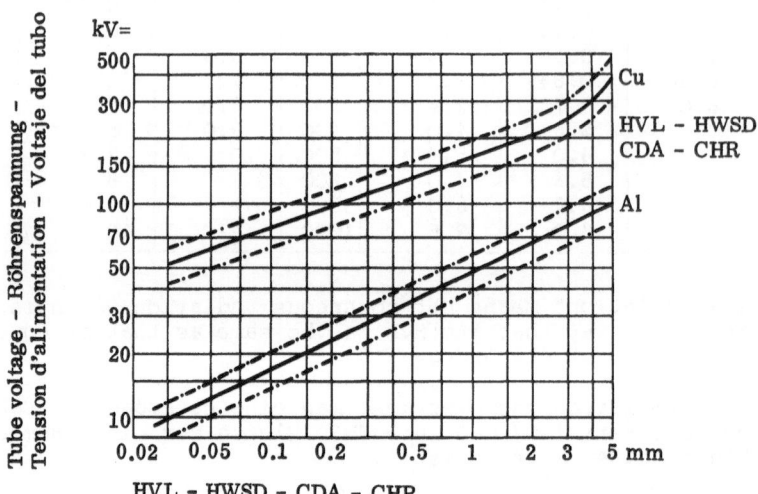

HVL - HWSD - CDA - CHR

The radiations used for calibration should be similar to those used
in therapy. To accomplish this, one must choose those tube voltages
and filtrations which result in calibration radiations with HVL values that lie between the dashed curves.

Kalibrierstrahlungen sollen den in der Therapie verwendeten Strahlungen ähnlich sein. Um dies zu erreichen, müssen Röhrenspannungen und
Filterungen so gewählt werden, daß die erzielten HWSD der Kalibrierstrahlungen zwischen den strichpunktierten Kurven liegen.

Les rayonnements utilisés pour les étalonnages devraient être voisins
de ceux utilisés en thérapie. Dans,ce but, les tensions des tubes,
et les filtrations doivent être determinées de telle sorte que la CDA
se trouve dans la zône limitée par les courbes en pointillé sur la
figure.

Las radiaciones usadas para la calibración deben ser similares a las
usadas en terapia. Para obtenerlo, deben seleccionarse los voltajes
del tubo y ajustar la filtración hasta que la CHR se encuentre dentro
del área limitada por las líneas interrumpidas de la figura.

3.3.1.2 Radionuclides - Radionuklide - Radionuclides - Radionúclidos

^{137}Cs; ^{60}Co

See also page - Siehe auch Seite - Voir aussi page - Ver también pagina 73

3.3.2   Radiation protection dosimeters
         Strahlenschutzdosimeter
         Dosimetres pour la protection
         Dosímetros de protección

3.3.2.1 Narrow spectra (highly filtered radiation) - Hart gefilterte
         Strahlung - Spectres étroits - Espectros estrechos

Tube voltage Röhrenspannung Tension au tube Voltaje del tubo	Total filtration Gesamtfilter Filtration totale Filtracion total mm				Mean energy Mittlere Energie Energie moyenne Energia média	First HVL Erste HWSD Première CDA Primera CHR
kV=	Al	Pb	Sn	Cu	keV	mm
20	1	-	-	-	16	0.35 Al
30	4	-	-	-	25	1.20 Al
40	4	-	-	0.21	29	0.09 Cu
60	4	-	-	0.6	48	0.24 Cu
80	4	-	-	2.0	66	0.59 Cu
100	4	-	-	5.0	83	1.16 Cu
120	4	-	1.0	5.0	99	1.73 Cu
150	4	-	2.5	-	119	2.40 Cu
200	4	-	3.0	2.0	157	3.90 Cu
250	4	-	2.0	-	205	5.20 Cu
300	4	-	3.0	-	248	6.30 Cu

3.3.2.2 Wide spectra (radiation with low filtration) - Wenig gefil-
         terte Strahlung - Spectres larges - Amplio espectro

Tube voltage Röhrenspannung Tension au tube Voltaje del tubo	Total filtration Gesamtfilter Filtration totale Filtracion total mm			Mean energy Mittlere Energie Energie moyenne Energia média	First HVL Erste HWSD Premiere CDA Primera CHR
kV=	Al	Sn	Cu	keV	mm
60	4	-	0.3	45	0.18 Cu
80	4	-	0.5	58	0.35 Cu
110	4	-	2.0	79	0.94 Cu
150	4	1.0	-	104	1.86 Cu
200	4	2.0	-	134	3.11 Cu
250	4	4.0	-	169	4.3 Cu
300	4	6.5	-	202	5.0 Cu

3.3.2.3 Radionuclides - Radionuklide - Radionuclides - Radionuclidos

Nuclide Nuklid Nucléide Nucléido	Energy Energie Energie γ Energía	Half-life Halbwertzeit Période Periodo	Gamma-ray constant Gammastrahlenkonstante Γ Constante spécifique Constante específica	
			$R\ m^2h^{-1}Ci^{-1}$	$C\ m^2kg^{-1}$
$^{125}I\ ^{125}J$	35 keV	60.1 d	0.0044	$0.084 \cdot 10^{18}$
^{241}Am	60 keV	458 a	0.013	0.025 "
^{57}Co	122 keV	270.5 d	0.097	0.186 "
^{203}Hg	279 keV	47 d	0.119	0.285 "
^{137}Cs	662 keV	29.9 a	0.336	0.626 "
^{60}Co	1.25 MeV	5.272 a	1.31	2.52 "

Lit.: 1. DREXLER, G., GOSSRAU, M.: IAEA-SM 143, 16 (1971)
       2. ISO TC 62, Draft May 1974
       3. DIN 6818, Berlin: Beuth-Verlag, Entwurf Nov. 1974

3.4   Exposure rate for different voltages and filtrations
       Dosisleistungen bei verschiedenen Spannungen und Filterungen
       Débit d'exposition pour différentes tensions et filtrations
       Indice de exposición con diferentes voltajes y filtros

3.4.1 10 - 150 kV Voltage range - Spannungsbereich - Domaine de
       tensions - Gama de kilovoltaje

       0.02 - 8 mm Al Filtration-Filterung-Filtration-Filtración

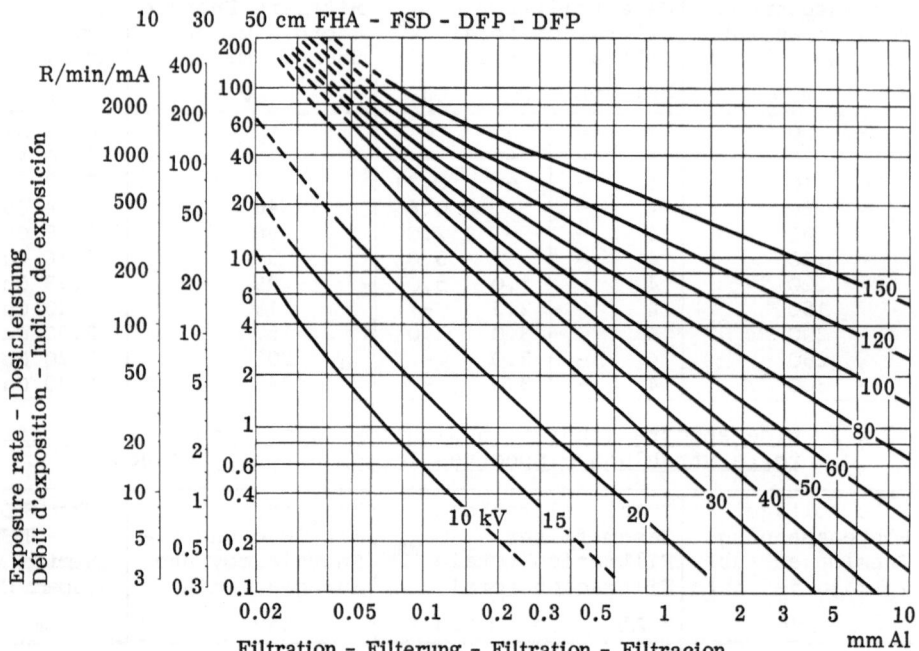

The average values given are for DC voltage and for an anode
angle of 45° (therapy tubes). For voltages with greater fluctuation
(see also page 79), and for smaller anode angles (diagnostic tubes),
the exposure rates are 20 - 40 % lower (also valid for page 76).

Die angegebenen Richtwerte gelten für Gleichspannung und Anodenwin-
kel von 45° (Therapieröhren). Bei Spannungen größerer Welligkeit
(siehe auch Seite 79) und kleineren Anodenwinkeln (Diagnostikröhren)
liegen die Dosisleistungen um 20 - 40 % niedriger (gilt auch für
Seite 76).

Valeurs moyennes données pour des tensions constantes et pour une
anode à 45° (tubes de thérapie). Pour des tensions pulsatoires et
pour des anodes avec des angles plus faibles (tubes de diagnostic)
les débits d'exposition sont 20 à 40 % plus faibles (vaut également
pour page 76).

Los valores estimativos indicados son válidos para corriente continua y ángulo de ánodo de 45° (tubos de terapía). Para voltajes de
mayor fluctuación (véase también página 79) y ángulos anódicos
menores (tubos de diagnóstico) las intensidades de dosis son un
20 - 40 % inferiores (vale también para página 76).

Lit.: 1. JENNINGS, W.A.: Cathode Press 7, 28 (1949/50)
      2. WACHSMANN, F.: Strahlenther. 83, 41 (1950)
      3. Mc CULLOUGH, E.C., CAMERON, R.: Brit.J.Radiol. 43,448 (1970)

FSD FHA DFP DFP	Filter Filter Filtre Filtro mm Al	Exposure rate - Dosisleistung Débit d'exposition - Indice de exposición Tube voltage - Röhrenspannung Tension d'alimentation - Voltaje del tubo							R/min mA kV=
		10	20	40	60	80	100	120	150
10 cm	0.02	(275)	(1600)	–	–	–	–	–	–
	0.03	(300)	(750)	(3300)	–	–	–	–	–
	0.04	(60)	(470)	(2100)	(2800)	–	–	–	–
	0.06	(30)	250	1100	(1600)	(2000)	–	–	–
	0.08	20	160	770	1100	1400	–	–	–
	0.1	12	110	580	880	1050	(1300)	–	–
	0.2	(5.0)	45	225	400	550	700	–	–
	0.3	–	25	140	250	375	500	(720)	–
	0.4	–	18	100	190	275	375	570	–
	0.6	–	10	58	125	200	275	450	(670)
	0.8	–	7.0	40	90	150	225	360	560
	1	–	5.0	30	72	125	200	300	500
	2	–	–	12	35	68	110	190	350
	3	–	–	7.5	23	48	85	140	250
	4	–	–	5.2	18	35	70	110	220
	6	–	–	3.2	12	25	50	85	170
	8	–	–	–	8.2	20	40	68	145
30 cm	0.02	(15)	(130)	–	–	–	–	–	–
	0.03	(17)	(70)	(310)	–	–	–	–	–
	0.04	(4.0)	(45)	(200)	(260)	(320)	(380)	–	–
	0.06	2.0	22	110	160	(200)	225	(320)	–
	0.08	1.5	13	75	110	130	160	(240)	–
	0.1	0.9	11	60	95	105	140	(200)	(275)
	0.2	(0.5)	4.7	24	45	60	75	(110)	(180)
	0.3	–	2.9	15	28	42	54	80	110
	0.4	–	2.0	11	21	30	42	62	92
	0.6	–	1.1	6.2	14	22	30	48	75
	0.8	–	0.8	4.4	10	16	25	40	62
	1	–	0.5	3.3	8.0	14	22	34	55
	2	–	–	1.3	3.8	7.5	12	21	40
	3	–	–	0.8	2.5	4.2	9.5	16	28
	4	–	–	0.5	2.0	3.8	7.8	12	24
	6	–	–	0.3	1.3	2.7	5.5	10	19
	8	–	–	–	0.9	2.2	4.4	8.0	16
50 cm	0.02	(3.5)	(32)	–	–	–	–	–	–
	0.04	(1.0)	(16)	(60)	(90)	(110)	(150)	–	–
	0.06	0.5	(11)	(36)	(52)	(66)	90	105	150
	0.08	0.4	5.5	25	36	47	64	80	105
	0.1	0.25	3.8	15	28	35	45	64	90
	0.2	(0.15)	1.2	7.5	14	20	25	38	62
	0.3	–	0.9	5.0	9.4	14	19	28	40
	0.4	–	0.6	3.8	7.0	11	14	22	33
	0.6	–	0.4	2.2	4.7	7.8	10	17	26
	0.8	–	0.3	1.5	3.5	5.8	8.6	14	22
	1	–	0.2	1.3	2.8	4.8	7.8	12	20
	2	–	–	0.4	1.3	2.7	4.2	7.2	14
	3	–	–	0.3	0.9	2.0	3.4	5.7	10
	4	–	–	0.2	0.7	1.4	2.8	4.3	8.5
	6	–	–	0.1	0.5	1.0	2.0	3.5	6.8
	8	–	–	–	0.3	0.8	1.6	2.8	5.8

3.4.2 60 - 500 kV Voltage range - Spannungsbereich - Domaine de tensions - Gama de kilovoltaje

Cu Filtration - Filterung - Filtration - Filtración

30 - 50 - 80 cm FSD - FHA - DFP - DFP

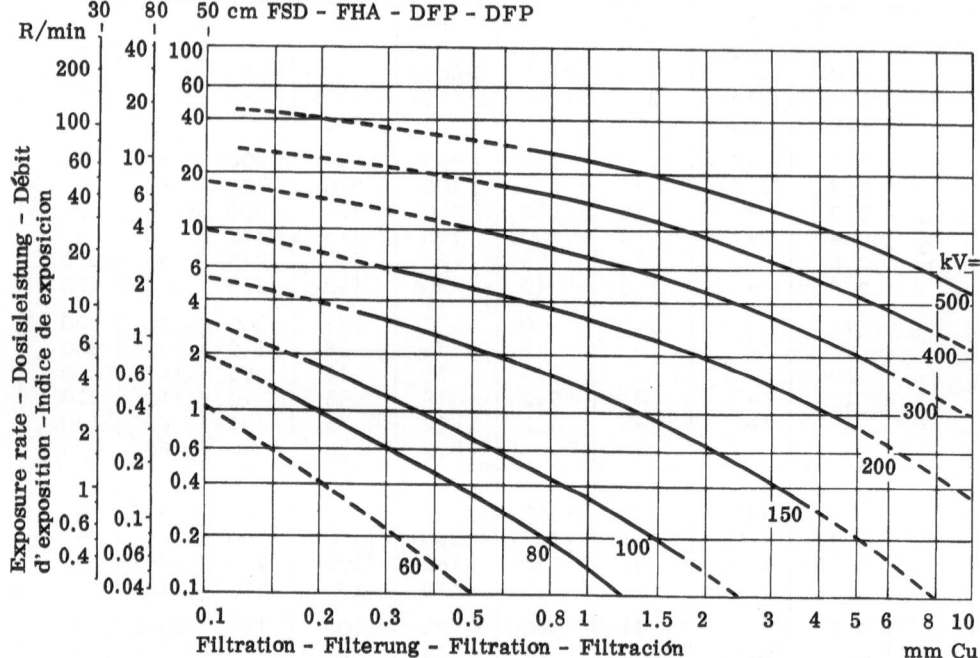

In half wave and fully rectified operation, the exposure rates on the same peak voltages are approximately half of the values given above.

Im Ein- oder Zweipulsbetrieb der Röntgenröhre sind die Dosisleistungen bezogen auf gleiche Scheitelspannungen etwa halb so groß wie angegeben.

Pour le fonctionnement en une ou deux alternances les débits d'exposition sont environ la moitié de ceux indiqués pour la même tension de crête.

En el caso de que el aparato trabaje con semi-onda, los indices de exposición se reducen, aceptando los mismos voltajes pico, aproximadamente a la mitad de aquellos dados.

Lit.: 1. DRESSER, R., COSMAN, B.J.: Am.J.Roentgenol. 39, 972 (1938)
       2. TRUMP, J.G., van de GRAAF: Phys.Rev. 55, 676 (1939)
       3. TAYLOR, L.S.: Medical Physics 2, 901 (1950)
       4. FARR, R.F.: Acta Radiol. 43, 152 (1955)
       5. ICRP Publication 3, Pergamon Press (1960)
       6. OSBORNE, S.B.: X-ray Focus 3, 22 (1962)
       7. NCRP Publications, Report No. 33, Washington D.C. (1968)
       8. Mc CULLOUGH, E.C., CAMERON, J.R.: Br.J.Radiol. 43,448 (1970)
       9. The Hospital Physicists' Association, Report No. 7 (1972)
      10. ICRP Publication 21, External Sources, Pergamon Press (1973)
      11. DIN 6812, Berlin: Beuth-Verlag, Entwurf Februar 1974

FSD FHA DFP DFP	Filter Filtre Filtro	Exposure rate - Dosisleistung Débit d'exposition - Indice de exposition						R/min 1 mA
	mm Cu	Tube voltage - Röhrenspannung Tension d'alimentation - Voltaje del tubo						kV
		80	100	150	200	300	400	500
30 cm	0.1	(5.3)	(8.2)	(14.5)	(25)	(48)	-	-
	0.2	2.6	4.8	(12.3)	(20)	(39)	(66)	(105)
	0.3	1.8	3.3	8.6	16	(34)	(56)	(98)
	0.4	1.2	2.6	7.2	14	(32)	(52)	(88)
	0.5	0.97	2.0	6.0	13	28	50	(80)
	0.6	0.77	1.6	5.2	11.5	25	47	75
	0.8	0.52	1.2	4.4	10.2	22	42	68
	1	0.38	0.96	3.7	8.8	19	39	62
	1.5	-	0.55	2.4	6.6	15	32	53
	2	-	(0.39)	1.8	5.2	13	25	43
	2.5	-	0.28	1.4	4.4	10.7	21	40
	3	-	-	1.15	3.8	9.1	18	36
	4	-	-	0.80	3.0	7.2	15	30
	5	-	-	0.57	2.3	5.5	12	24
	6	-	-	0.44	(1.8)	4.7	10.5	21
	8	-	-	0.28	(1.3)	(3.6)	7.7	16
	10	-	-	-	(0.94)	(2.8)	(6.4)	13
50 cm	0.1	(1.9)	(3.0)	(5.2)	(9.2)	(17.5)	-	-
	0.2	0.95	1.75	(4.5)	(7.2)	(14.0)	(24)	(44)
	0.3	0.63	1.20	3.1	5.9	(12.5)	(20)	(36)
	0.4	0.45	0.92	2.6	5.1	(11.5)	(19)	(33)
	0.5	0.35	0.72	2.2	4.8	10.0	18	31
	0.6	0.28	0.58	1.9	4.2	9.0	17	29
	0.8	0.19	0.43	1.6	3.7	7.8	15	26
	1	0.14	0.35	1.35	3.2	7.0	14	24
	1.5	-	0.20	0.88	2.4	5.4	11.5	19
	2	-	(0.14)	0.65	1.9	4.6	8.8	16
	2.5	-	(0.10)	0.52	1.6	3.9	7.6	14.5
	3	-	-	0.42	1.4	3.3	6.6	13.0
	4	-	-	0.29	1.1	2.6	5.2	11.0
	5	-	-	0.21	0.85	2.0	4.4	8.6
	6	-	-	0.16	(0.67)	1.7	3.8	7.5
	8	-	-	0.10	(0.48)	(1.3)	2.8	5.6
	10	-	-	-	(0.34)	(1.0)	(2.3)	4.6
80 cm	0.1	(0.74)	(1.2)	(2.1)	(3.7)	(6.9)	-	-
	0.2	0.37	0.70	(1.8)	(2.9)	(5.5)	(9.4)	(19)
	0.3	0.25	0.47	1.2	2.3	(5.0)	(8.0)	(15)
	0.4	0.17	0.36	1.0	2.0	(4.5)	(7.4)	(14)
	0.5	0.14	0.28	0.86	1.9	4.0	7.0	(13)
	0.6	0.11	0.24	0.74	1.6	3.5	6.6	12
	0.8	0.07	0.17	0.63	1.5	3.1	6.0	10
	1	0.05	0.14	0.53	1.3	2.8	5.5	9.4
	1.5	-	0.08	0.35	0.94	2.1	4.5	7.4
	2	-	(0.05)	0.26	0.74	1.8	3.5	6.2
	2.5	-	(0.04)	0.21	0.63	1.5	3.0	5.7
	3	-	-	0.16	0.55	1.3	2.6	5.2
	4	-	-	0.11	0.43	1.0	2.1	4.3
	5	-	-	0.08	0.33	0.80	1.7	3.4
	6	-	-	0.06	(0.26)	0.66	1.5	3.0
	8	-	-	0.04	(0.19)	(0.50)	1.1	2.2
	10	-	-	-	(0.13)	(0.40)	(0.9)	1.8

3.5

Mean energy and dose rate of X-rays for various filtrations (approximate values).
Mittlere Energie und Dosisleistung von Röntgenstrahlen bei verschiedener Filterung (Richtwerte).
Énergie moyenne et débit de dose des rayons X pour différentes filtrations (valeurs moyennes).
Energía promedio e índice de dosis de rayos-X para diferentes filtraciones (valores aproximados).

Mean energy/peak energy - Mittlere Energie/Grenzenergie
Energie moyenne/énergie maximale - Energía promedio/energía pico

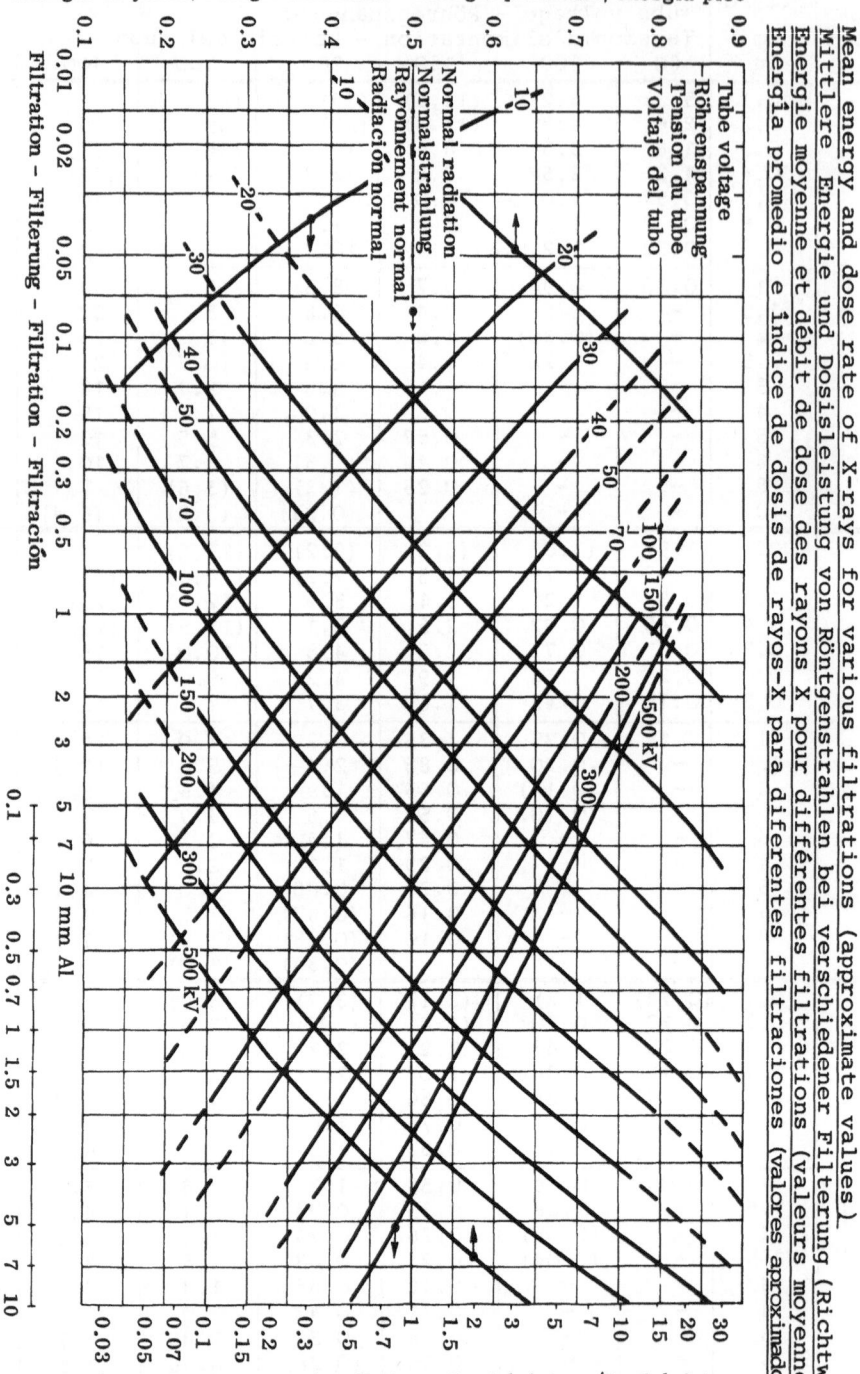

Tube voltage
Röhrenspannung
Tension du tube
Voltaje del tubo

Normal radiation
Normalstrahlung
Rayonnement normal
Radiación normal

Filtration – Filterung – Filtration – Filtración

Dose rate/dose rate for normal radiation - Dosisleistung/Dosisleistung
Normalstrahlung - Débit de dose/débit de dose du rayonnement normal -
Indice de dosis/índice de dosis para radiación normal

See pages – Siehe Seiten – Voir pages – Ver páginas 68 – 69, 74 – 77

3.6   Conversion of pulsed voltages into constant potential
       Umrechnung von pulsierenden Spannungen in Gleichspannung
       Conversion de tension pulsée en tension constante
       Conversión de voltaje pulsatil a voltaje constante

Pulsed voltages (kV∿ and kV⩟) required to produce radiation approximately equivalent with respect to HVL and exposure rate to radiation from an X-ray tube operated with constant potential (kV=).

Pulsierende Spannungen (kV∿ und kV⩟), die eingestellt werden müssen, um bezüglich HWSD und Dosisleistung einer mit Gleichspannung (kV=) betriebenen Röntgenröhre etwa äquivalente Strahlungen zu erhalten.

Tensions pulsées (kV∿ et kV⩟) produisant des rayonnements équivalents à celui fourni par une tension constante (kV=) en ce qui concerne la CDA et le débit d'exposition.

Voltajes pulsantes de tubo (kV∿ y kV⩟) para obtener radiaciones aproximadamente equivalentes en relación de CHR y exposición a las obtenidas por un tubo que opere con potencial constante (kV=).

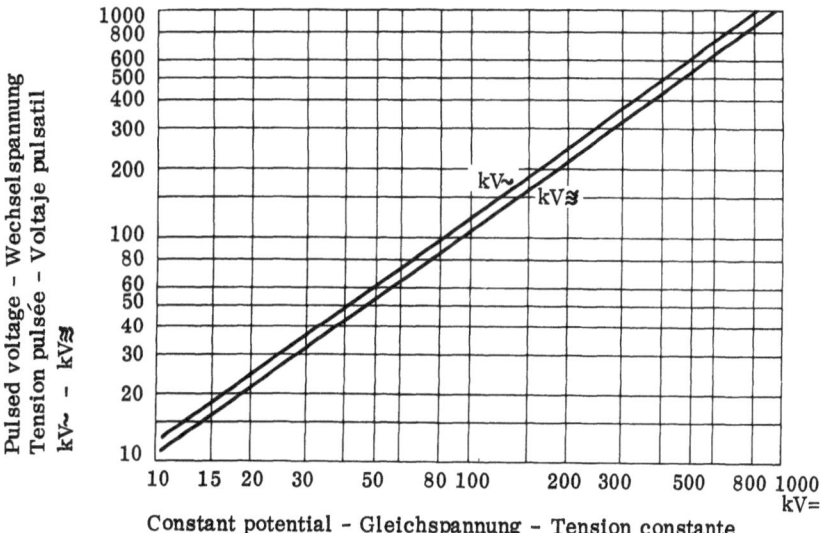

Constant potential - Gleichspannung - Tension constante
Voltaje constante

Equivalent tube voltages - Äquivalente Röhrenspannungen - Tensions équivalentes - Voltajes equivalentes en el tubo										
kV=	kV∿	kV⩟	kV=	kV∿	kV⩟	kV=	kV∿	kV⩟	kV=	kV∿	kV⩟
10	12	10.5	40	49	42	90	110	95	300	365	315
15	18	16	50	61	53	100	122	105	400	490	420
20	24	21	60	73	63	150	183	157	500	610	525
25	30	26	70	85	74	200	244	210	700	850	735
30	37	32	80	98	84	250	305	262	1000	1220	1050

Lit.: 1. Mc CULLOUGH, E.C., CAMERON, J.R.:Brit.J.Radiol.43,448(1970)
      2. KELLEY, J.P., TROUT, D.E.: Radiation Physics 100,653(1971)
      3. Authors' measurements - Eigene Messungen - Mesures
         personnelles - Medidas propias

3.7   Attenuation of X-rays in air
      Schwächung von Röntgenstrahlen in Luft
      Atténuation des rayons X dans l'air
      Atenuación de los rayos X en el aire

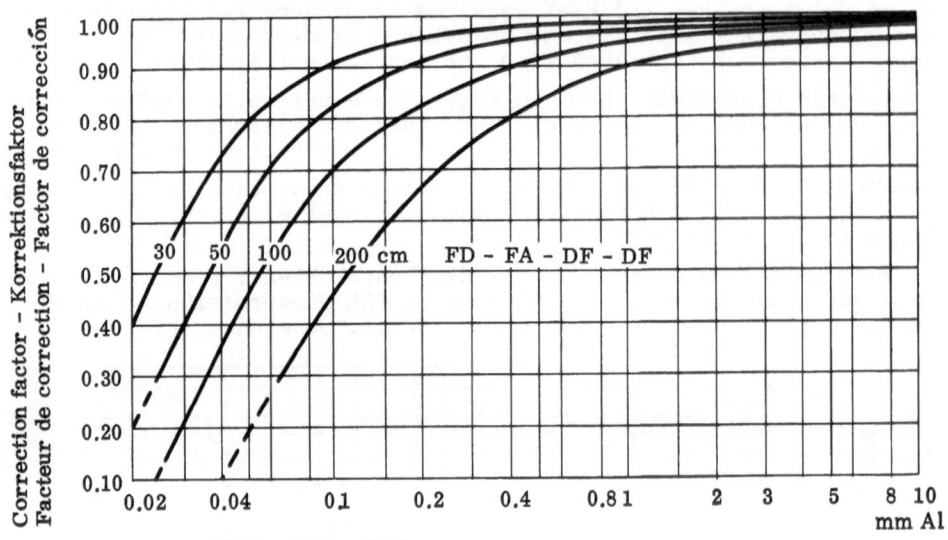

HVL - HWSD - CDA - CHR

Correction factor for the exposure calculated according to the inverse square low from the exposure at 10 cm FD - Korrektionsfaktor
für die aus der Dosis in 10 cm FA nach dem Quadratgesetz berechne-
ten Dosis - Facteur de correction de l'exposition calculée par
l'inverse carré des distances à partir d'une DF de 10 cm - Factor
de corrección de la exposición calculada conforme la ley del cuadrado para la exposición a partir de 10 cm DF

HVL-HWSD-CDA-CHR mm Al	FD - FA - DF - DF			cm
	30	50	100	200
0.02	0.40	0.20	-	-
0.03	0.62	0.41	0.21	-
0.05	0.80	0.65	0.45	(0.20)
0.07	0.87	0.74	0.59	0.33
0.1	0.91	0.82	0.70	0.45
0.15	0.94	0.88	0.78	0.59
0.2	0.96	0.92	0.82	0.67
0.3	0.97	0.93	0.87	0.75
0.5	0.98	0.94	0.91	0.82
0.7	0.98	0.96	0.93	0.87
1.0	0.99	0.97	0.95	0.90
1.5	0.99	0.97	0.96	0.91
2.0	0.99	0.98	0.96	0.92
3.0	1.00	0.99	0.97	0.94
5.0	1.00	0.99	0.98	0.96
10.0	1.00	1.00	0.99	0.97

Lit.: 1. WACHSMANN, F.: Hdb. Haut- und Geschlechtskrankheiten, Er-
         gänzungsband V/2, Berlin: Springer 1959
      2. See page 61 - Siehe Seite 62 - Voir page 63 - Ver página 64

3.8   Examples of X-ray spectra (narrow beam)
      Beispiele von Röntgenspektren (enges Bündel)
      Exemples de spectres de rayons X (faisceaux étroits)
      Ejemplos de espectros de rayos-X (haz estrecho)

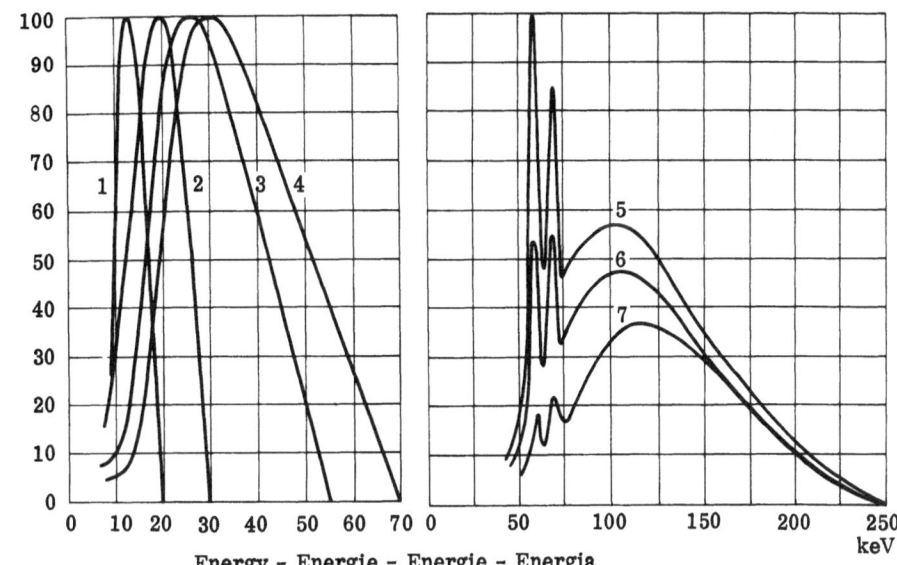

Fluence – Fluenz – Fluence – Flujo (rel.)

Energy - Energie - Energie - Energia

1. 20 kV=; 0.14 mm Al *)
2. 30 kV=; 0.3 mm Al
3. 55 kV=; 0.8 mm Al
4. 70 kV=; 1.25 mm Al

5. 250 kV=; 1.5 mm Cu *)
6. 250 kV=; 2.0 mm Cu
7. 250 kV=; 2.7 mm Cu

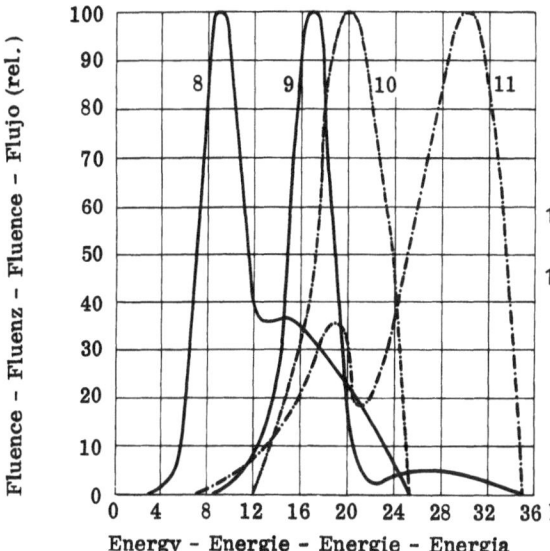

Fluence – Fluenz – Fluence – Flujo (rel.)

8. W-Anode; 25 kV= 1 mm Be*)

9. Idem behind – hinter –
   après – detras 8 cm H_2O

10. Mo Anode; 35 kV=
    0.05 mm Mo *)

11. Idem behind – hinter –
    après – detras 8 cm H_2O

*) Filtration – Filterung
   Filtration – Filtración

Energy - Energie - Energie - Energia

Lit.: 1. PEAPLE, L.H.J., BURT, A.K.: Phys.Med.Biol. 11, 225 (1966)
      2. DREXLER, G.: Proceedings of the XIII Intern. Congress of
         Rad. Madrid 1973, International Congress Series No. 339,
         Excerpta Medica, Amsterdam

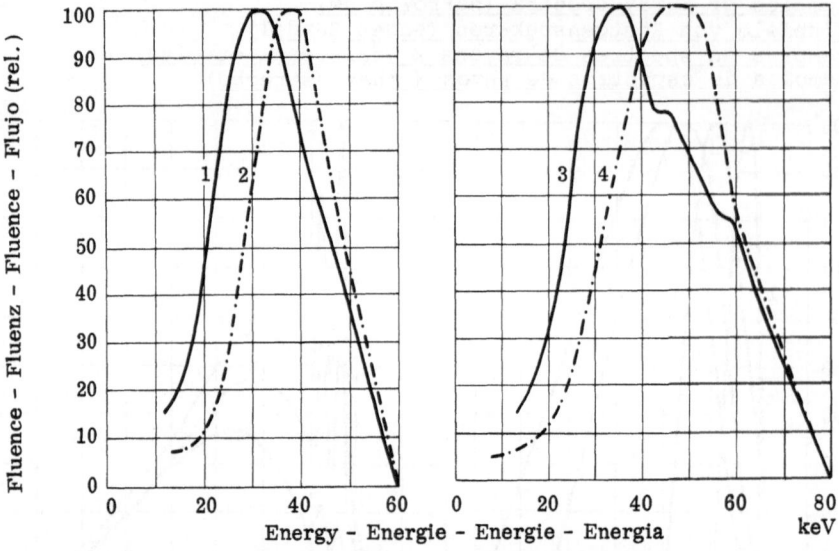

1. 60 kV=; 2 mm Al

2. Idem behind-hinter-après-
   detras 20 cm H_2O **)

3. 80 kV=; 2 mm Al

4. Idem behind-hinter-après-
   detras 20 cm H_2O **)

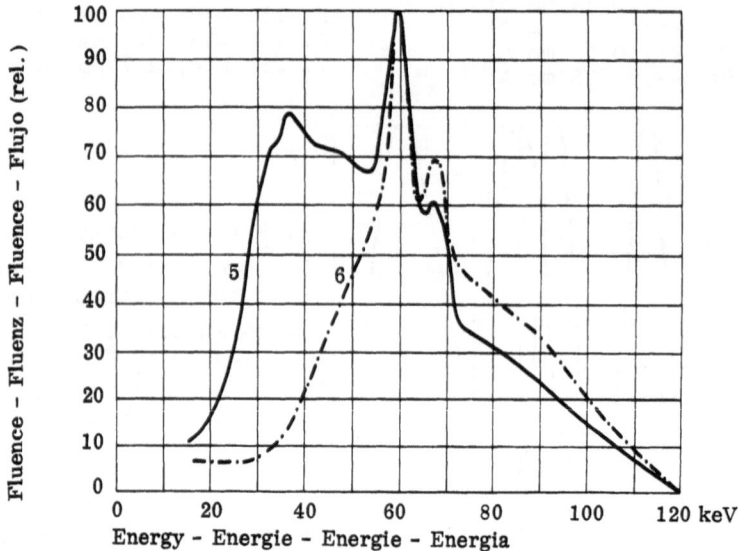

5. 120 kV=; 2 mm Al

6. Idem behind - hinter - après -
   detras 20 cm H_2O **)

**) Spectra 1-6 show clearly that, in X-ray diagnosis, only the ener-
getic radiation reaches the image recorder, and that low-energy components only cause unnecessary exposure to the patient.

Die Spektren 1-6 zeigen deutlich, daß in der Röntgendiagnostik
nur die energiereichen Anteile bis zum Bildempfänger gelangen
und daß die weichen den Patienten nur unnötig belasten.

Les spectres no 1-6 montrent clairement qu'en radiodiagnostic
seuls les rayonnements des plus hautes ênergies atteignent
le detecteur tandis que les rayonnements de plus faible énergie
ne font que délivrer une dose inutile au malade.

Los esprectros muestran claramente que en el radiodiagnostico
solamente los rayos energéticos alcanzan el detector de imagen
y que los blandos solo cargan inutilmente al paciente.

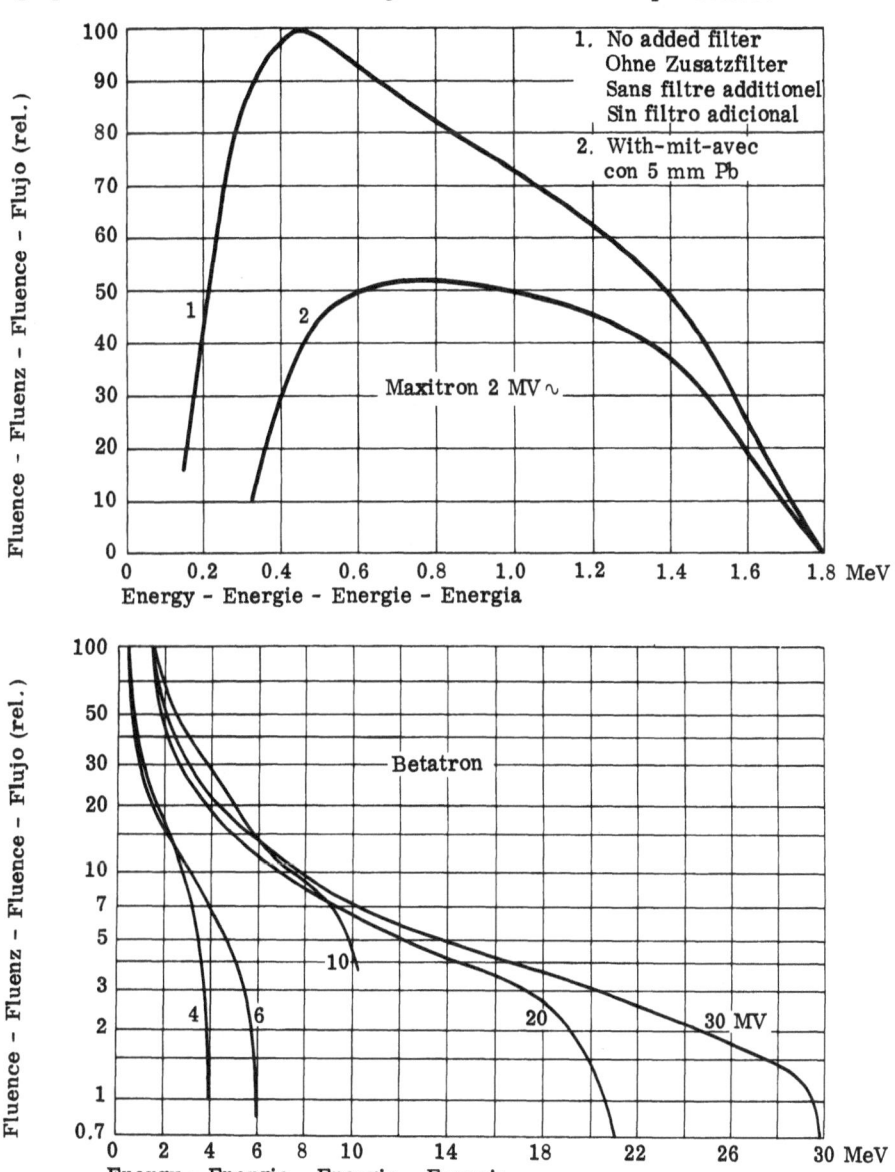

Lit.: 1. SAYLOR, W.L.: Phys.Med.Biol. 14, 87 (1969)
      2. MARUYAMA, T., SAKATA, S., KUMAMOTO, Y., HASHIZUME, T.,
        HATTORI, H., KANAMORI, H., YAMAMOTO, M.: Health Phys. 28,
        777 (1975)

3.9   Attenuation processes of X rays in a 10 cm layer of water
       Schwächungsprozesse von Röntgenstrahlung in 10 cm Wasser
       Modes d'atténuation des rayons X dans 10 cm d'eau
       Procesos por disminuir los rayos X en 10 cm de agua

100 cm^2 Field size - Feld - Champ - Campo

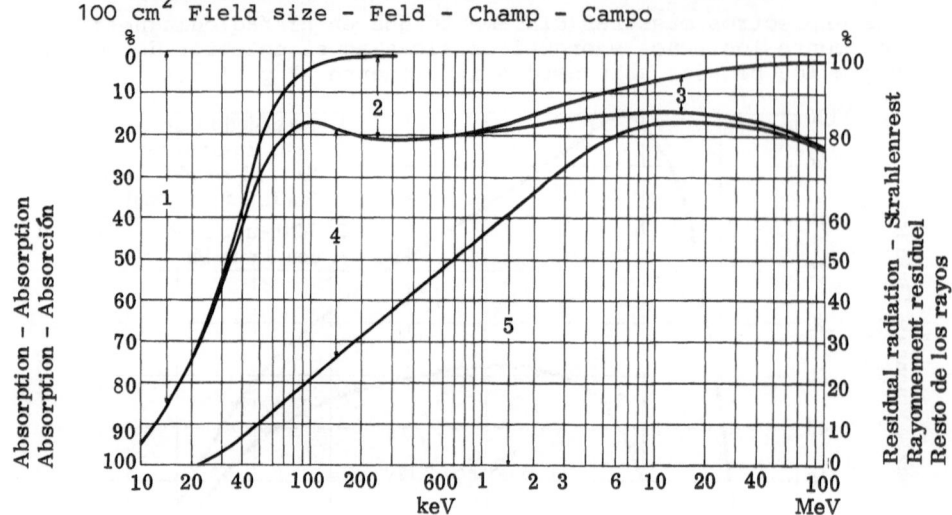

Energie - Energy - Energie - Energía

1. Photoelectric absorption - Photoabsorption - Absorption photoélectrique - Absorción fotoeléctrica
2. Compton absorption - Absorption compton - Absorption compton -
   Absorción compton
3. Pair production - Paarbildung - Formation de paires - Formación
   de pares
4. Scattering - Streuung - Diffusion - Dispersión
5. Transmitted primary radiation - Unbeeinflußter Strahlenrest -
   Rayonnement primaire résiduel - Radiación residual inalterada

E keV/ MeV	Proportion of the incident radiation - Anteile an der Einfallstrahlung - Pourcentage du rayonnement incident - Participación en la radiación incidente %				
	1	2	3	4	5
10	95	0	0	5	∿0
20	75	∿0	0	25	∿0
30	55	2.5	0	40	2.5
50	21	9	0	60	10
100	4.0	13	0	63	20
200	1.0	19	0	48	32
300	0	20	0	42	38
500	0	20	0	34	46
1	0	18	0	25	57
2	0	14	3	16	67
3	0	12	4	11	73
5	0	9.5	5.5	6.5	79
10	0	6.0	7.5	2.5	84
20	0	4.0	10	2.0	84
30	0	2.0	12	2.0	84
50	0	2.0	15	1.0	82
70	0	1.2	18	0.8	80
100	0	1.0	21	∿0	78

Table of contents - Inhaltsverzeichnis
Table des matières - Tabla de materias

4.1 Central axis relative depth doses for X-rays
Relative Tiefendosen im Zentralstrahl für Röntgenstrahlen
Rendements relatives en profondeur sur l'axe pour les rayons X
Dosis relativas en profundidad en el eje central para rayos X

General information - Allgemeine Erklärungen - Explications générales - Explicaciónes generales

The values given on the following pages for the "relative depth doses" based on the surface or maximum dose are for the quality of radiation (HVL), focus-skin distance (FSD), and field size (cm^2) indicated, for measurements in "infinite" phantoms. The numbers in the tables are rounded off, since more precise values are uncertain and of no practical significance. Unreliable data are indicated in the graphs by dashed lines, and in the tables, by parentheses.

Die auf den folgenden Seiten angegebenen Werte für die auf die Oberflächen- bzw. Maximaldosen bezogenen "relativen Tiefendosen" gelten für die jeweils angegebenen Strahlenqualitäten (HWSD), Fokus-Hautabstände (FHA) und Feldgrößen (cm^2) für Messungen in "unendlich großen" Phantomen. In den Tabellen sind abgerundete Zahlen angegeben, da genauere Werte unsicher und für die Praxis ohne Bedeutung sind. Nicht zuverlässige Angaben sind in den Kurven gestrichelt und in den Tabellen eingeklammert angegeben.

Les valeurs données dans les pages suivantes pour les "rendements relatifs en profondeur" sont rapportées à la dose à la surface ou à la dose maximale, pour différentes qualités de rayonnement (CDA), distances foyer-peau (DFP) et dimensions de champ (cm^2) et correspondent à des mesures dans un fantôme "semi-infini". Les valeurs données dans les tables sont arrondies car le chiffre suivant serait imprécis et sans signification pratique. Les valeurs qui ne sont pas sûres sont mises entre parenthèses dans les tables et sont representées par des courbes pointillées dans les figures.

Los valores de las "dosis en profundidad relativas" referidas a la dosis superficial o máxima, que se indican en las páginas se refieren a la calidad de la radiación (CHR), distancia foco-piel (DFP) y amplitud de campo (cm^2) para medidas en fantomas de "tamano infinito". Los números que figuran en las tablas estan redondeados a ya que valores más exactos son inseguros y carecen de importancia práctica. Los datos que no son de total confianza aparecen plumeados en las curvas y entre paréntesis en las tablas.

Lit.: 1. IAEA, Atlas of Radiation Dose Distribution, Vol. 1, Vienna 1965
2. RUDERMAN, A.J., BIBEGAL, A.A., VAINBERG, M.Sh.: Atlas of Dose Fields, 1, SSSR: Moscow 1968
3. JOHNS, H.E., CUNNINGHAM, J.R.: The Physics of Radiology, 3th Edit., Springfield: C.C.Thomas 1969
4. Brit.J.Radiol., Suppl. 11, London 1972
5. Authors' measurements - Eigene Messungen - Mesures personnelles - Medidas propias

These references also apply to pages - Diese Literaturstellen gelten auch für die Seiten - Ces références se rapportent aussi aux pages - Estas indicaciones bibliográficas valen también para las páginas 87, 104, 118, 126, 128.

4.2 Low energy X-rays - Weiche Röntgenstrahlen - Rayons X mous - Rayos X blandos

4.2.1 0.02 - 0.8 mm Al HVL - HWSD - CDA - CHR

(10) - 30 - (50) cm FSD - FHA - DFP - DFP

(10) - 100 - (400) cm^2 Field size - Feldgröße - Champ - Campo

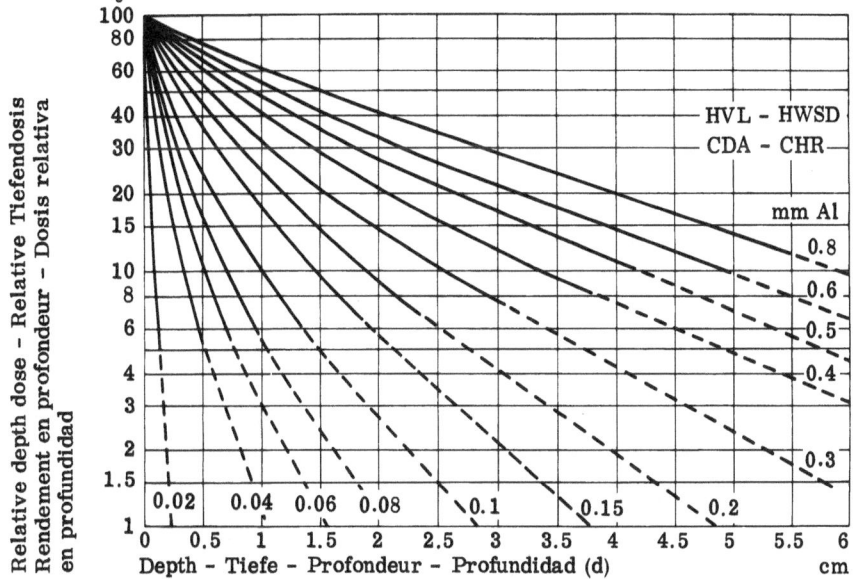

Relative depth dose - Relative Tiefendosis
Rendement en profondeur - Dosis relativa en profundidad

Depth - Tiefe - Profondeur - Profundidad (d)

d cm	Depth doses - Tiefendosen - Rendement en profondeur - Dosis en profundidad %							
	HVL - HWSD - CDA - CHR: mm Al				d cm			
cm	0.02	0.04	0.06	0.08	cm	0.04	0.06	0.08
0.02	50	76	86	78	0.4	(7.8)	14.5	21
0.04	30	66	72	90	0.5	(5.4)	10.5	16.5
0.06	20	52	62	67	0.6	(4.0)	(7.8)	13.5
0.08	13	46	59	66	0.8	(2.1)	(4.6)	(8.0)
0.10	(9)	38	54	62	1.0	(1.1)	(3.0)	(5.5)
0.15	(3.7)	27	36	45	1.2	-	(2.0)	(4.0)
0.20	(1.5)	20	33	41	1.4	-	(1.5)	(2.8)
0.25	-	15.0	26	34	1.6	-	(< 1)	(2.0)
0.30	-	12.0	21	29	1.8	-	-	(1.5)

d cm	0.1	0.15	0.2	0.3	0.4	0.5	0.6	0.8
0.1	62	78	81	85	88	92	95	97
0.2	50	62	68	76	80	84	88	91
0.4	30	43	49	59	66	72	77	82
0.6	20	31	38	48	56	62	68	75
0.8	14.5	24	29	39	48	54	60	68
1	10.0	17.5	24	32	41	48	54	62
1.5	(5.0)	9.7	14.5	21	29	36	42	50
2	(2.7)	(5.6)	(9.0)	14.5	21	27	33	41
2.5	(1.6)	(3.4)	(6.5)	10.5	16.0	21	26	35
3	(< 1)	(2.1)	(4.1)	(7.6)	12.0	17.0	22	29
4	-	-	(1.9)	(4.2)	(7.5)	11.5	14.5	20
5	-	-	(< 1)	(2.4)	(4.8)	(7.0)	9.6	14.0

<u>1 mm Al HVL - HWSD - CDA - CHR</u>
       15 - 30 - 50 cm FSD - FHA - DFP - DFP
       10 - 400 cm^2 Field size - Feldgröße - Champ - Campo

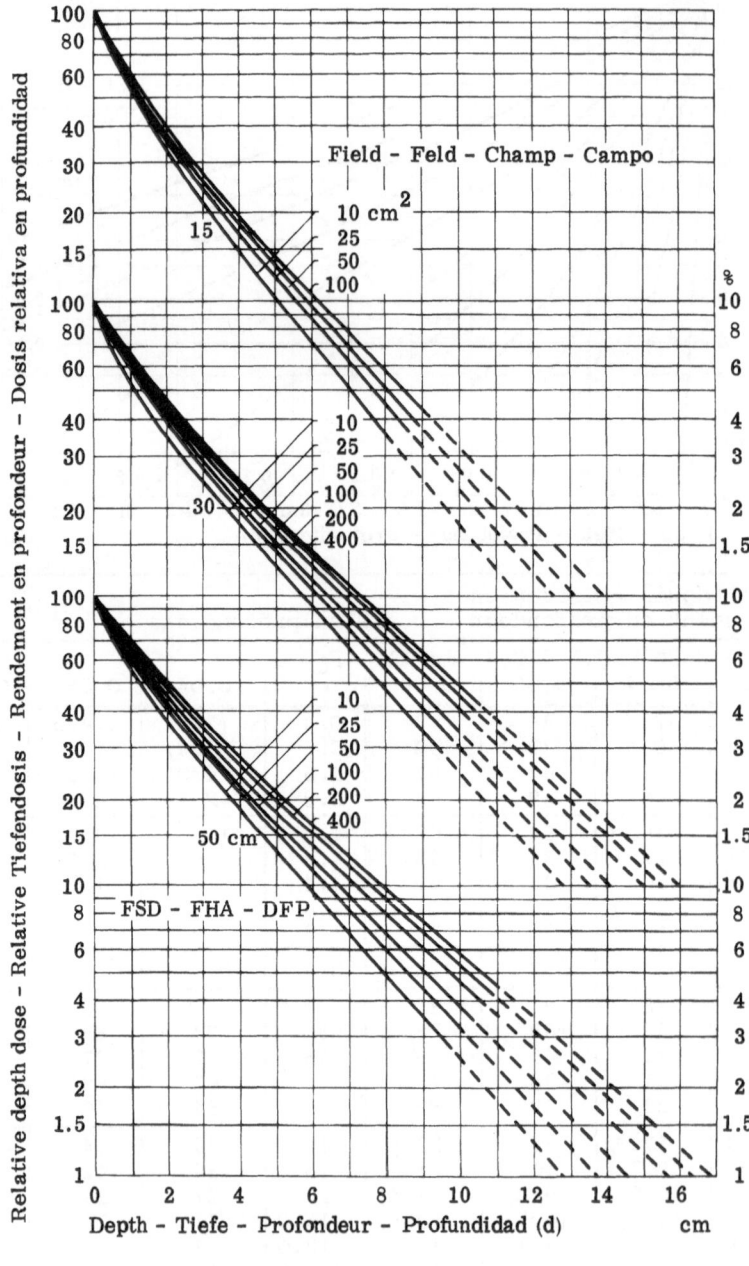

FSD FHA DFP	d cm	Field size - Feldgröße - Champ - Campo: cm²					
		10	25	50	100	200	400
15 cm	0	100	100	100	100		
	0.5	65	68	70	73		
	1	53	55	57	60		
	1.5	40	44	46	50		
	2	32	35	37	40		
	3	21	24	26	28		
	4	15.0	17.0	18.5	20		
	5	10.5	12.5	13.5	14.5		
	6	7.3	8.8	9.4	11.0		
	7	5.2	6.3	7	7.8		
	8	3.6	4.6	5.1	5.8		
	9	2.5	3.2	(3.6)	(4.3)		
	10	1.8	(2.3)	(2.7)	(3.2)		
	11	(1.2)	(1.7)	(2.0)	(2.4)		
	12	-	(1.4)	(1.5)	(1.8)		
	13	-	-	(1.0)	(1.3)		
30 cm	0	100	100	100	100	100	100
	0.5	65	71	75	77	79	81
	1	53	60	62	64	67	70
	1.5	44	50	52	55	56	58
	2	35	39	41	43	45	46
	3	25	27	29	31	33	34
	4	18.0	19.5	21	23	24	25
	5	13.5	14.5	15.5	16.5	18.0	18.5
	6	9.2	10.5	11.5	12.5	13.5	14.0
	7	6.8	7.8	8.3	9.6	10.5	11.5
	8	4.8	5.7	6.3	7.3	7.9	8.4
	9	3.5	4.2	4.7	5.6	6.1	6.4
	10	(2.5)	(3.0)	(3.5)	4.2	4.5	5.0
	11	(1.8)	(2.2)	(2.6)	(3.1)	(3.4)	(3.7)
	12	(1.4)	(1.7)	(1.9)	(2.4)	(2.7)	(2.9)
	13	-	(1.2)	(1.4)	(1.7)	(2.0)	(2.2)
	14	-	-	(1.0)	(1.3)	(1.5)	(1.7)
	15	-	-	-	(1.0)	(1.2)	(1.3)
	16	-	-	-	-	-	(1.1)
50 cm	0	100	100	100	100	100	100
	0.5	70	74	76	78	80	82
	1	56	60	63	66	68	70
	1.5	46	49	51	54	56	58
	2	38	42	44	46	48	50
	3	18.5	29	41	43	45	47
	4	13.5	21	23	24	26	28
	5	14	15.5	17.0	18.5	20	22
	6	9.6	11.5	12.5	14.0	15.5	16.5
	7	7.0	8.4	9.4	10.5	12.0	13.0
	8	5.0	6.0	7.0	8.2	9.2	10.0
	9	3.6	4.5	5.2	6.2	7.1	7.7
	10	(2.6)	3.2	3.9	4.8	5.4	6.0
	11	(1.8)	(2.4)	(2.9)	(3.6)	4.2	4.6
	12	(1.4)	(1.8)	(2.2)	(2.8)	(3.2)	(3.6)
	13	(1.0)	(1.2)	(1.6)	(2.1)	(2.4)	(2.7)
	14	-	-	-	(1.6)	(1.9)	(2.1)
	15	-	-	-	(1.2)	(1.4)	(1.6)
	16	-	-	-	-	(1.1)	(1.3)

2 mm Al HVL – HWSD – CDA – CHR

15 – 30 – 50 cm FSD – FHA – DFP – DFP

10 – 400 cm^2 Field size – Feldgröße – Champ – Campo

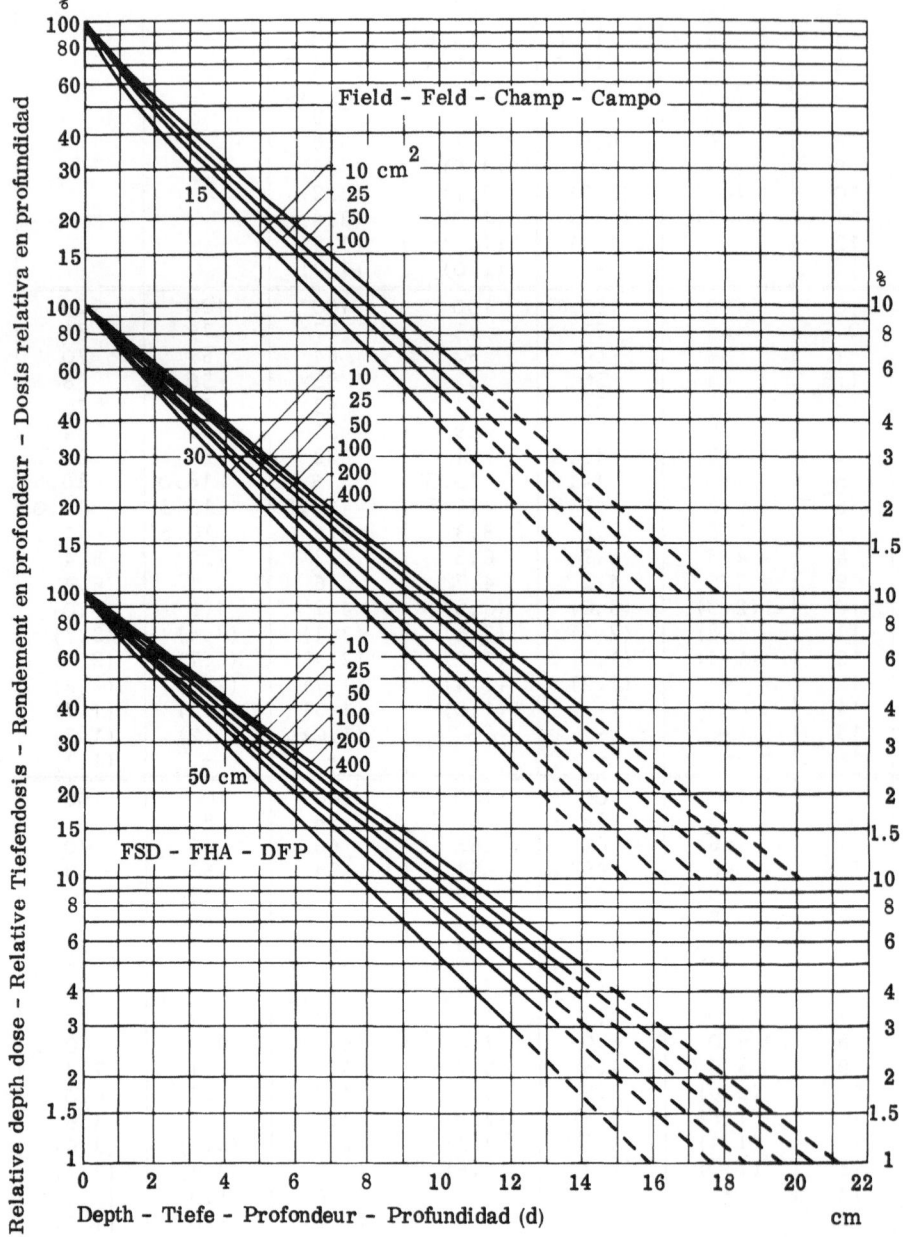

FSD FHA DFP	d cm	Field size - Feldgröße - Champ - Campo: 10	25	50	100	200	400 cm²
15 cm	0.5	76	80	82	84		
	1	60	68	70	73		
	1.5	50	58	60	63		
	2	42	48	50	54		
	3	32	37	39	43		
	4	23	27	29	32		
	5	17.5	20	22	25		
	6	12.5	15.0	17.0	19.0		
	7	9.4	12.0	13.5	15.0		
	8	6.4	8.6	9.8	11.5		
	9	5.2	6.6	7.6	9.0		
	10	(3.8)	4.0	5.8	6.9		
	12	(2.2)	(2.9)	(3.5)	(4.3)		
	14	(1.2)	(1.5)	(2.0)	(2.5)		
	16	–	–	(1.4)	(1.5)		
	18	–	–	–	(1.0)		
30 cm	0.5	84	87	88	89	90	91
	1	70	74	76	78	79	80
	1.5	60	64	66	68	70	72
	2	50	55	57	60	63	65
	3	37	41	43	46	48	50
	4	27	30	33	36	38	39
	5	20	23	25	28	30	32
	6	15.0	17.5	19.5	22	23	25
	7	11.5	13.5	15.0	17.0	18.5	19.5
	8	8.4	10.0	11.5	13.5	14.5	15.5
	9	6.2	7.6	8.9	10.5	11.5	12.5
	10	4.6	5.7	6.8	8.2	9.0	10.0
	12	2.6	3.3	4.0	5.0	5.6	6.3
	14	(1.4)	(1.9)	(2.4)	(2.9)	3.5	4.0
	16	–	(1.1)	(1.4)	(1.8)	(2.2)	(2.5)
	18	–	–	–	(1.1)	(1.3)	(1.6)
	20	–	–	–	–	–	(1.0)
50 cm	0.5	79	83	87	89	91	93
	1	69	74	75	77	81	83
	1.5	59	64	66	68	72	73
	2	52	57	60	62	65	67
	3	38	43	45	48	52	54
	4	29	33	35	38	41	44
	5	22	26	28	31	33	35
	6	16.5	20	22	24	26	28
	7	12.5	15.5	17.0	19.0	21	22
	8	9.2	12.5	13.5	15.0	16.5	18.5
	9	7.0	9.1	10.5	12.0	13.5	14.5
	10	5.2	7.1	8.1	9.8	11.0	12.0
	12	3.0	4.2	5.0	6.0	6.7	7.6
	14	(1.7)	(2.5)	(3.2)	(3.7)	(4.3)	5.9
	16	(1.0)	(1.5)	(1.9)	(2.3)	(2.7)	(3.1)
	18	–	–	(1.1)	(1.4)	(1.7)	(2.0)
	20	–	–	–	–	(1.1)	(1.3)

<u>3 mm Al HVL - HWSD - CDA - CHR</u>
15 - 30 - 50 cm FSD - FHA - DFP - DFP
10 - 400 cm^2 Field size - Feldgröße - Champ - Campo

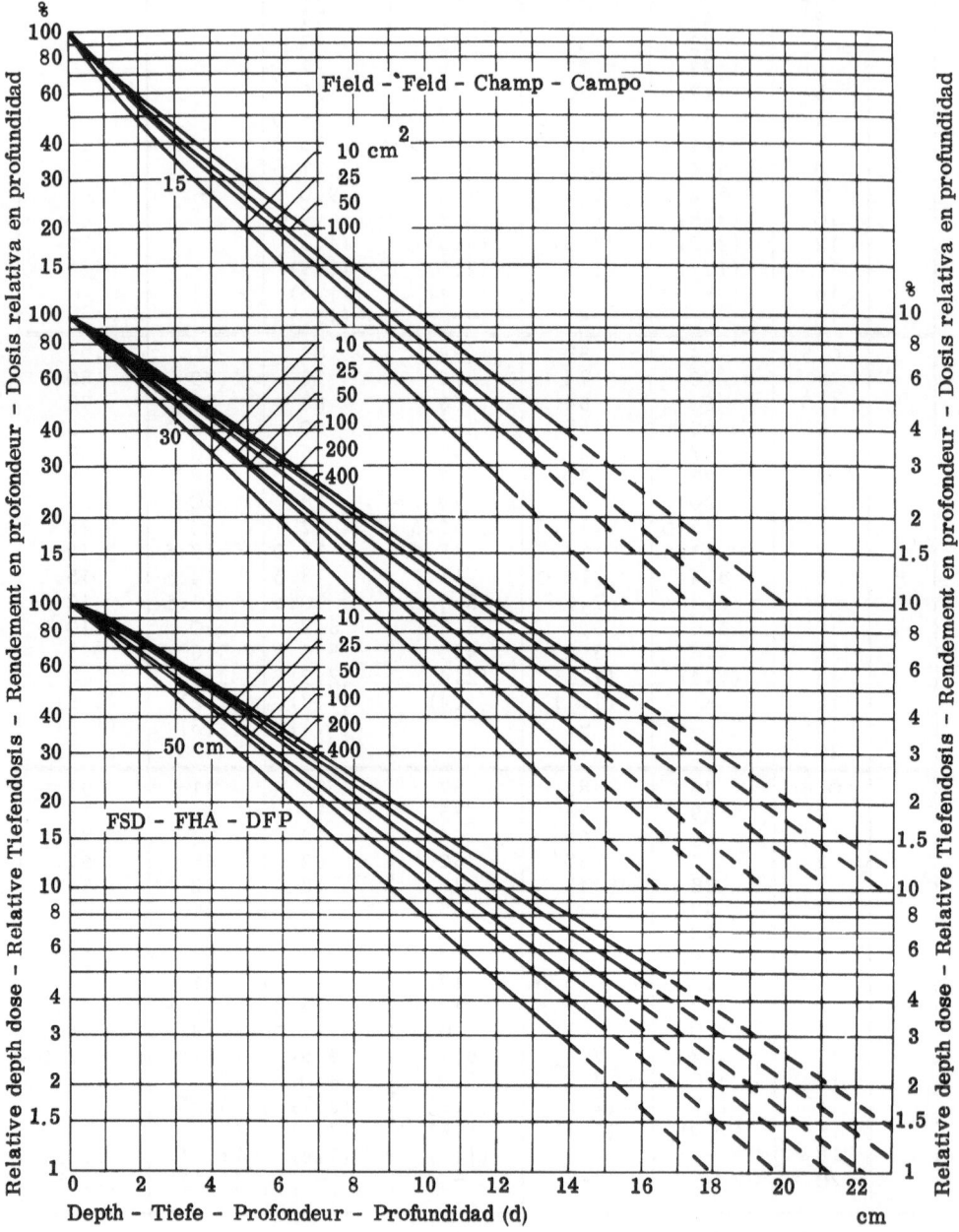

FSD FHA DFP	d	Field size - Feldgröße - Champ - Campo:					cm^2
	cm	10	25	50	100	200	400
15 cm	0.5	80	82	84	86		
	1	66	72	74	76		
	1.5	56	62	64	66		
	2	47	54	56	58		
	3	35	41	43	47		
	4	26	31	33	36		
	5	19.5	24	26	29		
	6	15.0	19.0	20	24		
	7	12.5	15.0	16.5	18.5		
	8	8.3	11.5	12.5	15.0		
	9	6.4	8.7	9.8	12.0		
	10	4.8	6.7	7.7	9.5		
	12	2.7	4.0	4.7	6.1		
	14	(1.5)	(2.3)	(2.9)	(3.7)		
	16	–	(1.4)	(1.7)	(2.4)		
	18	–	–	(1.1)	(1.5)		
	20	–	–	–	(1.0)		
30 cm	0.5	87	89	90	92	93	94
	1	76	79	81	84	85	87
	1.5	65	68	70	72	74	76
	2	57	61	63	66	68	70
	3	44	49	51	54	56	58
	4	33	37	39	43	45	46
	5	25	29	31	34	36	38
	6	19.0	23	25	28	30	32
	7	14.0	18.0	20	23	25	27
	8	11.0	13.5	15.5	18.0	20	21
	9	8.0	11.5	12.0	14.5	16.5	17.5
	10	6.1	8.2	9.7	12.0	13.5	14.5
	12	3.5	5.0	6.0	7.8	9.0	10.0
	14	(2.0)	(3.0)	(3.7)	4.9	6.0	6.7
	16	(1.1)	(1.7)	(2.2)	(3.0)	(3.9)	4.4
	18	–	(1.0)	(1.4)	(2.0)	(2.6)	(3.0)
	20	–	–	–	(1.3)	(1.8)	(2.1)
	22	–	–	–	–	(1.2)	(1.4)
50 cm	0.5	88	92	93	95	96	97
	1	78	83	85	88	90	91
	1.5	68	74	75	78	81	83
	2	60	65	68	72	74	76
	3	47	53	55	60	62	64
	4	36	42	44	48	50	52
	5	28	33	35	40	41	43
	6	22	26	28	33	35	36
	7	17.0	21	23	26	28	30
	8	13.0	16.5	18.5	21	23	25
	9	10.0	13.5	15.0	17.5	19.0	21
	10	7.6	10.5	12.0	14.0	15.5	17.0
	12	4.6	6.3	7.5	9.0	10.5	12.0
	14	2.8	3.9	4.9	5.8	7.0	8.0
	16	(1.6)	(2.4)	(3.0)	3.7	4.6	5.4
	18	(1.0)	(1.5)	(2.0)	(2.4)	(3.1)	(3.7)
	20	–	(1.0)	(1.3)	(1.6)	(2.0)	(2.5)
	22	–	–	–	(1.0)	(1.4)	(1.7)

<u>4 mm Al HVL - HWSD - CDA - CHR</u>

   15 - 30 - 50 cm FSD - FHA - DFP - DFP

   10 - 400 cm^2 Field size - Feldgröße - Champ - Campo

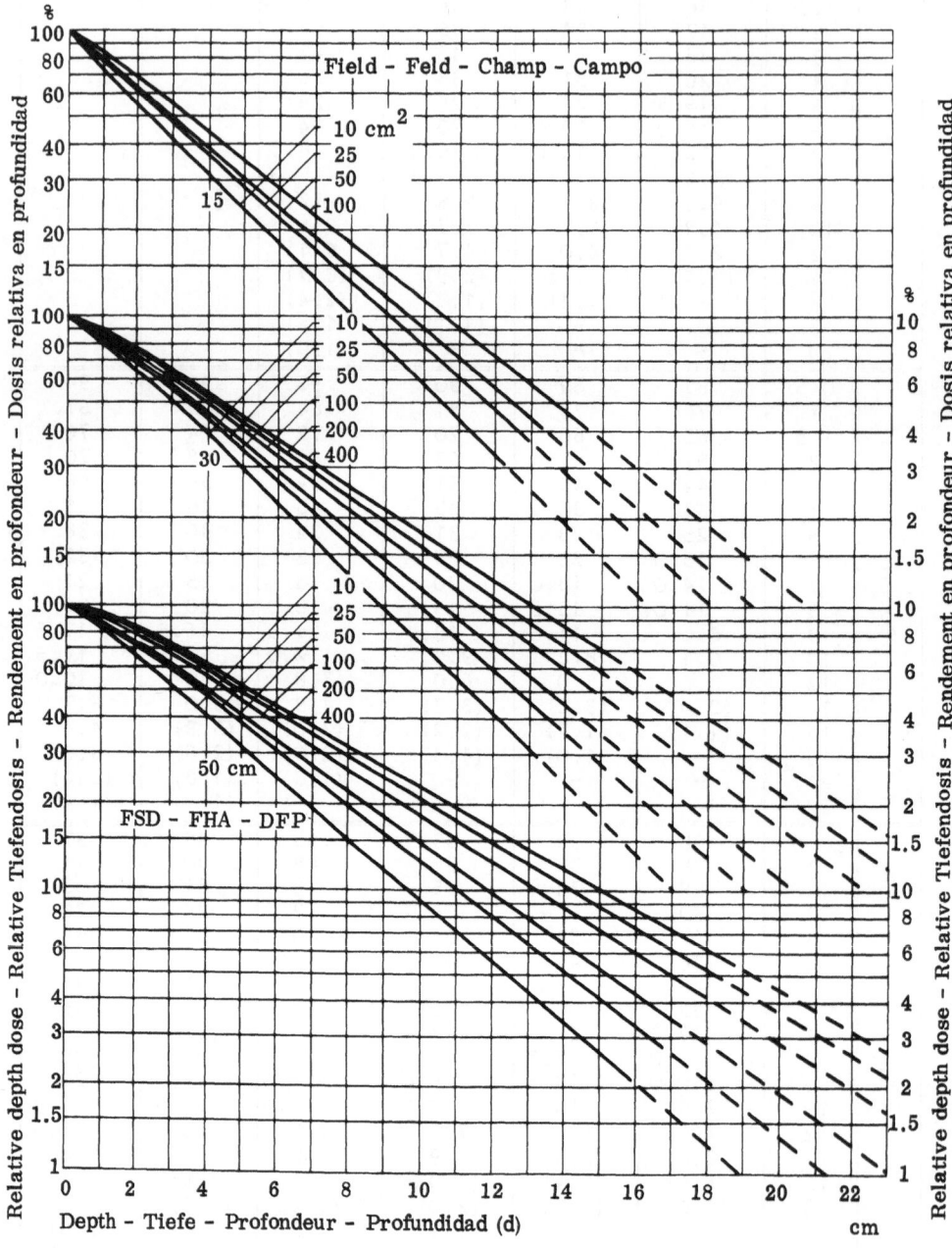

FSD FHA DFP	d cm	Field size - Feldgröße - Champ - Campo:					cm^2
		10	25	50	100	200	400
15 cm	0.5	84	87	89	92		
	1	72	76	78	84		
	1.5	63	68	70	76		
	2	54	60	62	68		
	3	41	46	48	54		
	4	31	36	38	44		
	5	24	28	30	35		
	6	17.5	22	24	28		
	7	13.5	17.0	19.0	22		
	8	10.5	13.0	15.0	18.0		
	9	7.7	10.0	11.5	14.5		
	10	5.8	7.8	9.0	11.5		
	12	3.4	4.8	5.8	7.3		
	14	(1.9)	(2.8)	(3.5)	4.6		
	16	(1.1)	(1.7)	(2.2)	(2.9)		
	18	-	(1.0)	(1.3)	(1.9)		
	20	-	-	-	(1.2)		
30 cm	0.5	89	91	93	95	96	97
	1	79	82	84	86	88	90
	1.5	71	75	77	78	79	83
	2	64	69	70	74	75	77
	3	50	54	57	60	62	64
	4	38	43	46	49	52	54
	5	29	34	36	39	42	44
	6	22	27	29	32	35	37
	7	17.0	21	23	26	29	31
	8	13.0	16.5	17.5	21	23	25
	9	9.6	12.5	14.5	17.5	19.5	22
	10	7.2	9.8	11.5	14.0	16.0	18.0
	12	4.1	5.8	7.1	9.0	10.5	12.0
	14	(2.4)	3.6	4.5	6.0	7.2	8.6
	16	(1.3)	(2.1)	(2.8)	3.8	4.7	5.8
	18	-	(1.3)	(1.7)	(2.6)	(3.3)	(4.0)
	20	-	-	(1.1)	(1.7)	(2.2)	(2.8)
	22	-	-	-	(1.1)	(1.5)	(1.9)
50 cm	0.5	91	93	94	96	97	98
	1	83	87	89	92	94	96
	1.5	74	78	82	85	88	90
	2	66	71	73	77	81	84
	3	52	58	62	66	70	73
	4	40	48	50	56	59	62
	5	32	38	41	46	49	52
	6	25	30	33	38	42	44
	7	19.5	25	28	32	35	38
	8	15.0	20.0	22	26	29	32
	9	12.5	16.0	18.0	23	26	28
	10	9.4	12.5	14.5	18.5	21	23
	12	5.4	8.0	9.7	12.5	15.0	17.0
	14	3.5	5.2	6.7	8.6	10.5	12.0
	16	(2.1)	(3.4)	(4.4)	6.0	7.4	8.6
	18	(1.2)	(2.1)	(2.8)	(4.2)	5.2	6.2
	20	-	(1.3)	(1.8)	(2.8)	(3.6)	(4.4)
	22	-	-	(1.3)	(2.0)	(2.6)	(3.2)

4.2.6   6 mm Al HVL - HWSD - CDA - CHR

15 - 30 - 50 cm FSD - FHA - DFP - DFP

10 - 400 cm^2 Field size - Feldgröße - Champ - Campo

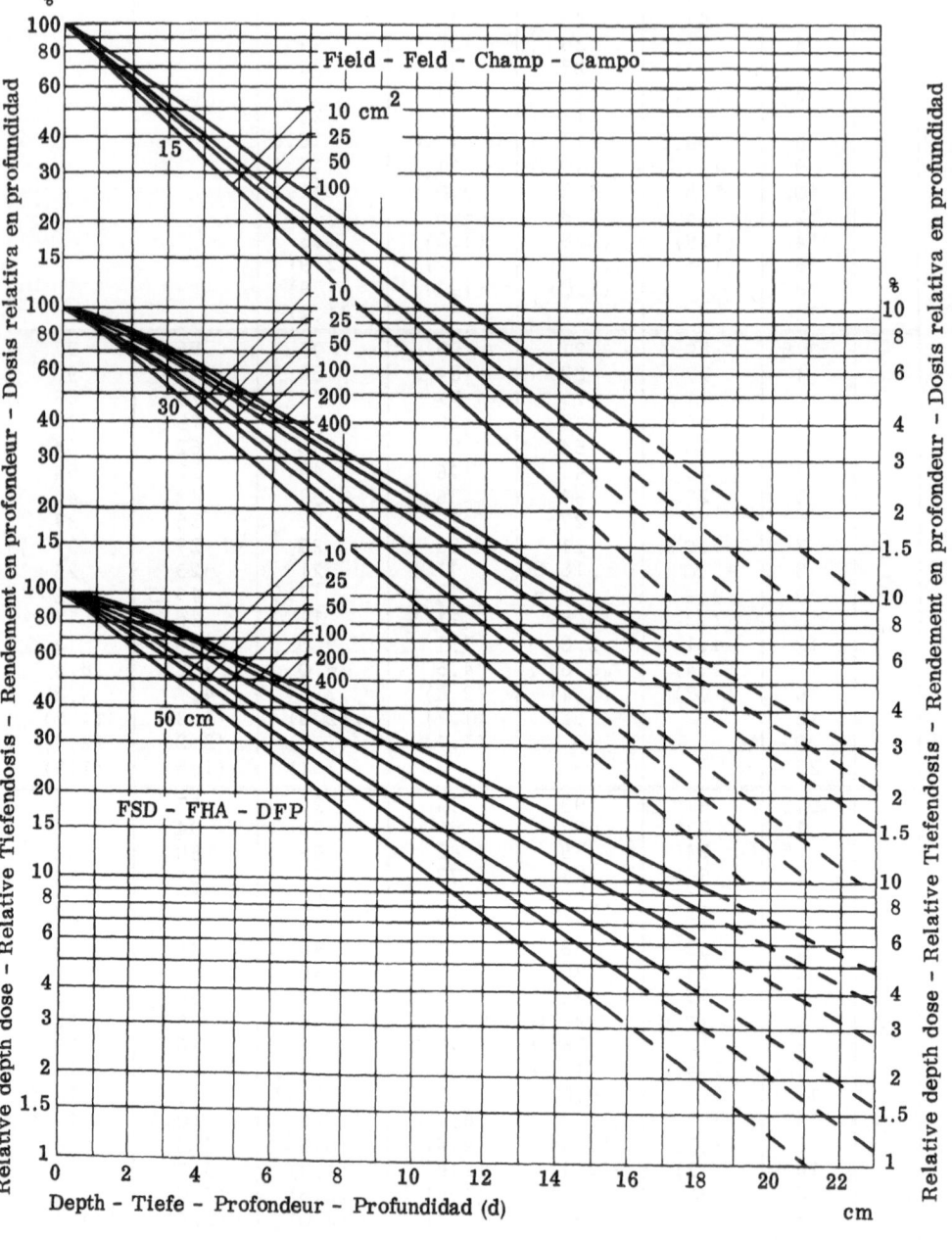

FSD FHA DFP	d cm	Field size - Feldgröße - Champ - Campo:					cm²
		10	25	50	100	200	400
15 cm	0.5	87	88	90	93		
	1	76	78	80	83		
	1.5	66	69	72	76		
	2	58	62	64	69		
	3	44	48	50	56		
	4	34	38	40	46		
	5	26	30	33	38		
	6	19.5	24	26	31		
	7	15.0	18.5	21	25		
	8	11.0	14.5	16.5	20		
	9	8.8	11.0	13.0	16.5		
	10	6.7	9.0	10.5	13.0		
	12	4.0	5.6	6.8	9.0		
	14	(2.3)	(3.4)	(4.3)	6.0		
	16	(1.4)	(2.1)	(2.8)	(4.0)		
	18	-	(1.3)	(1.8)	(2.7)		
	20	-	-	(1.1)	(1.7)		
	22	-	-	-	(1.2)		
30 cm	0.5	90	92	93	95	97	98
	1	83	86	88	91	93	96
	1.5	75	78	81	84	86	88
	2	66	70	73	77	80	83
	3	52	58	61	66	70	73
	4	42	48	51	56	59	62
	5	32	38	42	47	50	53
	6	25	31	34	39	42	45
	7	20	25	28	33	36	38
	8	15.5	19.5	22	27	29	32
	9	12.0	15.5	18.5	23	25	27
	10	9.5	12.5	14.5	18.0	21	23
	12	6.0	8.2	9.7	12.5	15.0	16.5
	14	3.7	5.2	6.4	8.8	10.0	11.5
	16	(2.2)	3.2	4.1	6.0	7.3	8.6
	18	(1.4)	(2.0)	(3.6)	(4.1)	(5.1)	(6.1)
	20	-	(1.3)	(1.8)	(2.8)	(3.6)	(4.4)
	22	-	-	(1.1)	(1.9)	(2.6)	(3.1)
50 cm	0.5	92	94	96	97	98	99
	1	84	89	90	93	96	98
	1.5	74	80	82	86	90	96
	2	67	74	78	82	86	90
	3	52	60	64	70	74	78
	4	43	49	54	61	66	70
	5	35	40	45	52	57	60
	6	28	33	37	44	50	53
	7	22	27	31	33	43	46
	8	17.5	22	25	31	36	39
	9	14.0	18.0	21	27	31	34
	10	11.5	15.0	17.5	23	27	30
	12	7.4	10.0	12.0	16.0	20	23
	14	4.8	6.7	8.5	11.5	14.5	17.0
	16	(3.0)	(4.5)	5.8	8.4	10.5	12.5
	18	(1.9)	(3.0)	(4.0)	(6.1)	(7.8)	9.7
	20	(1.2)	(2.0)	(2.8)	(4.5)	(5.8)	(7.3)
	22	-	(1.4)	(1.9)	(3.2)	(4.3)	(5.2)

4.2.7   <u>8 mm Al HVL – HWSD – CDA – CHR</u>

        15 – 30 – 50 cm FSD – FHA – DFP – DFP

        10 – 400 cm^2 Field size – Feldgröße – Champ – Campo

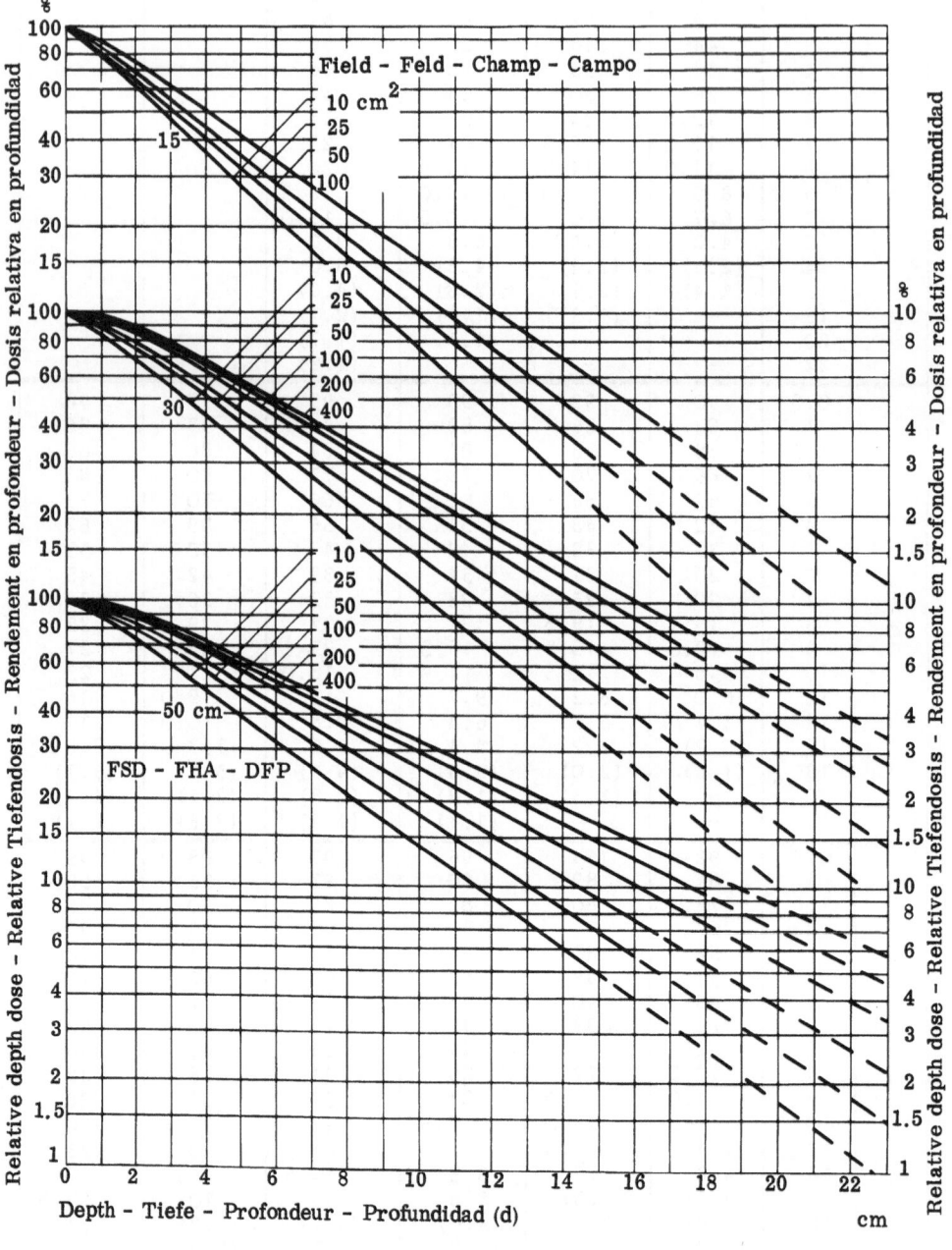

FSD FHA DFP	d cm	Field size - Feldgröße - Champ - Campo:					cm²
		10	25	50	100	200	400
15 cm	0.5	90	92	94	97		
	1	79	82	84	89		
	1.5	70	73	76	82		
	2	62	66	70	76		
	3	47	51	55	62		
	4	36	40	45	50		
	5	28	32	35	42		
	6	22	25	28	34		
	7	16.5	20	23	28		
	8	13.0	16.0	18.5	23		
	9	9.7	12.5	15.0	19.0		
	10	7.7	9.8	11.5	15.5		
	12	4.6	6.2	7.8	10.5		
	14	(2.7)	3.8	4.9	7.0		
	16	(1.6)	(2.4)	(3.2)	4.7		
	18	-	(1.5)	(2.0)	(3.0)		
	20	-	-	(1.3)	(2.1)		
	22	-	-	-	(1.4)		
30 cm	0.5	90	94	95	97	98	99
	1	83	88	90	93	95	97
	1.5	77	83	86	90	93	95
	2	68	75	78	84	87	90
	3	54	61	66	72	75	78
	4	44	51	55	62	66	68
	5	36	40	45	52	55	58
	6	27	33	37	44	47	50
	7	22	27	32	37	40	43
	8	17.0	22	26	30	34	37
	9	13.5	17.5	21	26	28	31
	10	10.5	14.0	17.0	21	24	26
	12	6.6	9.4	12.0	15.0	17.0	19.5
	14	4.2	6.2	8.2	10.5	12.0	14.0
	16	(2.5)	(4.0)	5.5	7.5	8.7	10.0
	18	(1.6)	(2.6)	(3.6)	(5.2)	(6.2)	7.5
	20	(1.0)	(1.7)	(2.5)	(3.8)	(4.5)	(5.5)
	22	-	(1.1)	(1.7)	(2.6)	(3.3)	(4.0)
50 cm	0.5	93	95	96	98	99	100
	1	88	93	94	96	97	98
	1.5	80	86	88	92	94	96
	2	73	80	83	88	90	92
	3	60	68	72	78	80	82
	4	49	56	62	67	70	73
	5	40	47	52	57	60	63
	6	32	38	43	49	52	55
	7	26	32	36	42	45	48
	8	21	26	30	35	40	42
	9	17.0	22	26	32	35	38
	10	14.0	18.0	21	26	30	32
	12	9.4	12.0	15.0	19.0	22	25
	14	6.1	8.3	11.0	14.0	17.0	19.0
	16	(4.0)	5.7	7.5	10.0	12.5	14.5
	18	(2.6)	(3.8)	(5.2)	(7.4)	9.2	11.0
	20	(1.8)	(2.6)	(3.7)	(5.4)	(7.0)	8.8
	22	(1.1)	(1.8)	(2.6)	(3.9)	(5.2)	(6.5)

4.2.8   Therapy with low energy X-rays, short distance- and half
deep therapy
Weichstrahltherapie, Nahbestrahlung und Halbtiefentherapie
Thérapie avec rayons mous, thérapie de contact et thérapie
superficielle
Terapia con rayos blandos, proximal y semiprofunda

4.2.8.1   Radiation qualities and dose rates obtained at 10 cm FSD
Strahlenqualitäten und in 10 cm FHA erreichte Dosisleistungen
Qualités de rayonnement et débits à une DFP de 10 cm
Calidad de la radiaciónes e intensidades obtenidas a 10 cm DFP

HVL - HWSD - CDA - CHR and - und - et - y									
Exposure rate-Dosisleistung-Débit d'exposition-Indice de exposición									
Tube voltage - Röhrenspannung - Tension d'alimentation - Voltaje del tubo: kV=								mm Al - Cu R/min/mA	
		10	20	30	40	50	60	80	100
Filtro - Filtre - Filter - Filter	1 mm Be	0.024 (200)	0.045 (1800)	0.050 -	0.055 -	0.057 -	0.060 -	0.065 -	0.07 -
	0.1 mm Al	0.042 15	0.074 80	0.085 380	0.098 580	0.10 750	0.11 900	0.12 1150	0.13 1300
	0.2 mm Al	0.06 (5)	0.11 45	0.14 150	0.15 225	0.16 340	0.17 400	0.18 530	0.21 700
	0.3 mm Al	0.08 -	0.15 25	0.18 80	0.21 140	0.22 190	0.25 260	0.30 380	0.37 500
	0.5 mm Al	0.13 -	0.24 12	0.32 40	0.38 80	0.42 115	0.48 155	0.62 200	0.80 320
	0.8 mm Al	0.17 -	0.37 6	0.50 23	0.62 40	0.72 65	0.81 90	1.15 150	1.5 290
	1.0 mm Al	0.20 -	0.45 5	0.62 17	0.80 30	0.90 48	1.00 70	1.35 130	1.70 200
	1.5 mm Al	0.29 -	0.62 -	0.82 10	1.2 18	1.3 32	1.4 46	1.8 90	2.3 145
	2.0 mm Al	- -	0.75 -	1.0 6.5	1.4 12	1.6 22	1.7 36	2.2 70	3.1 120
	0.2 mm Cu	- -	- -	- -	- -	2.8 2.0	3.3 9.0	4.4 23	(0.2) 42
	0.5 mm Cu	- -	- -	- -	- -	- -	3.7 2.5	4.9 8.0	(0.4) 16

Lit.: 1. OOSTERKAMP, W.J.: Acta Radiol. 33, 491 (1950)
      2. CHAOUL, H., WACHSMANN, F.: Die Nahbestrahlung, Stuttgart:
         Thieme 1953
      3. WACHSMANN, F.: Jadassohn Hdb. Haut- und Geschlechtskrankh.,
         Band V/2, Berlin-Göttingen-Heidelberg-New York:
         Springer 1959
      4. See pages - Siehe Seiten - Voir pages - Ver paginas 75 - 76

4.2.8.2   Approximate HVD obtained - Etwa erreichte GHWT
PDA approximative - PHR aproximadamente obtenida

HVD - GHWT - PDA - PHR								mm
with - mit - avec - con:				HVL - HWSD - CDA - CHR				
mm Al	0.025	0.1	0.2	0.3	0.4	0.5	0.8	1.0
FSD-FHA-DFP cm 1.5	0.22	-	-	-	-	-	-	-
3	0.22	0.4	0.7	1.4	1.6	1.8	-	-
5	0.22	0.6	1.2	2.4	3.0	3.2	3.5	5.0
10	0.22	1.0	2.4	3.8	4.7	6.0	7.0	9.0
15	0.22	1.4	3.0 [1]	4.8	6.2 [1]	7.6	9.5	12 [1]
20	0.22	1.7	3.5	5.4	7.0	8.7	12	14
30	0.23 [1]	2.0	4.2 [1]	6.2	8.2 [1]	10	15	17 [1]
50	0.23	2.2	4.4	6.6	8.6	10.7	16	19
100	0.23	-	-	6.7	8.8	11	17	20
200	0.23	-	-	-	-	11	17	20
mm Al	1.5	2	3	4	5	6	8	10
mm Cu					0.16	0.20	0.3	0.5
FSD-FHA-DFP cm 1.0	-	-	-	3-4 [2]	-	-	-	-
3	-	-	-	7-9	-	-	-	-
5	8.0	13	-	10-13	-	-	-	-
10	14	20	22	26	30	35	40	42
15	18	23	27	32	35	40	43	45
20	21	24	29	35	38	43	46	48
30	23	27	33	38 [3]	42	46	50	52
50	26	29	36	43	45	50	54	57
100	27	32	41	47	48	54	58	62
200	28	34	43	50	52	56	61	65

1) Values commonly used in low-energy-therapy
   In der Weichstrahltherapie häufig benützte Werte
   Valeurs souvent utilisées en radiothérapie par rayons X mous
   Valores generalmente usados en la terapía con rayos blandos

2) Short distance therapy - Nahbestrahlung - Thérapie de contact -
   Terapía a distancia corta (proximal)

3) Values recommended for subcutaneous- and half deep therapy
   Für die Unterhaut- und Halbtiefentherapie empfohlene Werte
   Valeurs recommandées pour la radiothérapie semiprofonde
   Valores recomendados para la terapía subcutánea y semiprofunda

Röhren - Tubes - Siemens tubes - Tubos	d cm	Relative depth doses - Relative Tiefendosen - Rendements en profondeur - Dosis relativa en profundidad %								
		kV and FSD - kV und FHA - kV et DFP - kV y DFP								
		Monopan			Dermopan					
		1*)	2	3	4	5	6	7	8	9
	kV	60	60	60	10	29	43	50	50	50
	cm	1.5	3	5	15	15	15	15	30	200
	0.5	48	64	74	23	41	58	69	80	83
	1	31	43	48	8.8	25	39	50	68	70
	1.5	21	32	46	-	16	27	36	56	60
	2	15	23	37	-	11	20	28	46	50
	2.5	11	17	29	-	8.0	15	21	39	43
	3	8.2	13	23	-	5.8	11	17	33	36
	3.5	6.3	10	18	-	-	8.3	13	28	31
	5	-	5.0	10	-	-	-	6.4	17	19

*) 1-9 See page - Siehe Seite - Voir page - Ver página 102

4.2.8.3 Siemens Dermopan and - und - et - y Monopan

Usual operating conditions - Gebräuchliche Betriebsbe-
dingungen - Conditions normales d'utilisation - Condiciones normales de utilización

Method Methode Méthode Metodo (Therapy)	Step Stufe Reglage Grado	kV	Filter Filter Filtre Filtro mm	FSD FHA DFP DFP cm	Field Feld Champ Campo Ø cm	Dose rate Dosisleistg. Débit Intensidad R/min	Curve Kurve Courbe Curva No.
Dermopan							
Grenz rays Grenzstrahlen Rayons Bucky Rayos Grenz	I I	10∿ 10∿	∿1 Be ∿1 Be	15 30	2-4 10	∿1000/25 mA ∿1000/25 mA	1 1
	II	29∿	0.3 Al	15	2-4	∿400/25 mA	2
	II	29∿	0.3 Al	30	∿10	∿100/25 mA	3
Soft X-rays	III	43∿	0.6 Al	15	2-4	∿400/25 mA	4
Weichstrahlen	III	43∿	0.6 Al	30	∿10	∿100/25 mA	5
Rayons mous	IV	50∿	1 Al	15	2-4	∿400/25 mA	6
Rayos blandos	IV	50∿	1 Al	30	∿10	∿100/25 mA	7
	IV	50∿	1 Al	200	>1000	∿5/25 mA	8
Monopan (Chaoul)							
Short distance or contact Nahbestrahlung Irradiation de contact Terapia proximal		60= 60= 60=	∿0.2 Cu ∿0.2 Cu ∿0.2 Cu	1.5 3 5	2-3 2-3 2-4.5	∿2000/8 mA ∿700/8 mA ∿300/8 mA	9 10 11
(van der Plaats)		50	∿0.2-3 Al	2-4	1-2.5	∿150-8000/2 mA	12

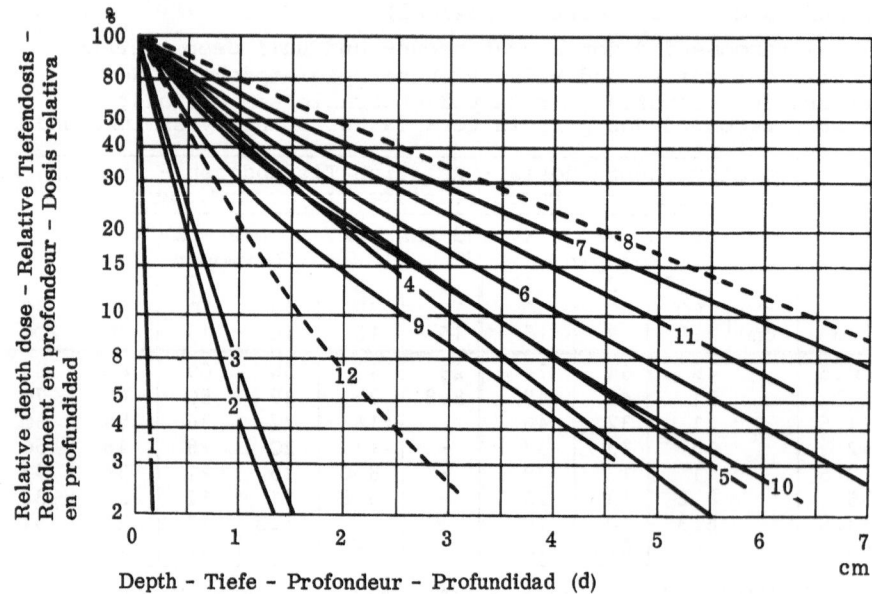

Depth - Tiefe - Profondeur - Profundidad (d)

4.2.8.4 Philips - Müller RT 100

Since many variations are possible, with this apparatus (as with similar equipment), the following numbers must be regardet only examples.

Da mit diesem Apparat - ebenso wie mit anderen ähnlichen - sehr viele Variationen möglich sind, stellen folgende Zahlen nur Beispiele dar.

Puisque de nombreuses variations sont possibles avec cet équipement (ou avec des équipements semblables), les exemples suivants sont donnés seulement à titre indicatif.

Puesto que con este aparato, lo mismo que con otros similares, son posibles muchas variaciones, los siguientes ejemplos serán tomados solamente como guía.

Method Methode Méthode Método	Tension Spannung Tension Tensión	Filter Filter Filtre Filtro	HVL HWSD CDA CHR	FSD FHA DFP DFP	Dose rate Dosisleistung Débit Intensidad	Curve Kurve Courbe Curva
(Therapy)	kV=	mm	mm Al	cm	R/min/mA	No
Grenz (Bucky) rays	10	∿1 Be	0.024	10	(100)	1
Grenzstrahlen	10	∿1 Be	0.024	30	12	1
Low energy Weichstrahl Rayons mous Rayos blandos	40	0.2 Al	0.15	15	110	2
	40	0.2 Al	0.15	30	28	3
	50	0.5 Al	0.48	15	50	4
	50	0.5 Al	0.48	30	12	5
	60	1.0 Al	1.0	15	32	6
Half deep Halbtief Semi profunde Semi profunda	60	1.0 Al	1.0	30	8	7
	100	0.5 Al	0.8	200	0.8	8
	100	0.2 Cu	0.2Cu	15	18	9
	100	0.2 Cu	0.2Cu	30	4.5	10

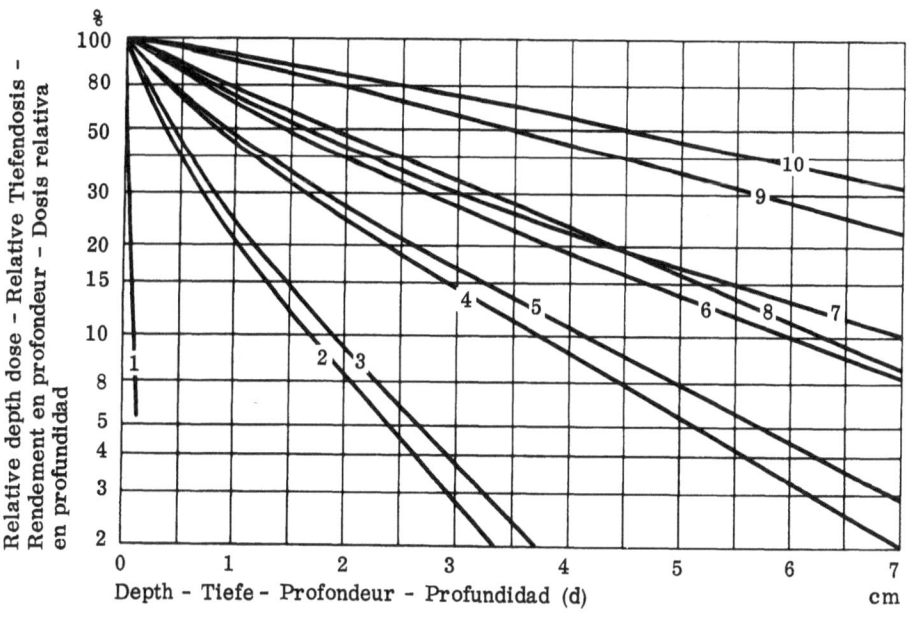

Relative depth dose - Relative Tiefendosis - Rendement en profondeur - Dosis relativa en profundidad

Depth - Tiefe - Profondeur - Profundidad (d)   cm

4.3 Orthovoltage X-rays – Harte Röntgenstrahlen
Rayons X classiques – Rayos X duros

4.3.1 Relative depth doses – Relative Tiefendosen – Rendements en profondeur – Dosis relativas en profundidad

0.5 mm Cu HVL – HWSD – CDA – CHR

30 – 50 – 80 cm FSD – FHA – DFP – DFP

10-25-50-100-200-400 cm^2 Field size – Feld – Champ – Campo

FSD FHA DFP	d cm	Field size - Feldgröße - Champ - Campo:					cm^2
		10	25	50	100	200	400
30 cm	0	100	100	100	100	100	100
	0.5	88	93	95	97	98	99
	1	80	85	91	94	96	97
	1.5	72	77	85	89	91	93
	2	65	70	78	84	86	89
	3	52	58	65	73	75	77
	4	43	48	54	61	64	66
	5	35	39	45	52	54	57
	6	28	32	38	43	46	49
	7	23	26	31	36	40	43
	8	18.5	22	26	31	34	37
	9	15.0	18.0	22	26	29	32
	10	12.5	15.0	18.0	21	25	28
	12	8.1	10.0	12.5	15.0	18.0	21
	14	5.4	6.8	8.8	11.0	13.5	14.0
	16	3.5	4.6	6.1	7.6	9.7	12.0
	18	2.4	3.1	4.3	5.3	7.2	8.9
	20	(1.5)	(2.1)	(3.0)	(3.7)	5.3	6.7
50 cm	0	100	100	100	100	100	100
	0.5	91	95	96	97	98	99
	1	83	88	92	95	97	98
	1.5	75	81	85	90	93	96
	2	68	76	80	85	90	93
	3	56	63	69	74	81	86
	4	46	53	59	65	72	77
	5	38	45	50	57	63	68
	6	32	38	43	48	55	59
	7	26	31	36	41	48	51
	8	22	26	30	35	41	45
	9	18.0	21	26	30	35	40
	10	15.0	18.0	22	26	31	35
	12	10.0	12.5	15.5	19.0	23	26
	14	6.6	8.4	11.5	13.5	17.0	20
	16	4.4	5.8	7.6	9.9	13.0	15.0
	18	3.0	4.0	5.5	7.1	9.3	11.5
	20	(2.0)	(2.8)	(3.9)	5.2	6.8	8.6
80 cm	0	100	100	100	100	100	100
	0.5	92	95	97	98	99	100
	1	86	89	92	95	97	99
	1.5	80	85	88	91	95	98
	2	73	79	83	87	91	94
	3	62	68	73	78	81	87
	4	52	58	63	69	73	79
	5	42	50	55	60	66	72
	6	35	42	46	52	58	66
	7	28	34	39	44	51	58
	8	24	29	33	38	45	51
	9	19.0	24	28	33	39	47
	10	16.0	20	24	28	34	41
	12	11.0	14.0	17.0	21	26	32
	14	7.4	9.8	12.5	15.0	19.5	25
	16	4.9	6.8	8.8	11.5	15.0	19.0
	18	(3.4)	(4.8)	(6.5)	(8.4)	11.5	15.0
	20	(2.2)	(3.3)	(4.6)	(6.1)	(8.7)	(12)

4.3.2 1 mm Cu HVL – HWSD – CDA – CHR

30 – 50 – 80 cm FSD – FHA – DFP – DFP

10-25-50-100-200-400 cm^2 Field size – Feld – Champ – Campo

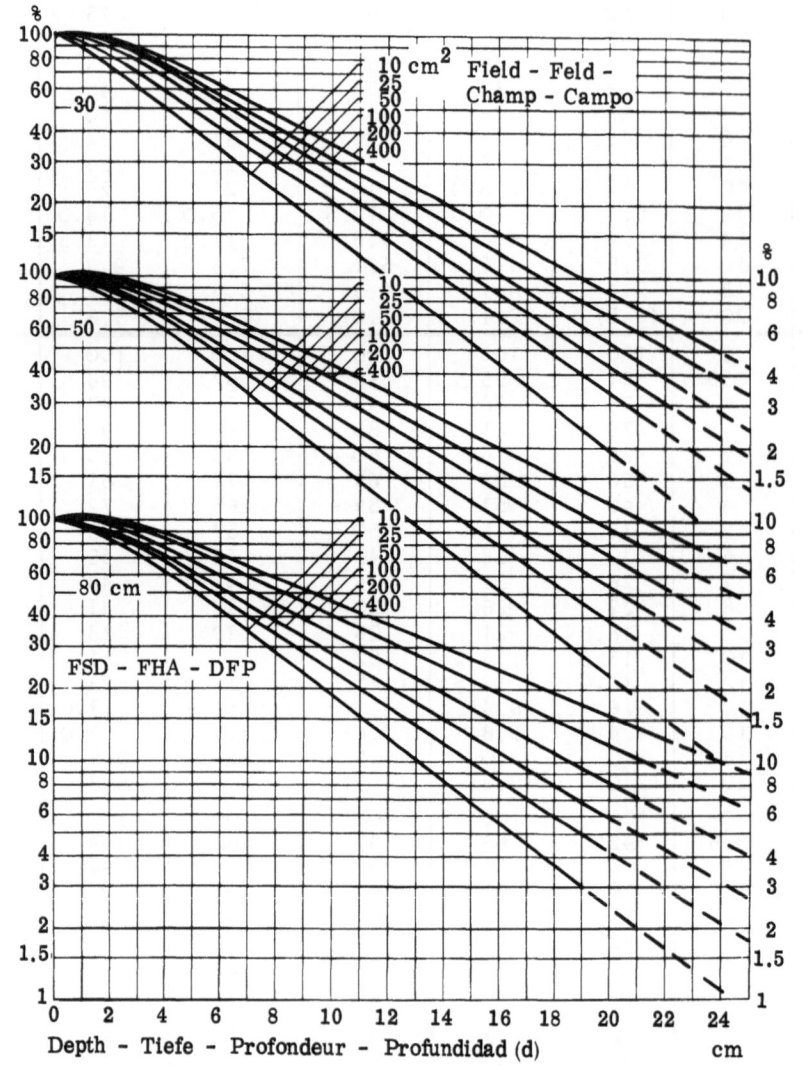

Relative depth dose – Relative Tiefendosis – Rendement en profondeur – Dosis relativa en profundidad

Depth – Tiefe – Profondeur – Profundidad (d)   cm

FSD FHA DFP	d cm	Field size - Feldgröße - Champ - Campo: 10	25	50	100	200	400 cm^2
30 cm	0	100	100	100	100	100	100
	0.5	94	97	99	100	101	102
	1	89	93	97	99	101	102
	1.5	80	88	94	97	99	100
	2	73	82	88	93	94	97
	3	60	70	77	83	86	88
	4	50	58	66	73	76	80
	5	41	49	56	62	66	71
	6	34	42	47	53	57	62
	7	27	35	40	45	49	55
	8	22	29	34	38	42	48
	9	18.5	24	28	33	36	41
	10	15.0	20	24	28	31	36
	12	10.0	14.0	17.0	20	23	27
	14	6.6	9.8	12.5	14.5	17.0	20
	16	4.3	6.8	8.6	10.5	13.0	15.0
	18	2.9	4.8	6.1	7.6	9.5	11
	20	1.9	3.3	4.3	5.4	6.0	8.7
50 cm	0	100	100	100	100	100	100
	0.5	96	98	99	100	101	104
	1	91	95	97	99	101	104
	1.5	86	91	93	96	100	102
	2	81	86	89	94	97	100
	3	70	76	80	85	90	94
	4	60	67	70	77	82	86
	5	49	56	62	67	74	78
	6	40	47	52	60	66	70
	7	33	40	44	52	58	63
	8	27	33	37	45	50	56
	9	22	27	32	38	44	50
	10	17.5	23	27	33	38	44
	12	12.0	16.0	20	24	29	34
	14	7.8	11.5	14.0	18.0	22	26
	16	5.1	7.5	10.0	13.0	16.0	20
	18	3.4	5.3	7.4	9.8	12.5	15.0
	20	2.3	3.8	5.4	7.2	9.4	12.0
80 cm	0	100	100	100	100	100	100
	0.5	97	99	100	101	103	104
	1	94	97	99	101	104	105
	1.5	88	91	94	99	100	103
	2	84	88	90	95	98	101
	3	72	78	81	87	92	96
	4	61	67	71	77	85	88
	5	51	58	61	67	76	81
	6	42	48	52	59	67	72
	7	35	40	45	52	59	66
	8	28	34	38	45	52	58
	9	23	28	33	39	46	52
	10	19.0	24	28	34	41	47
	12	12.5	17.0	21	26	32	38
	14	8.4	12.0	15.0	19.5	25	30
	16	5.6	8.5	11.0	14.5	19.0	24
	18	3.4	6.0	8.0	11.0	15.0	19.5
	20	2.4	4.2	5.8	8.2	12.0	15.5

<u>2 mm Cu HVL – HWSD – CDA – CHR</u>

30 – 50 – 80 cm FSD – FHA – DFP – DFP

10-25-50-100-200-400 cm^2 Field size – Feld – Champ – Campo

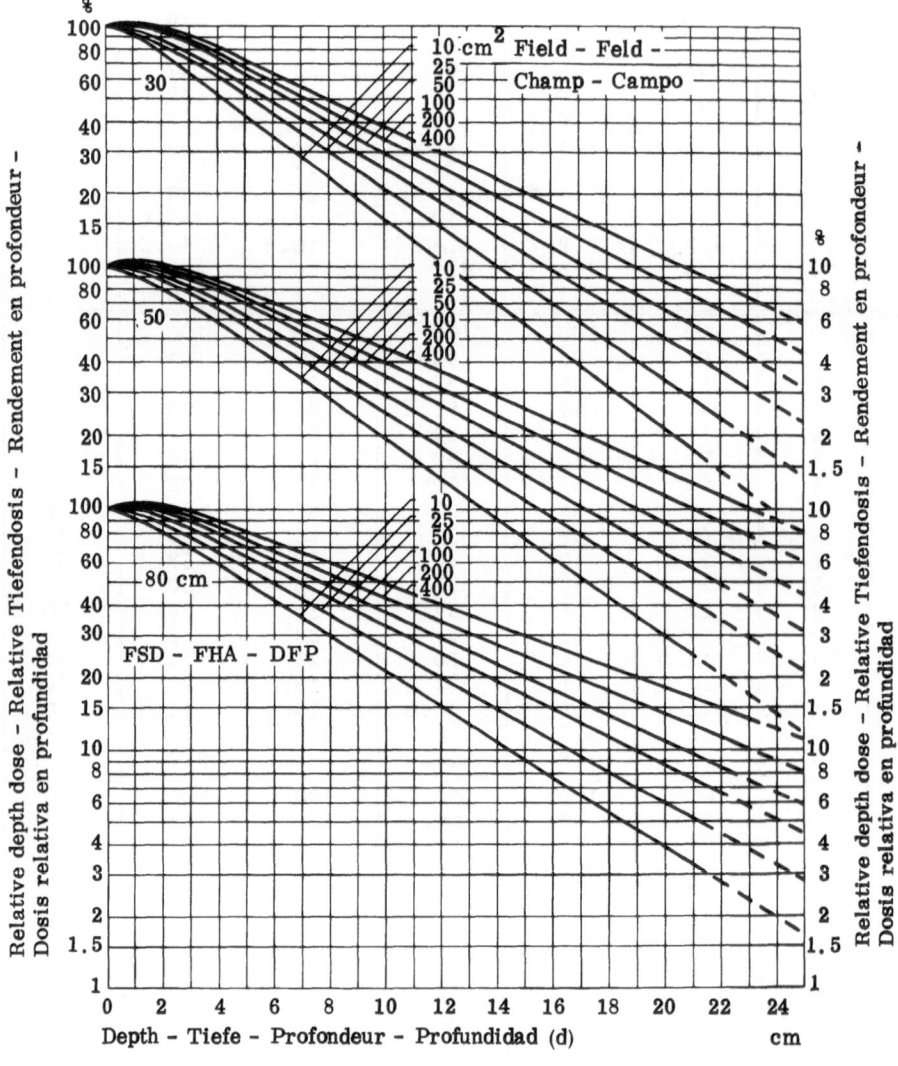

FSD FHA DFP	d	Field size - Feldgröße - Champ - Campo:					cm²
	cm	10	25	50	100	200	400
30 cm	0	100	100	100	100	100	100
	0.5	95	96	97	100	102	104
	1	90	93	96	99	101	103
	1.5	83	88	92	97	99	102
	2	76	82	87	94	96	100
	3	63	72	76	84	88	92
	4	52	62	66	74	78	82
	5	43	51	57	63	67	72
	6	35	43	48	54	59	64
	7	28	36	41	46	52	56
	8	23	30	36	40	45	50
	9	19.5	25	30	34	39	44
	10	15.5	21	26	29	34	38
	12	10.5	14.5	19.0	22	26	30
	14	7.0	10.0	13.5	16.0	20	23
	16	4.7	7.0	9.7	12.5	15	18.0
	18	3.2	4.9	7.2	9.0	12	14.0
	20	2.2	3.4	5.1	6.6	8.8	11.0
50 cm	0	100	100	100	100	100	100
	0.5	95	98	100	102	104	105
	1	90	94	96	100	103	106
	1.5	85	92	95	98	101	105
	2	79	86	90	94	98	101
	3	68	76	80	87	92	96
	4	58	66	71	78	83	88
	5	49	56	62	68	74	79
	6	40	47	53	60	66	71
	7	33	40	46	53	58	64
	8	28	34	39	46	51	57
	9	23	29	34	40	45	51
	10	19.0	25	29	35	40	46
	12	13.0	18.0	22	26	31	37
	14	9.2	13.0	16.0	20	24	29
	16	6.3	9.3	12.0	15.0	19.0	33
	18	4.3	6.8	9.0	11.5	14.5	18.0
	20	3.0	4.9	6.6	7.7	11.5	14.5
80 cm	0	100	100	100	100	100	100
	0.5	96	98	100	102	104	106
	1	91	94	96	101	104	107
	1.5	86	92	98	100	104	107
	2	80	87	92	96	102	105
	3	69	75	83	89	94	99
	4	58	65	73	79	84	90
	5	49	57	64	70	75	80
	6	42	49	56	62	67	83
	7	35	42	49	54	60	66
	8	30	36	43	48	54	60
	9	25	31	38	42	48	54
	10	21	27	33	38	43	49
	12	15.0	20	25	29	34	40
	14	11.0	15.0	19.5	23	28	33
	16	7.8	11.0	15.0	18.0	22	27
	18	5.6	8.2	11.5	14.0	18.0	22
	20	3.9	6.0	8.8	11.0	14.0	18.0

4.3.4 <u>4 mm Cu HVL – HWSD – CDA – CHR</u>

30 – 50 – 80 cm FSD – FHA – DFP – DFP

10-25-50-100-200-400 cm^2 Field size – Feld – Champ – Campo

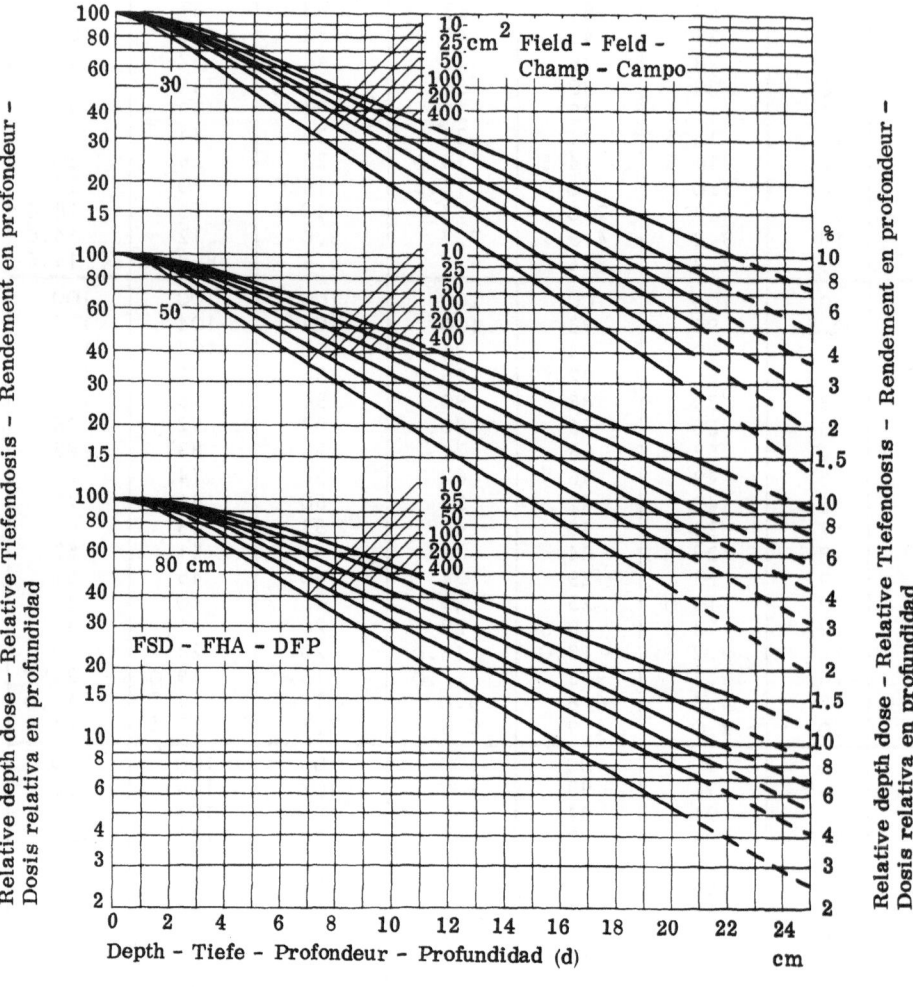

FSD FHA DFP	d cm	Field size - Feldgröße - Champ - Campo:					cm^2
		10	25	50	100	200	400
30 cm	0	100	100	100	100	100	100
	0.5	95	96	97	98	99	100
	1	90	92	93	94	96	98
	1.5	85	88	90	92	94	96
	2	79	83	86	88	90	93
	3	66	74	77	79	83	87
	4	56	64	68	71	75	79
	5	47	54	60	63	66	71
	6	39	47	52	56	59	63
	7	33	40	44	48	51	57
	8	27	34	38	43	47	51
	9	23	28	33	37	41	45
	10	19.0	24	28	32	36	40
	12	13.5	17.0	21	24	28	32
	14	9.4	12.5	15.5	18.0	22	25
	16	6.6	8.4	11.5	13.5	16.5	20
	18	4.6	6.4	8.1	10.0	13.0	16.5
	20	(3.2)	4.5	5.9	6.6	9.6	13.0
50 cm	0	100	100	100	100	100	100
	0.5	98	98	99	99	100	100
	1	94	95	96	97	98	99
	1.5	86	90	92	94	96	98
	2	80	86	89	92	94	96
	3	68	75	80	84	87	90
	4	57	64	72	76	80	84
	5	49	56	63	68	73	77
	6	41	48	55	60	66	70
	7	35	42	48	54	59	65
	8	30	36	42	48	53	59
	9	25	31	37	43	48	53
	10	22	27	32	38	43	48
	12	16.0	20	25	29	34	38
	14	11.5	15.0	19.0	23	27	31
	16	8.1	11.5	14.5	17.5	21	25
	18	6.0	8.6	11.0	13.5	17.0	21
	20	(4.3)	6.3	8.4	10.5	13.0	16.0
80 cm	0	100	100	100	100	100	100
	0.5	98	98	99	99	100	101
	1	95	96	97	98	99	100
	1.5	91	94	96	97	99	100
	2	84	90	93	95	97	98
	3	74	80	85	88	91	93
	4	63	70	77	80	86	88
	5	54	62	68	73	78	83
	6	46	54	60	66	72	77
	7	40	47	53	59	65	70
	8	34	41	46	52	60	65
	9	29	36	41	46	53	58
	10	25	31	36	41	47	52
	12	18.0	24	28	33	38	44
	14	13.5	18.0	21	26	30	36
	16	9.8	13.5	16.5	20	24	29
	18	7.2	11.0	13.0	15.5	19.0	24
	20	5.2	8.0	9.8	12.5	15.0	19.0

4.3.5 <u>Tissue-air ratio for orthovoltage X-rays</u>
<u>Gewebe/Luft-Verhältnis für harte Röntgen-Strahlung</u>
<u>Rapports tissu – air pour rayons X classiques</u>
<u>Relación tejido/aire para rayos-X duros</u>

<u>1 mm Cu HVL – HWSD – CDA – CHR</u>

0 – 400 cm^2 Field size – Feldgröße – Champ – Campo

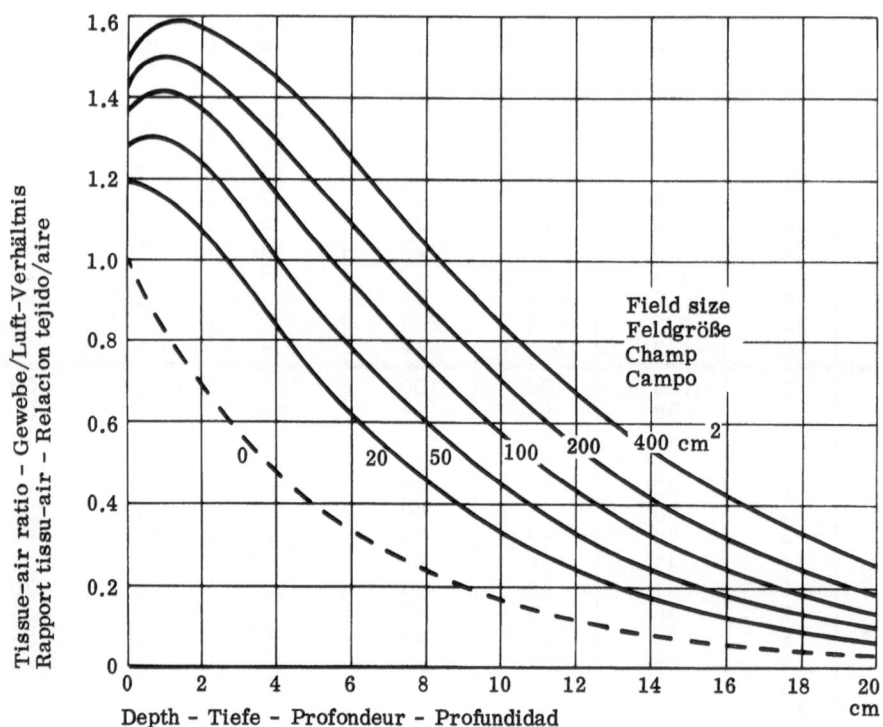

Depth – Tiefe – Profondeur – Profundidad

Depth Tiefe Profondeur Profundidad cm	Tissue-air ratio – Gewebe/Luft-Verhältnis – Rapport tissu – air – Relación tejido/aire					
	Field size – Feldgröße – Champ – Campo					cm^2
	0	20	50	100	200	400
0	1.0	1.19	1.23	1.33	1.41	1.50
1	0.81	1.16	1.30	1.42	1.50	1.59
2	0.69	1.08	1.24	1.37	1.46	1.57
3	0.58	0.96	1.14	1.27	1.38	1.53
4	0.48	0.83	1.00	1.16	1.28	1.46
5	0.39	0.72	0.89	1.05	1.19	1.36
6	0.33	0.63	0.79	0.95	1.09	1.25
7	0.28	0.54	0.70	0.85	0.98	1.14
8	0.24	0.46	0.60	0.75	0.88	1.04
9	0.20	0.39	0.53	0.66	0.78	0.94
10	0.17	0.34	0.45	0.58	0.70	0.85
12	0.12	0.24	0.33	0.44	0.55	0.68
14	0.08	0.18	0.24	0.33	0.41	0.54
16	0.06	0.12	0.18	0.25	0.33	0.43
18	0.04	0.09	0.14	0.18	0.25	0.33
20	0.03	0.06	0.10	0.13	0.18	0.26

2 mm Cu HVL - HWSD - CDA - CHR
0 - 400 cm^2 Field size - Feldgröße - Champ - Campo

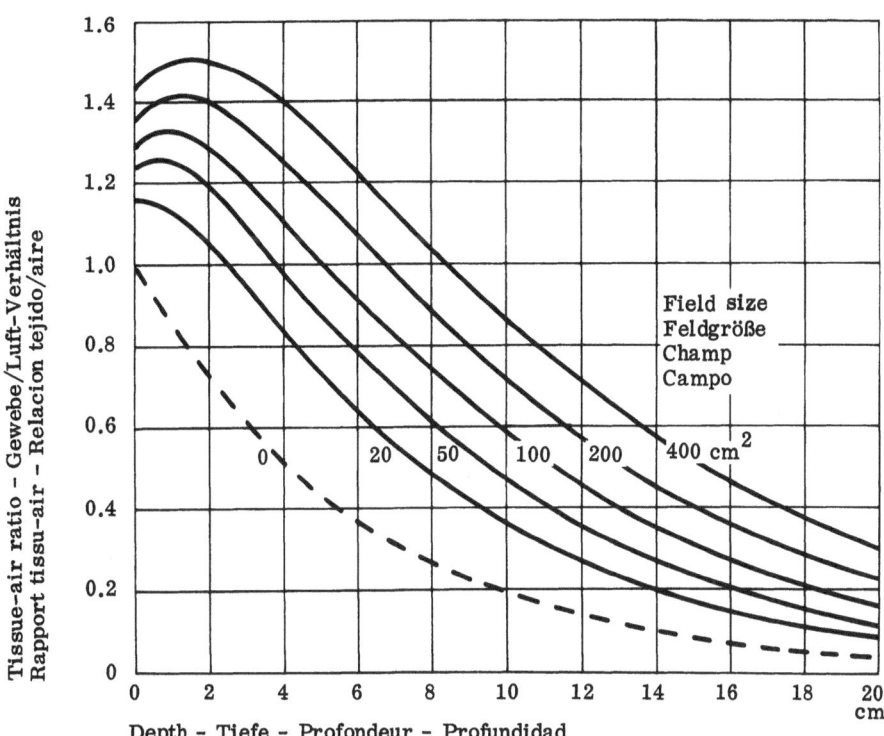

Depth - Tiefe - Profondeur - Profundidad

Depth Tiefe Profondeur Profundidad cm	Tissue-air ratio - Gewebe/Luft-Verhältnis - Rapport tissu - air - Relación tejido/aire					
	Field size - Feldgröße - Champ - Campo cm^2					
	0	20	50	100	200	400
0	1.0	1.16	1.23	1.29	1.35	1.42
1	0.85	1.13	1.25	1.33	1.42	1.49
2	0.73	1.05	1.19	1.29	1.39	1.49
3	0.61	0.94	1.08	1.20	1.33	1.47
4	0.51	0.83	0.98	1.10	1.24	1.40
5	0.43	0.73	0.88	1.00	1.16	1.32
6	0.37	0.64	0.79	0.91	1.07	1.22
7	0.31	0.56	0.70	0.83	0.98	1.12
8	0.27	0.49	0.62	0.75	0.88	1.04
9	0.23	0.42	0.54	0.66	0.80	0.95
10	0.19	0.36	0.47	0.59	0.72	0.87
12	0.14	0.27	0.36	0.46	0.57	0.71
14	0.10	0.20	0.27	0.35	0.45	0.58
16	0.07	0.15	0.21	0.27	0.36	0.46
18	0.05	0.11	0.16	0.21	0.28	0.38
20	0.04	0.09	0.12	0.16	0.23	0.30

Lit.: 1. ICRU, Rep. 10 a, Clin. Dosimetry, NBS-Handbook 87, Washington 1963
See page - Siehe Seite - Voir page - Ver página 114

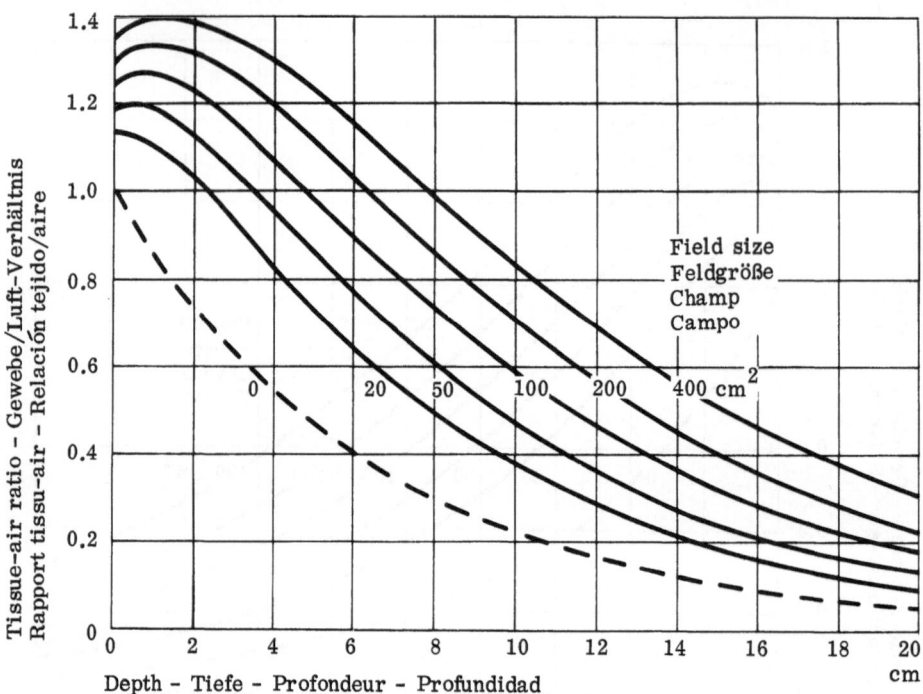

3 mm Cu HVL - HWSD - CDA - CHR

0 - 400 cm^2 Field size - Feldgröße - Champ - Campo

Tissue-air ratio - Gewebe/Luft-Verhältnis - Rapport tissu-air - Relación tejido/aire

Field size
Feldgröße
Champ
Campo

0   20   50   100   200   400 cm^2

Depth - Tiefe - Profondeur - Profundidad

Depth Tiefe Profondeur Profundidad cm	Tissue-air ratio - Gewebe/Luft-Verhältnis - Rapport tissu-air - Relación tejido/aire					
	Field size - Feldgröße - Champ - Campo					cm^2
	0	20	50	100	200	400
0	1.00	1.15	1.23	1.29	1.35	1.42
1	0.85	1.13	1.25	1.33	1.42	1.50
2	0.72	1.05	1.19	1.29	1.40	1.50
3	0.61	0.94	1.09	1.20	1.33	1.47
4	0.52	0.83	0.98	1.10	1.25	1.40
5	0.44	0.73	0.88	1.00	1.15	1.32
6	0.37	0.64	0.79	0.92	1.07	1.22
7	0.31	0.56	0.70	0.82	0.98	1.12
8	0.26	0.49	0.62	0.74	0.88	1.04
9	0.23	0.43	0.54	0.66	0.79	0.95
10	0.19	0.26	0.47	0.59	0.72	0.87
12	0.14	0.27	0.36	0.46	0.58	0.71
14	0.10	0.20	0.37	0.35	0.45	0.58
16	0.07	0.15	0.21	0.27	0.36	0.46
18	0.05	0.11	0.15	0.21	0.28	0.38
20	0.04	0.09	0.12	0.16	0.23	0.30

Lit.: 2. SCHOKNECHT, G.: Strahlenther. 132, 516 (1967); 136, 24 (1968)
      3. HOLT, J.G., LAUGHLIN, J.S., MORONEY, J.B.: Radiology 96, 437 (1970)

See page - Siehe Seite - Voir page - Ver pagina 115

4 mm Cu HVL - HWSD - CDA - CHR

0 - 400 m² Field size - Feldgröße - Champ - Campo

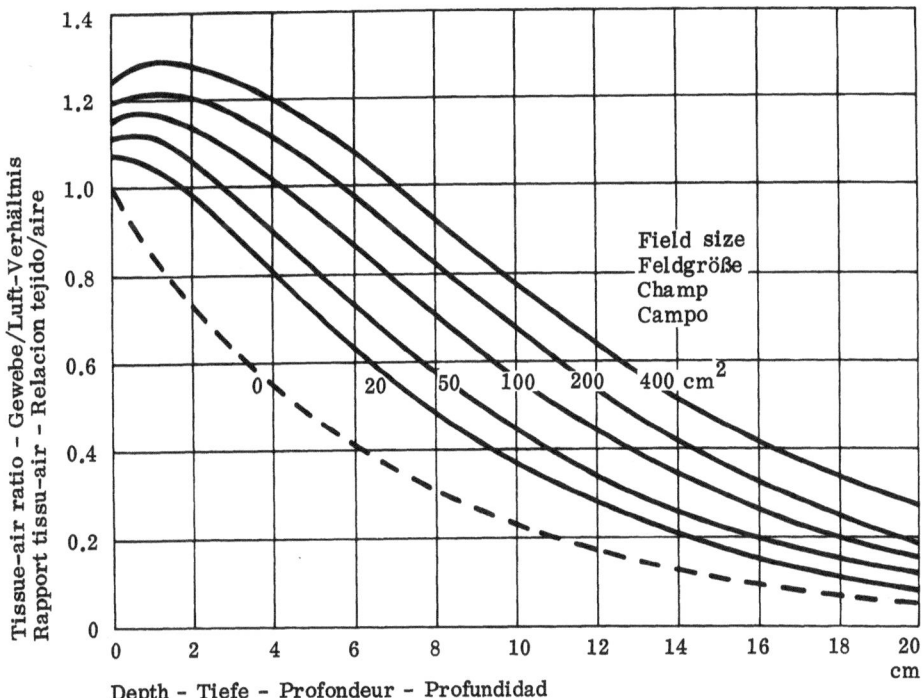

Depth - Tiefe - Profondeur - Profundidad

Depth Tiefe Profondeur Profundidad cm	Tissue-air ratio - Gewebe/Luft-Verhältnis - Rapport tissu-air - Relación tejido/aire					
	Field size - Feldgröße - Champ - Campo					cm²
	0	20	50	100	200	400
0	1.00	1.07	1.11	1.15	1.19	1.24
1	0.85	1.05	1.12	1.17	1.22	1.29
2	0.73	0.98	1.06	1.14	1.20	1.27
3	0.63	0.90	0.98	1.08	1.16	1.24
4	0.54	0.81	0.90	1.02	1.12	1.20
5	0.47	0.72	0.81	0.95	1.05	1.14
6	0.41	0.63	0.73	0.87	0.97	1.07
7	0.36	0.55	0.65	0.78	0.90	1.00
8	0.31	0.48	0.57	0.70	0.83	0.93
9	0.27	0.42	0.51	0.63	0.75	0.85
10	0.23	0.37	0.45	0.56	0.68	0.98
12	0.17	0.28	0.34	0.45	0.53	0.64
14	0.13	0.21	0.26	0.35	0.42	0.52
16	0.09	0.16	0.20	0.26	0.33	0.41
18	0.07	0.11	0.15	0.20	0.25	0.34
20	0.05	0.07	0.12	0.16	0.18	0.27

Lit.: 4. COHEN, M., JONES, D.E.A., GREENE, D.: Central Axis Depth Dose Data for Use in Radiotherapy, Brit.J.Radiol., Suppl. 11 (1972)

4.4 Conversion of relative depth dose from 50 cm to other FSD's
Umrechnung relativer Tiefendosen von 50 cm auf andere FHA
Conversion de rendements en profondeur de 50 cm à d'autres DFP
Conversión de las dosis relativas en profundidad para 50 cm a otras DFP

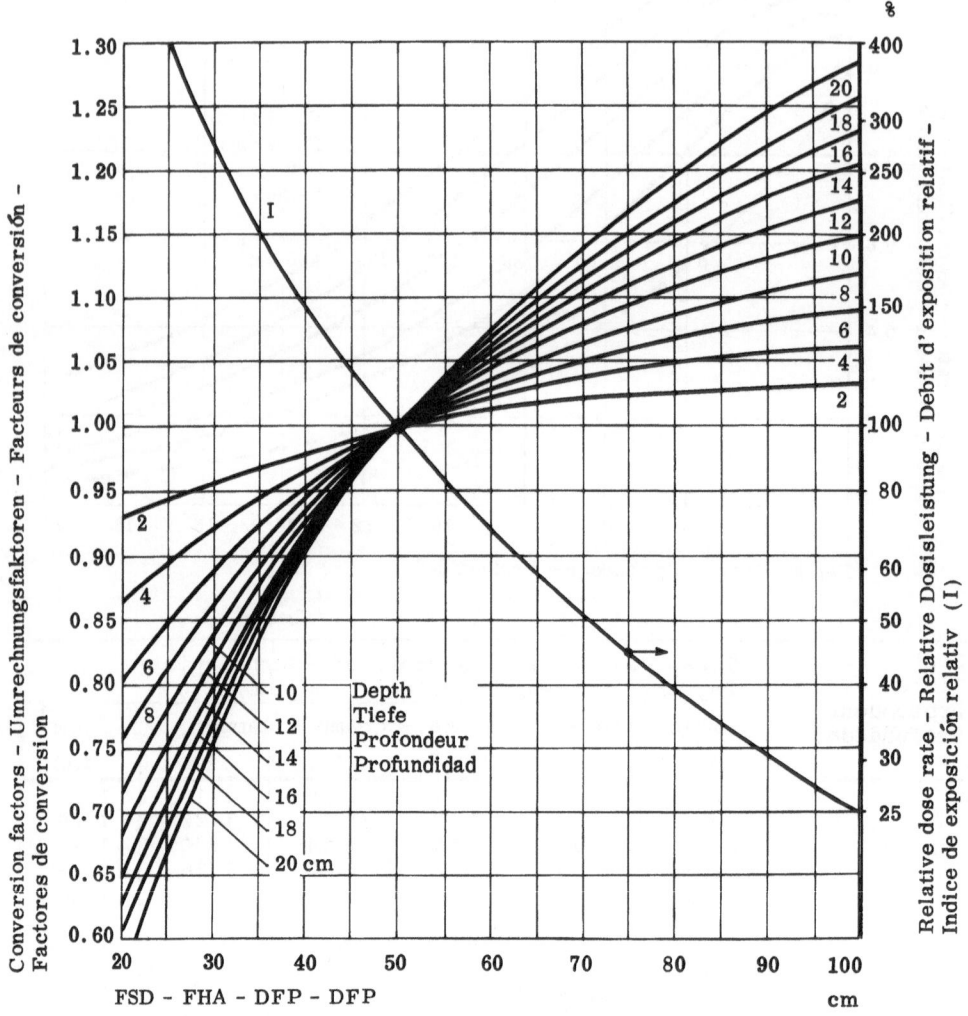

FSD - FHA - DFP - DFP   cm

Lit.: 1. PFALZNER, P.M.: Brit.J.Radiol. 34, 236 (1961)
2. WEBSTER, E.W., TSIEN, K.C.: Atlas of Radiation Dose Distributions, IAEA, Vienna 1965
3. JOHNS, H.E., CUNNINGHAM, J.R.: The Physics of Radiology, 3th Edition, Springfield: Thomas 1969
4. BURNS, J.E., in: Depth Dose Data for Use in Radiotherapy, Brit.J.Radiol., Suppl. 11, Appendix B, London 1972

FSD FHA DFP DFP	Conversion factors for tissue depths of Umrechnungsfaktoren für Gewebetiefen von Facteurs de conversion pour des profondeurs de Factores de conversión para profundidades en el tejido cm									
cm	2	4	6	8	10	12	14	16	18	20
20	0.93	0.86	0.81	0.76	0.72	0.68	0.65	0.63	0.60	-
25	0.95	0.90	0.85	0.82	0.78	0.75	0.73	0.71	0.69	0.66
30	0.96	0.92	0.89	0.86	0.80	0.82	0.80	0.79	0.77	0.76
35	0.97	0.95	0.93	0.91	0.89	0.88	0.86	0.86	0.85	0.84
40	0.98	0.96	0.95	0.95	0.94	0.93	0.92	0.92	0.91	0.91
45	0.99	0.98	0.98	0.97	0.97	0.97	0.97	0.96	0.96	0.96
50	1.00	1.00	1.00	1.00	1.00	1.00	1.00	1.00	1.00	1.00
55	1.01	1.01	1.01	1.02	1.02	1.03	1.03	1.03	1.04	1.04
60	1.01	1.02	1.03	1.04	1.04	1.05	1.06	1.06	1.07	1.08
65	1.02	1.03	1.04	1.05	1.06	1.07	1.08	1.09	1.10	1.11
70	1.02	1.04	1.05	1.06	1.08	1.09	1.11	1.12	1.13	1.14
75	1.03	1.05	1.06	1.08	1.10	1.11	1.13	1.14	1.15	1.17
80	1.03	1.05	1.07	1.09	1.11	1.13	1.14	1.16	1.18	1.20
85	1.03	1.06	1.08	1.10	1.12	1.14	1.16	1.18	1.20	1.22
90	1.03	1.06	1.08	1.11	1.13	1.16	1.18	1.20	1.25	1.25
95	1.03	1.06	1.09	1.11	1.14	1.17	1.20	1.22	1.24	1.27
100	1.03	1.06	1.09	1.12	1.15	1.18	1.21	1.23	1.26	1.29

Dose rate-Dosisleistung-Débit d'exposition-Indice de exposición: I

FSD - FHA - DFP cm (50 cm = 100 %)								
cm	20	25	30	35	40	45	55	60
I %	625	400	278	204	156	123	82.6	69.4
cm	65	70	75	80	85	90	95	100
I %	59.1	51.0	44.4	39.1	34.6	30.9	27.4	25

The conversion factors shown represent values which may be encountered in practice at different depths in tissue, when secondary effects (scattering, finite focal spot size, etc.) are taken into account. The conversion factors calculated from the inverse square law differ to a small extend from those given above.

Die angegebenen Umrechnungsfaktoren stellen die in der Praxis unter Berücksichtigung von sekundären Einflüssen (Streuung, endliche Fokusgröße usw.) in verschiedenen Gewebetiefen etwa auftretenden Werte dar. Die aus dem Quadratgesetz errechneten Umrechnungsfaktoren weichen von den angegebenen geringfügig ab.

Les facteurs de conversion donnés, représentent des valeurs rencontrées en pratique lorsque l'on tient compte des phénomènes secondaires (diffusion, dimensions du foyer, etc.). Les facteurs de conversion calculés par l'inverse carré des distances diffèrent un peu des facteurs donnés ici.

Los factores de conversión indicados representan los valores practicos teniendo en cuenta factores secundarios (dispersión, tamaño focal, etc.) en diferentes profundidades de tejido. Los valores teóricos calculados a partir de la ley del cuadrado recíproco se apartan de los aquí indicados dentro de ciertos límites.

4.5 γ-Teletherapy units - γ-Fernbestrahlungsapparaturen - Appareils de télégammathérapie - Aparatos de telecurieterapia

4.5.1 Cs 137

15 - 20 - 30 - 40 - 50 cm SSD - QHA - DSP - DFP

100 cm^2 Field size - Feld - Champ - Campo

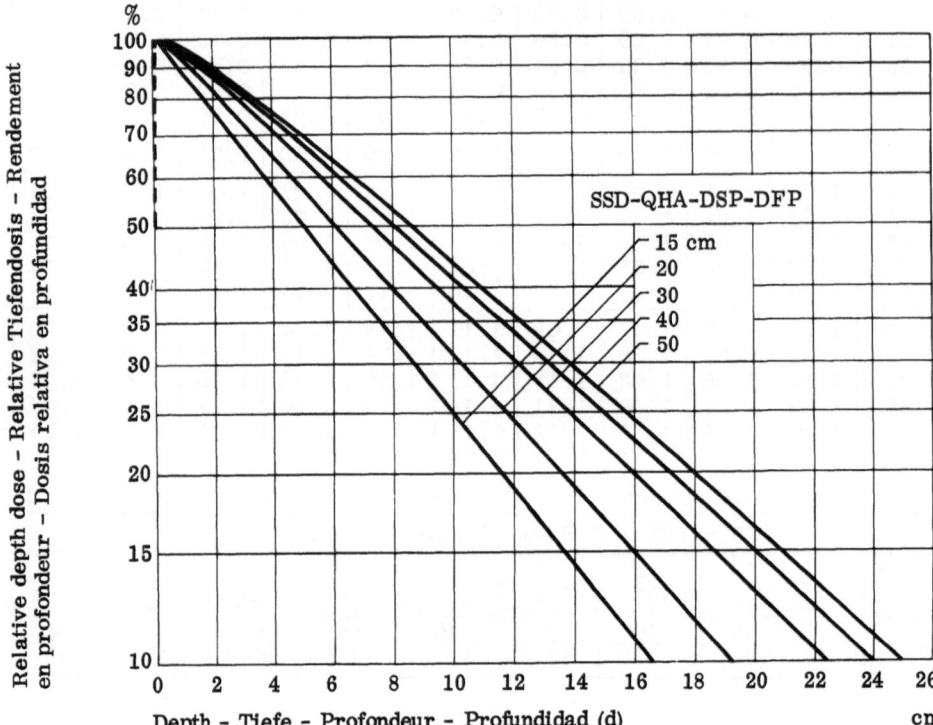

	SSD - QHA - DSP - DFP									
d cm	15	20	30	40	50	d cm	15	20	30	40	50
0	(50)	(50)	(50)	(50)	(50)	13	16.0	21	27	31	33
0.2	100	100	100	100	100	14	14.0	19.0	25	28	30
1	88	93	95	97	98	15	12.0	16.5	22	25	27
2	76	82	88	89	91	16	11.0	15.0	20	23	25
3	66	73	79	81	83	17	9.2	13.0	17.5	20	24
4	58	63	71	74	76	18	-	11.5	16.0	18.0	20
5	50	58	64	68	70	19	-	10.0	14.0	16.5	18.0
6	44	50	58	62	64	20	-	9.0	13.0	15.0	16.0
7	38	45	52	56	59	21	-	-	10.5	12.0	13.5
8	33	40	47	50	53	22	-	-	10.5	12.0	13.5
9	24	36	43	46	48	23	-	-	9.2	10.5	12.0
10	25	31	39	41	44	24	-	-	-	10.0	11.0
11	22	28	34	37	40	25	-	-	-	9.0	10.0
12	19	25	30	33	37						

Lit.: See page - Siehe Seite - Voir page - Ver página 119

4.5.2 Co 60

50 cm SSD - QHA - DSP - DFP

(0)-20-50-100-200-400 cm^2 Field size - Feld - Champ - Campo

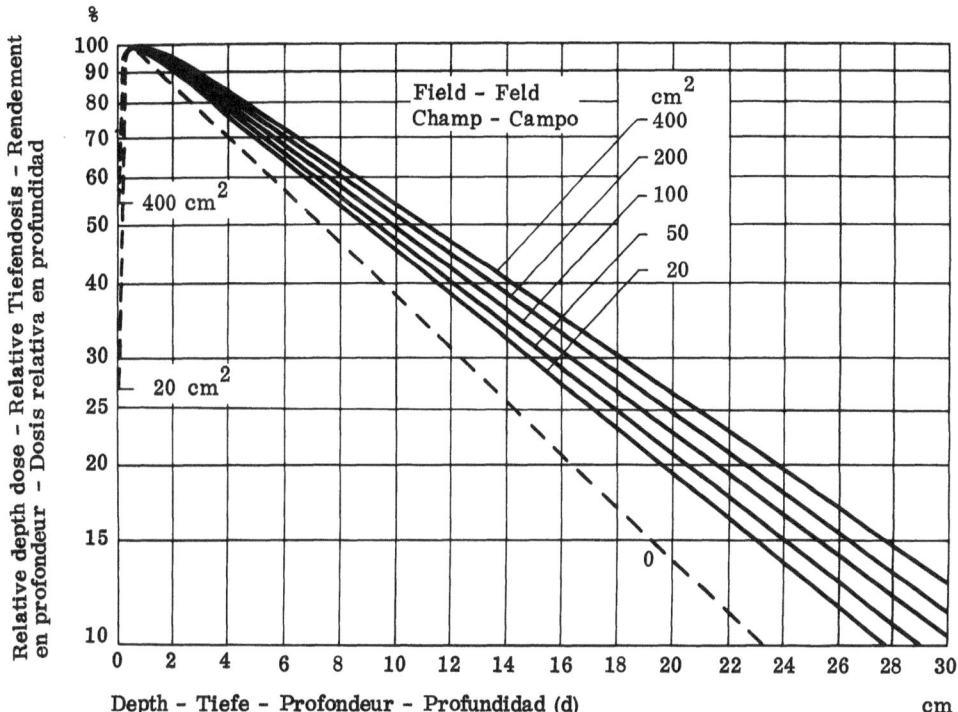

Relative depth dose - Relative Tiefendosis - Rendement en profondeur - Dosis relativa en profundidad

Depth - Tiefe - Profondeur - Profundidad (d)   cm

Field size - Feldgröße - Champ - Campo: cm^2												
d cm	0	20	50	100	200	400	d cm	0	20	50	100	200	400
0	-	(29)	(36)	(43)	(58)	(55)	11	(34)	42	44	46	49	50
0.5	100	100	100	100	100	100	12	(31)	38	40	42	45	48
1	95	97	97	98	98	99	13	(28)	34	36	39	41	43
2	86	90	91	93	94	95	14	(26)	32	34	36	38	40
3	77	83	84	86	88	90	15	(23)	30	31	33	36	38
4	70	75	77	79	81	83	16	(21)	27	29	31	33	35
5	63	70	71	73	76	78	17	(19)	25	26	28	30	32
6	57	64	65	67	70	72	18	(17)	22	25	26	28	30
7	52	59	60	62	65	67	19	(15)	21	23	25	27	28
8	47	54	55	57	60	62	20	(14)	19.5	21	23	24	26
9	43	50	51	53	56	59	22	(12)	17.5	18.0	19.0	21	23
10	38	45	47	49	52	54	24	(9)	13.5	15.0	17.0	18.0	20

Lit.: 1. WEBSTER, E.W., TSIEN, K.C.: IAEA Atlas I, Vienna 1965
      2. DREXLER, G., WACHSMANN, F.: Strahlenther.132,1-7 (1967)
      3. COHEN, M., JONES, D.E.A., GREENE, D.: Central Axis Depth Dose Data for Use in Radiotherapy, Brit.J.Radiol., Suppl. 11 (1972)

Co 60

60 cm SSD - QHA - DSP - DFP

(0)-20-50-100-200-400 cm^2 Field size - Feld - Champ - Campo

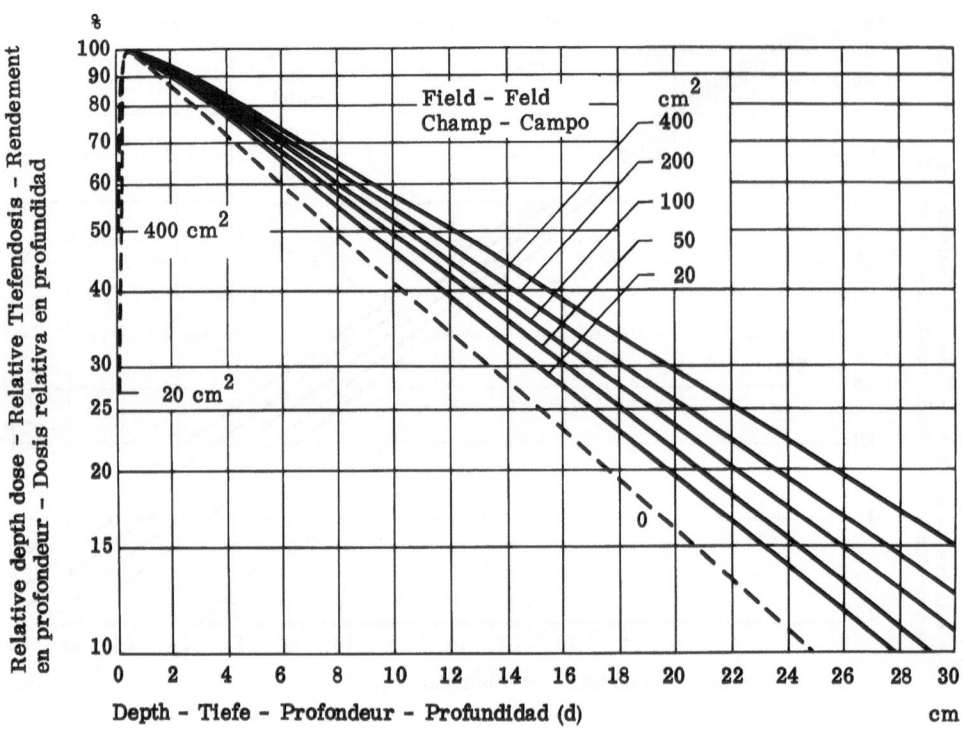

Relative depth dose - Relative Tiefendosis - Rendement en profondeur - Dosis relativa en profundidad (%)

Field - Feld — Champ - Campo

cm^2 — 400, 200, 100, 50, 20

400 cm^2

20 cm^2

0

Depth - Tiefe - Profondeur - Profundidad (d)   cm

d cm	0	20	50	100	200	400	d cm	0	20	50	100	200	400
0	–	(26)	(32)	(36)	(42)	(50)	11	(38)	42	45	47	50	54
0.5	(100)	100	100	100	100	100	12	(34)	39	42	45	48	51
1	(94)	95	96	97	98	99	13	(31)	35	38	41	44	47
2	(87)	90	91	92	93	94	14	(28)	33	35	38	41	44
3	(79)	82	83	85	87	89	15	(25)	30	33	36	39	42
4	(71)	77	79	80	82	84	16	(23)	28	30	33	36	39
5	(64)	71	74	76	78	80	17	(20)	21	28	29	33	37
6	(60)	65	68	70	71	73	18	(19)	23	25	27	30	35
7	(53)	60	63	65	67	70	19	(18)	21	23	25	28	31
8	(49)	54	57	59	62	65	20	(16)	20	22	24	26	30
9	(45)	50	53	55	58	61	22	(13)	16.5	18.0	20	22	26
10	(41)	46	50	53	55	58	24	(11)	13.5	16.5	17.5	19.5	23

Field size - Feldgröße - Champ - Campo: cm^2

Co 60

80 cm SSD - QHA - DSP - DFP

(0)-20-50-100-200-400 cm^2 Field size - Feld - Champ - Campo

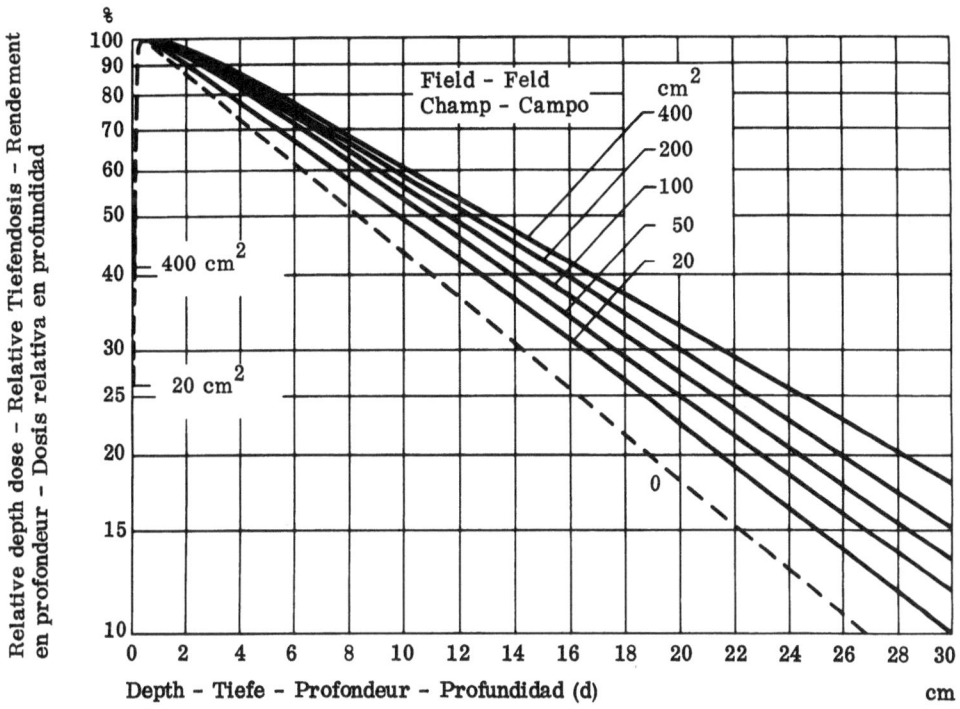

Relative depth dose - Relative Tiefendosis - Rendement en profondeur - Dosis relativa en profundidad

Depth - Tiefe - Profondeur - Profundidad (d)

Field size - Feldgröße - Champ - Campo: cm^2											
d cm	0	20	50	100	200	400	d cm	0	20	50	100	200	400
0	–	(26)	(28)	(31)	(36)	(41)	11	40	45	50	53	55	57
0.5	100	100	100	100	100	100	12	37	43	45	49	52	54
1	95	97	97	98	98	99	13	33	40	43	45	47	50
2	87	90	92	94	96	97	14	31	37	40	42	45	47
3	80	84	88	90	91	92	15	28	34	37	40	43	45
4	73	78	82	84	86	87	16	26	32	34	37	40	43
5	67	72	77	79	81	83	17	24	28	32	34	37	40
6	62	67	72	74	76	77	18	22	27	29	32	35	37
7	57	63	67	70	72	73	19	20	25	28	30	33	36
8	52	58	63	65	67	68	20	18.0	23	25	28	30	34
9	47	54	58	61	63	64	22	15.0	19.0	22	24	27	29
10	43	50	53	56	59	61	24	13.0	16.0	18.5	21	23	26

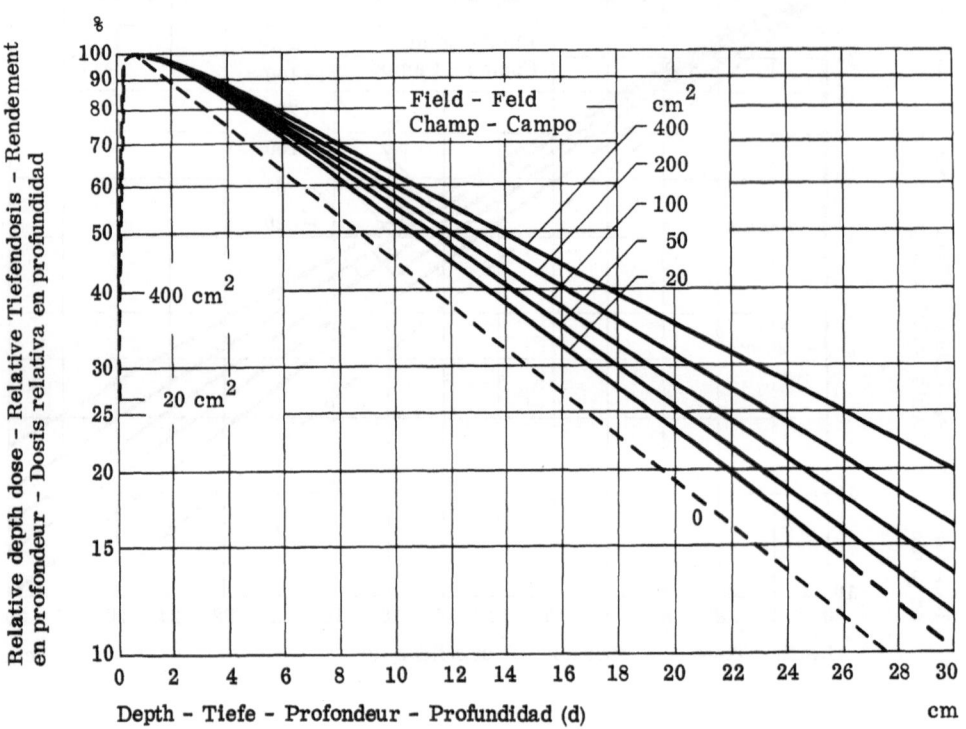

Co 60

100 cm SSD - QHA - DSP - DFP

(O)-20-50-100-200-400 cm^2 Field size - Feld - Champ - Campo

Relative depth dose – Relative Tiefendosis – Rendement en profondeur – Dosis relativa en profundidad

Depth - Tiefe - Profondeur - Profundidad (d)

cm

Field size - Feldgröße - Champ - Campo: cm^2												
d cm	0	20	50	100	200	400	d cm	0	20	50	100	200	400
0	–	(25)	(28)	(31)	(36)	(40)	11	42	49	52	55	58	60
0.5	100	100	100	100	100	100	12	37	45	48	50	53	56
1	97	98	98	99	99	100	13	35	41	44	47	50	53
2	89	95	96	97	98	98	14	32	38	42	44	47	50
3	82	90	91	92	92	93	15	29	35	38	40	43	47
4	75	83	85	86	87	88	16	27	32	35	37	40	44
5	69	77	79	81	83	84	17	25	30	32	35	38	42
6	63	71	73	75	77	78	18	23	28	30	32	35	40
7	58	67	70	72	74	74	19	21	25	27	30	33	37
8	53	62	64	66	68	70	20	19.0	24	25	27	31	35
9	49	57	60	62	65	67	22	16.0	20	22	24	27	32
10	45	53	55	57	60	63	24	13.5	17.0	18.5	21	24	28

4.5.3 Tissue-air ratio for γ teletherapy units
       Gewebe/Luft-Verhältnis für γ-Fernbestrahlungsapparaturen
       Rapport tissu - air pour des appareils de télégamma-thérapie
       Relación tejido/aire para aparatos tele-γ

4.5.3.1 Cs 137

$0 - 400 \text{ cm}^2$ Field size - Feldgröße - Champ - Campo

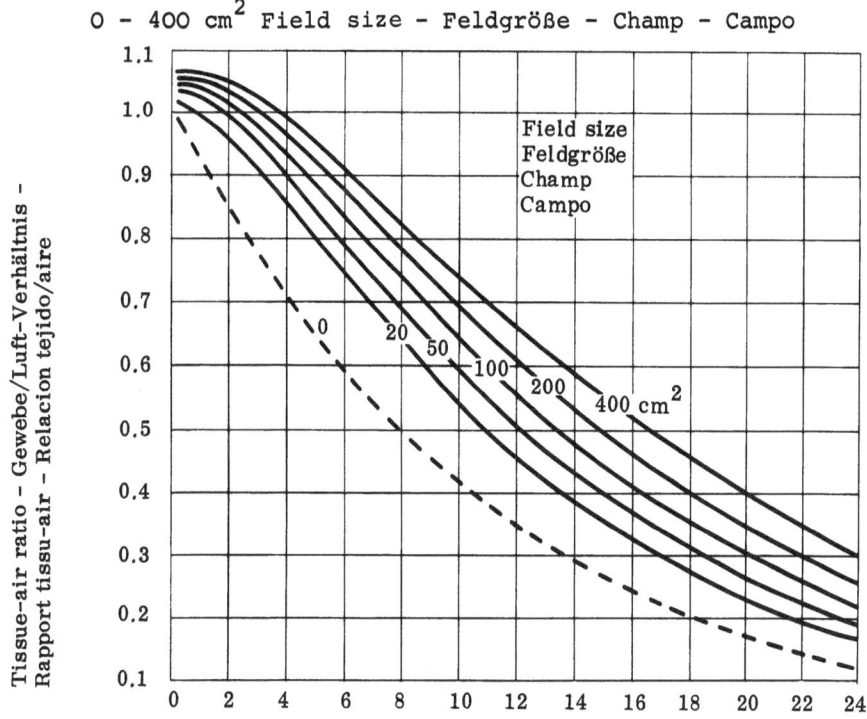

Depth - Tiefe - Profondeur - Profundidad

Depth Tiefe Profondeur Profundidad cm	Tissue-air ratio - Gewebe/Luft-Verhältnis - Rapport tissu-air - Relación tejido/aire					
	Field size - Feldgröße - Champ - Campo					cm^2
	0	20	50	100	200	400
0.2	1.00	1.02	1.04	1.05	1.06	1.07
1	0.93	1.00	1.02	1.04	1.05	1.06
2	0.85	0.96	0.99	1.02	1.04	1.05
3	0.78	0.91	0.95	0.98	1.00	1.03
4	0.72	0.86	0.90	0.93	0.97	0.99
5	0.65	0.80	0.85	0.89	0.92	0.95
6	0.59	0.75	0.79	0.84	0.88	0.91
7	0.55	0.70	0.74	0.79	0.83	0.87
8	0.50	0.64	0.69	0.74	0.78	0.83
9	0.46	0.59	0.64	0.69	0.74	0.78
10	0.42	0.54	0.59	0.65	0.69	0.74
12	0.35	0.46	0.51	0.56	0.61	0.66
14	0.29	0.39	0.44	0.48	0.54	0.59
16	0.25	0.33	0.37	0.41	0.47	0.52
18	0.21	0.27	0.32	0.36	0.41	0.46
20	0.17	0.23	0.27	0.30	0.35	0.40
22	0.14	0.19	0.23	0.26	0.30	0.35
24	0.12	0.16	0.18	0.22	0.26	0.30

4.5.3.2   Co 60

0 - 400 cm^2 Field size - Feldgröße - Champ - Campo

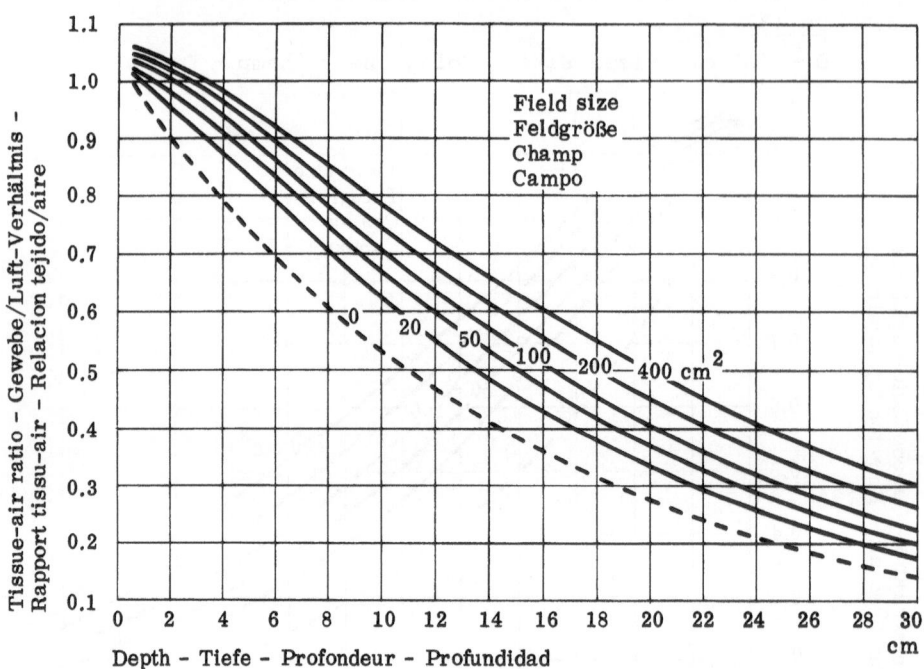

Depth - Tiefe - Profondeur - Profundidad

Depth Tiefe Profondeur Profundidad cm	Tissue-air ratio - Gewebe/Luft-Verhältnis - Rapport tissu-air - Relación tejido/aire					
	Field size - Feldgröße - Champ - Campo					cm^2
	0	20	50	100	200	400
0.5	1.00	1.02	1.03	1.04	1.05	1.06
2	0.91	0.96	0.98	1.00	1.02	1.03
4	0.79	0.86	0.91	0.94	0.96	0.98
6	0.69	0.79	0.83	0.86	0.89	0.92
8	0.61	0.71	0.75	0.78	0.82	0.85
10	0.54	0.62	0.67	0.71	0.75	0.78
12	0.47	0.55	0.60	0.64	0.68	0.72
14	0.42	0.48	0.53	0.57	0.62	0.66
16	0.36	0.43	0.48	0.51	0.56	0.60
18	0.32	0.38	0.42	0.46	0.50	0.55
20	0.28	0.34	0.38	0.41	0.45	0.60
22	0.24	0.30	0.33	0.37	0.41	0.46
24	0.21	0.26	0.29	0.33	0.37	0.41
26	0.18	0.23	0.26	0.29	0.33	0.37
28	0.16	0.20	0.23	0.26	0.29	0.34
30	0.14	0.18	0.20	0.22	0.26	0.31

Lit.: 1. COHEN, M., JONES, D.E.A., GREENE, D.: Central Axis Depth
          Dose Data for Use in Radiotherapy, Brit.J.Radiol., Suppl. 11
          (1972)

4.6   Dose distributions obtainable with rotational irradiation
Mit Rotationsbestrahlung erreichbare Dosisverteilungen
Distributions de doses obtenues en cyclothérapie
Distribución de la dosis asequible mediante radiación rotatoria

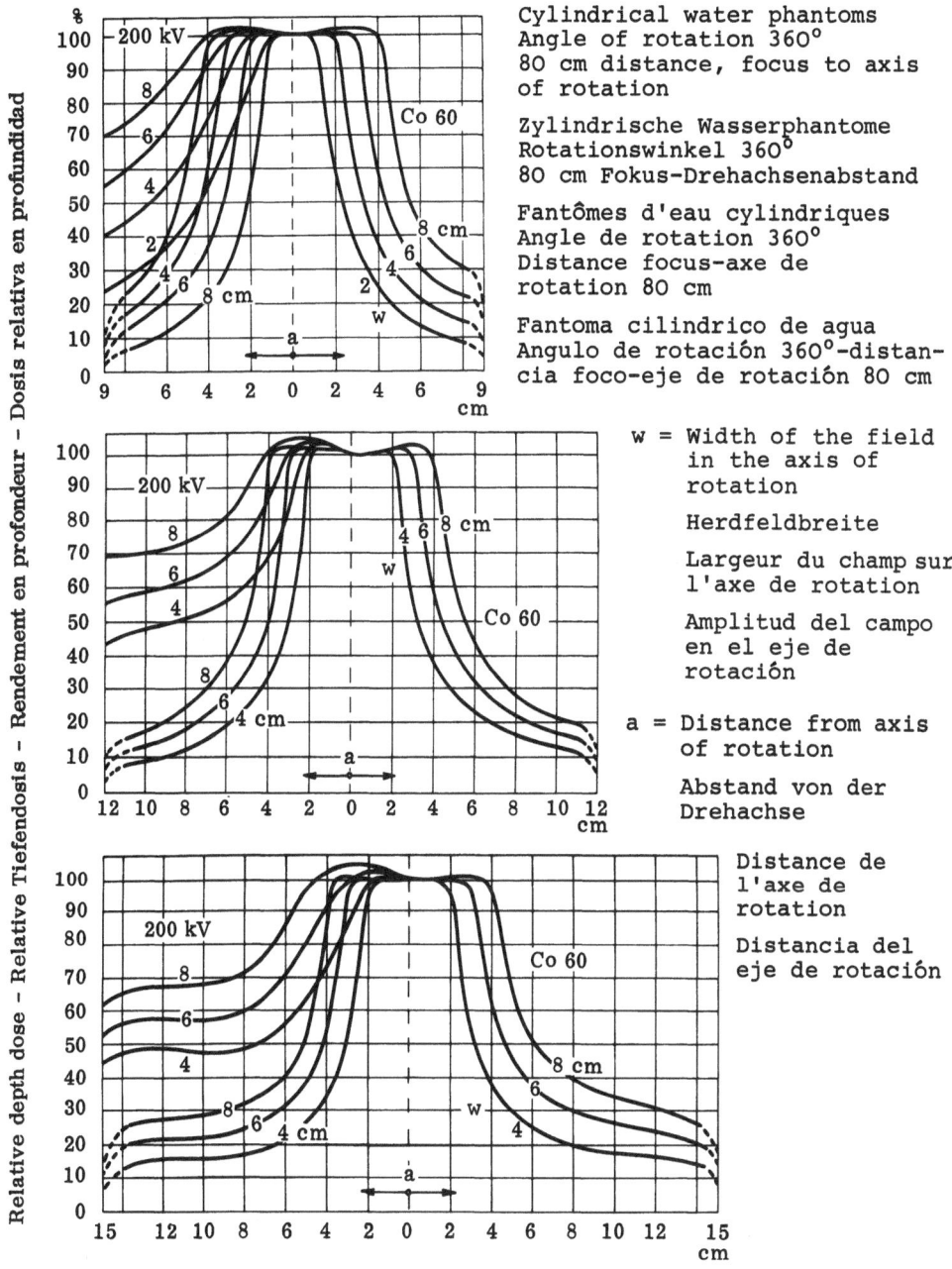

Cylindrical water phantoms
Angle of rotation 360°
80 cm distance, focus to axis
of rotation

Zylindrische Wasserphantome
Rotationswinkel 360°
80 cm Fokus-Drehachsenabstand

Fantômes d'eau cylindriques
Angle de rotation 360°
Distance focus-axe de
rotation 80 cm

Fantoma cilindrico de agua
Angulo de rotación 360°-distan-
cia foco-eje de rotación 80 cm

w = Width of the field
    in the axis of
    rotation

Herdfeldbreite

Largeur du champ sur
l'axe de rotation

Amplitud del campo
en el eje de
rotación

a = Distance from axis
    of rotation

Abstand von der
Drehachse

Distance de
l'axe de
rotation

Distancia del
eje de rotación

Lit.: 1. WACHSMANN, F., BARTH, G.: Bewegungsbestrahlung, Stuttgart:
          Thieme 1953
      2. WACHSMANN, F., BARTH, G., LANZL, L.H., CARPENDER, W.J.:
          Moving Field Therapy, University of Chicago Press 1962

125

Percentage depth doses with supervoltage X-rays
Relative Tiefendosen sehr harter Röntgenstrahlen
Rendements en profondeur, rayonnements de haute énergie
Dosis relativas en profundidad para radiaciones muy duras

1 - 2 - 5 - 10 MV

100 cm FSD - FHA - DFP - DFP

25 - 100 - 225 cm^2 Field size - Feld - Champ - Campo

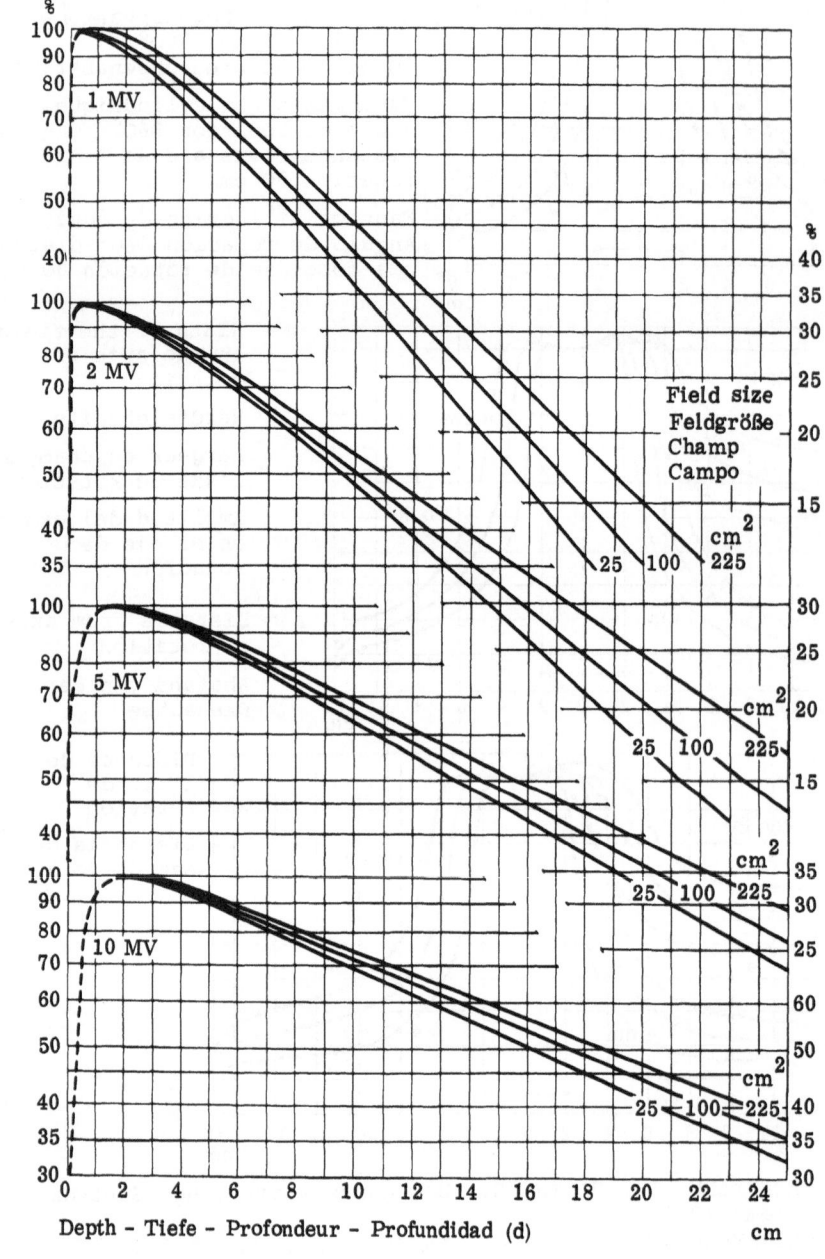

Relative depth dose – Relative Tiefendosis – Rendement en profondeur – Dosis relativa en profundidad

Depth - Tiefe - Profondeur - Profundidad (d)   cm

d cm	Relative depth dose - Relative Tiefendosis - Rendement en profondeur - Dosis relativa en profundidad %						
	Field size - Feld - Champ - Campo cm²						
	25	100	225		25	100	225
	1 MV				2 MV		
0	(45)	(55)	(70)		(29)	(39)	(55)
0.5	99	100	100		99	100	100
1	97	98	99		98	99	99
2	90	93	97		94	94	95
3	81	85	90		88	89	91
4	73	78	83		81	83	85
5	65	71	76		74	76	79
6	59	64	70		69	71	73
7	52	57	62		63	65	68
8	47	52	57		57	60	62
9	41	45	49		52	55	58
10	36	40	45		48	50	53
11	32	36	41		43	46	49
12	27	32	37		39	42	46
13	24	28	33		36	39	42
14	21	25	29		32	36	39
15	18.0	22	26		28	32	37
16	15.5	19.0	23		26	29	34
17	13.5	17.0	21		23	27	31
18	12.0	15.0	18.5		21	24	29
(19)	10.5	13.0	17.0		19.0	22	26
20	9.0	12.0	15.0		17.0	20	24
22	-	9.0	12.0		14.0	17.0	21
24	-	-	9.0		12.5	14.5	19.5
	5 MV				10 MV		
0	(20)	(28)	(35)		(16)	(22)	(27)
0.5	(78)	(80)	(84)		(67)	(75)	(78)
1	(97)	(98)	(99)		(90)	(92)	(94)
1.5	100	100	100		(96)	(97)	(98)
2	98	99	99		99	99	99
2.5	97	98	99		100	100	100
3	95	97	98		98	99	99
4	90	92	94		93	95	97
5	86	88	91		89	91	93
6	81	83	86		85	87	89
7	76	78	81		80	82	84
8	72	74	77		77	79	81
9	67	70	73		72	75	77
10	63	66	69		69	71	73
11	58	62	64		65	68	71
12	54	57	61		62	65	68
13	51	54	57		58	62	64
14	48	51	54		55	59	62
15	45	48	52		53	56	59
16	42	45	48		51	53	56
17	39	42	46		48	51	54
18	37	40	43		46	49	52
19	35	38	41		43	46	49

Lit.: 1. WEBSTER, E.W., TSIEN, K.C.: IAEA Atlas of Radiation Dose Distributions, Vol. I, Vienna 1965
2. COHEN, M., JONES, D.E.A., GREENE, D.: Brit.J.Radiol., Suppl. 11 (1972)

4.8.1 <u>Percentage depth doses for very high energy X-rays</u>
<u>Relative Tiefendosen ultraharter Röntgenstrahlen</u>
<u>Rendements en profondeur, rayonnements X de très haute energie</u>
<u>Dosis relativas en profundidad para radiaciones X ultraduras</u>

15 - 20 - 30 - 50 - 100 MV

50 - 75 - 100 cm FSD - FHA - DFP - DFP

(15-) 100 (-400) cm^2 Field size - Feldgröße - Champ - Campo

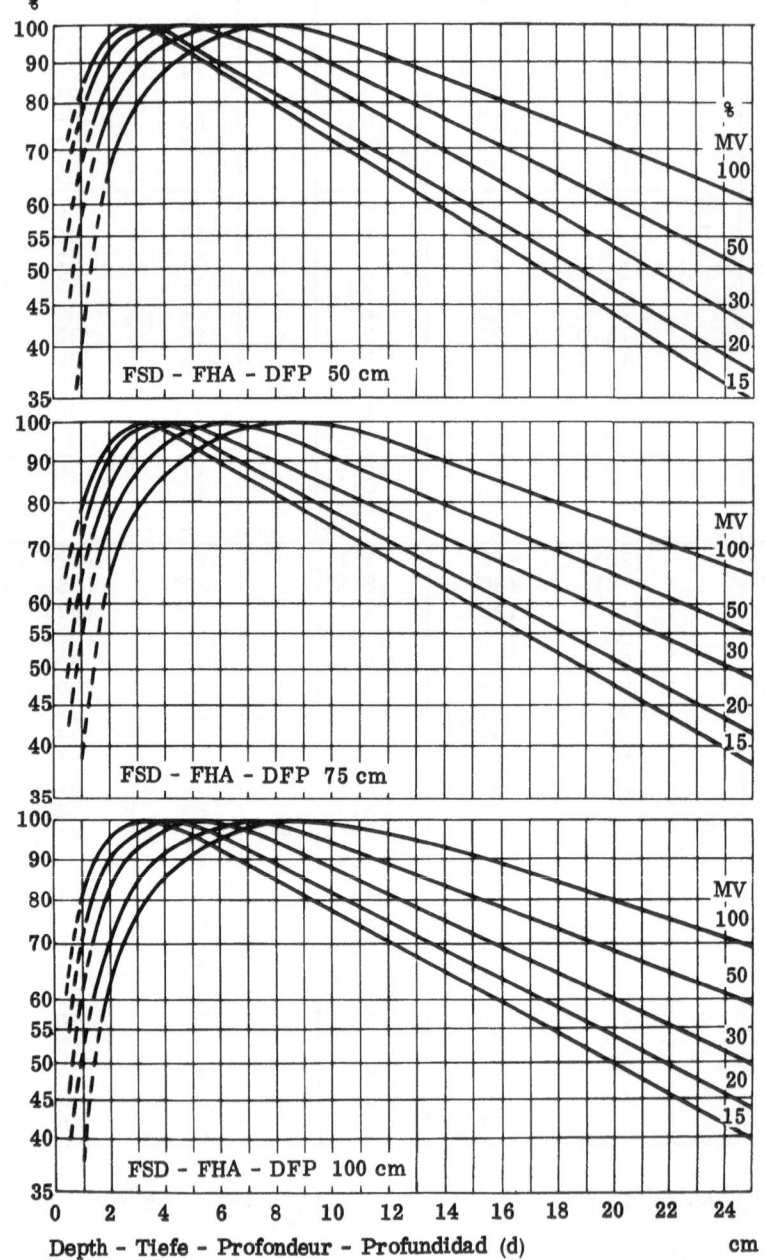

Depth - Tiefe - Profondeur - Profundidad (d)   cm

Relative depth dose - Relative Tiefendosis - Rendement en profondeur - Dosis relativa en profundidad

Relative depth dose - Relative Tiefendosis - Rendement en profondeur - Dosis relativa en profundidad %

Quality - Qualität - Qualité - Calidad — MV

FSD - FHA - DFP 50 cm (left group) and FSD - FHA - DFP 75 cm (right group)

d (cm)	15	20	30	50	100	15	20	30	50	100
0	(20)	(16)	(15)	(13)	(10)	(20)	(16)	(15)	(13)	(10)
0.5	(66)	(63)	(55)	(42)	(21)	(66)	(61)	(53)	(41)	(20)
1	(82)	(76)	(67)	(57)	40	78	(72)	(63)	(55)	(38)
1.5	90	85	75	(64)	(50)	88	82	74	(67)	(51)
2	97	93	85	77	65	94	90	82	75	64
2.5	99	97	90	83	72	97	95	90	81	72
3	100	98	94	88	78	100	98	94	87	78
3.5	98	100	98	92	84	99	99	97	91	87
4	97	99	99	94	88	98	100	99	94	86
4.5	94	97	100	97	91	96	98	100	96	89
5	92	94	100	98	92	93	97	99	98	92
6	88	90	98	100	97	90	92	97	100	97
7	84	86	95	99	99	85	89	92	98	98
8	80	82	92	97	100	82	86	90	97	100
9	76	78	88	93	99	78	82	87	94	100
10	72	75	84	90	97	75	78	84	91	99
11	68	72	80	87	95	72	75	80	88	98
12	65	68	76	83	92	68	72	78	85	95
13	62	65	73	80	88	65	68	85	87	92
14	59	62	70	77	86	63	66	72	80	90
15	56	59	67	74	83	60	63	70	77	88
16	53	57	64	70	80	57	61	67	74	85
17	51	54	61	68	78	55	58	65	72	82
18	48	52	58	65	75	52	56	63	69	80
19	46	49	56	63	73	50	53	61	67	78
20	44	47	53	60	72	48	52	58	75	85
21	42	45	51	58	68	46	49	57	63	74
22	40	43	48	56	67	43	47	54	61	71
23	38	41	46	58	65	42	45	52	59	68
24	37	39	44	52	63	40	43	51	57	67
25	35	37	42	50	60	38	42	48	55	65

Quality - Qualität - / Qualité - Calidad — MV

FSD - FHA - DFP 100 cm

d (cm)	15	20	30	50	100	d (cm)	15	20	30	50	100
0	(20)	(16)	(15)	(13)	(10)	11	74	78	94	92	98
0.5	(65)	(60)	(52)	(40)	(20)	12	71	75	82	89	96
1	81	(71)	(62)	(53)	(38)	13	68	73	78	86	95
1.5	90	80	71	60	(50)	14	65	69	75	83	93
2	95	90	82	70	62	15	62	66	72	81	91
2.5	98	93	88	76	69	16	60	64	69	78	89
3	99	97	92	84	76	17	57	62	67	76	87
3.5	100	98	95	88	81	18	54	58	65	73	84
4	98	100	97	92	85	19	52	56	62	71	82
4.5	97	99	99	94	88	20	50	54	60	79	80
5	96	98	100	96	91	21	47	52	58	67	77
6	92	95	99	98	95	22	46	50	55	65	75
7	89	92	97	100	98	23	44	48	53	63	73
8	85	89	95	99	100	24	42	46	52	61	71
9	81	85	91	97	100	25	40	43	49	59	69
10	78	82	88	94	99						

See page - Siehe Seite - Voir page - Ver página 126

4.8.2 <u>Angular distribution of megavoltage X-rays</u>
<u>Winkelverteilung ultraharter Röntgenstrahlen</u>
<u>Distribution angulaire des rayons X de très haute énergie</u>
<u>Reparto angular de radiaciones ultraduras</u>

Average values - Richtwerte - Valeurs moyennes -
Valores aproximados

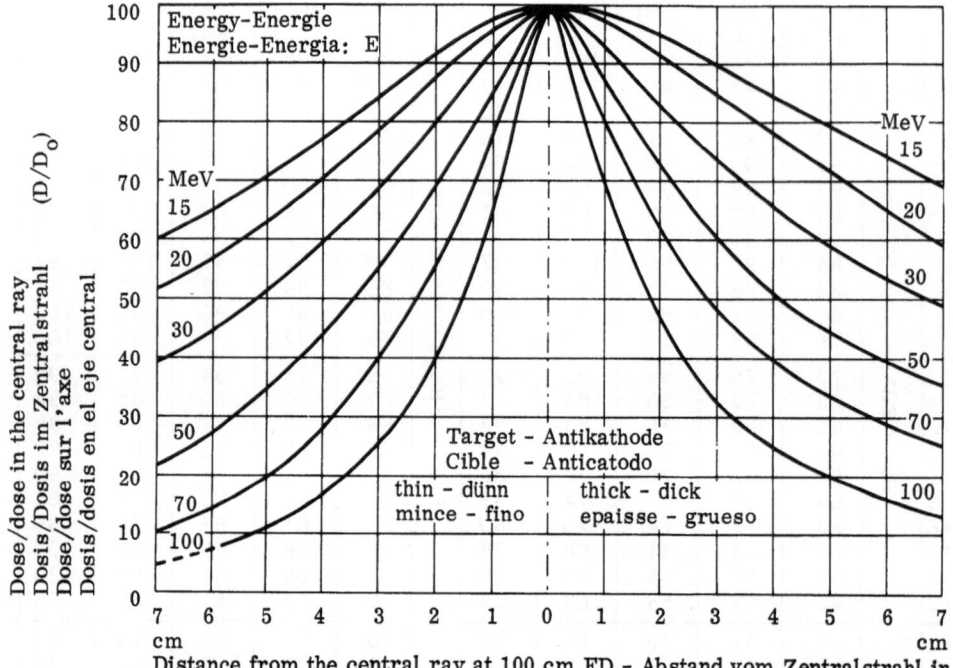

Distance from the central ray at 100 cm FD - Abstand vom Zentralstrahl in
100 cm FA - Distance à l'axe à DF 100 cm - Distancia del rayo central en
100 cm DF = d

d	D/Do % Target - Antikathode - Cible - Anticátodo											
	Thin – Dünn – Mince – Fino E MeV						Thick-Dick-Épaisse-Grueso E MeV					
cm	15	20	30	50	70	100	15	20	30	50	70	100
0	100	100	100	100	100	100	100	100	100	100	100	100
0.5	99	98	97	94	90	83	100	99	97	95	92	85
1	98	96	92	85	78	65	99	97	93	87	80	70
1.5	95	94	87	77	65	51	97	95	87	80	71	57
2	92	88	80	69	55	40	95	92	83	73	61	47
2.5	88	83	74	62	47	32	93	88	78	66	54	39
3	84	79	69	56	40	25	90	85	74	60	49	33
4	77	74	60	44	28	17	85	78	65	51	40	25
5	71	63	52	35	20	11	80	72	59	45	34	20
6	65	57	45	27	14	(7)	75	65	53	40	29	16
7	60	51	39	21	10	(5)	69	60	49	35	25	13

Lit.: 1. CHARLTON, E.K., BREED, H.E.: Am.J.Roentgenol. <u>60</u>, 158 (1948)
      2. GUND, K., SCHITTENHELM, R.: Strahlenther. <u>92</u>, 506 (1953)

4.8.3　Approximate relative depth dose of X- and γ-rays at a depth of O and O.5 cm, and depth of the dose maximum (summary)

Ungefähre rel. Tiefendosen von Röntgen- und γ-Strahlen in O und O,5 cm und Tiefenlage des Dosismaximums (Zusammenfassung)

Dose approximative de rayons X et γ à une profondeur de O et O,5 cm et profondeur de la dose maximale (résumé)

Dosis rel.en profundidad aproximada de rayos X y γ a profundidades de O y O,5 cm y profundidad de la dosis máxima (resumen)

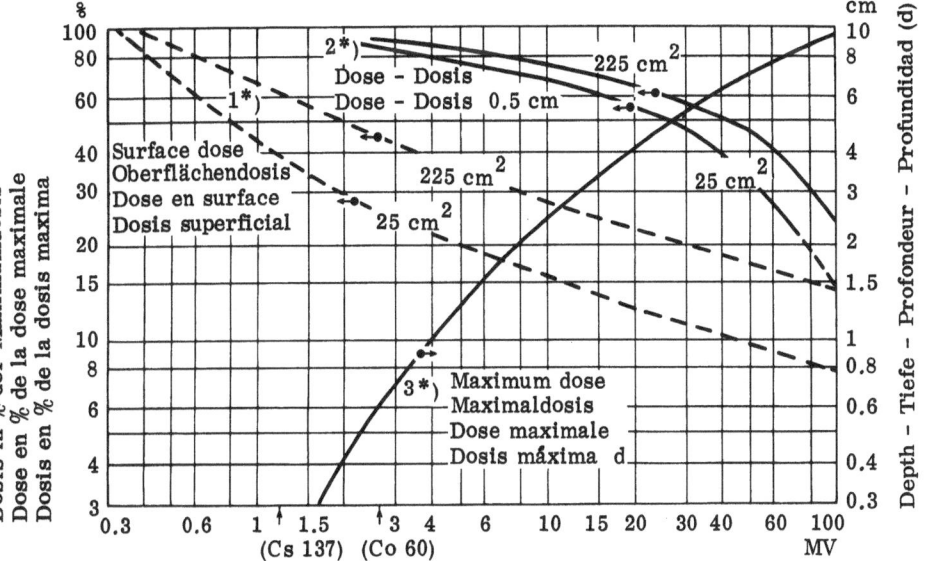

Energy - Energie - Energie - Energía

Energy Energie Energie Energía	1. Surface dose *) Oberfl. Dosis Dose en surface Dosis superficial		2. Dose at *) Dosis in Dose à Dosis en: 0.5 cm		3. Dose max. *) Max. Dosis Dose max. Dosis max.
MV	25 cm^2	% 225 cm^2	25 cm^2	% 225 cm^2	d cm
0.3	100	100	–	–	($\sim$O)
0.5	(70)	(92)	–	–	($\sim$O)
1.O	(44)	(65)	–	–	(O.1)
Cs 137	(39)	(61)	–	–	(0.17)
1.5	(34)	(55)	–	–	0.26
Co 60	(26)	(45)	87	90	0.60
5	(20)	(38)	77	84	1.35
10	(16)	(29)	68	77	2.5
20	(13)	(23)	58	67	4.1
30	(12)	(20)	47	58	5.5
50	(8)	(17)	32	47	7.O
100	(7)	(15)	24	(15)	9.5

Lit.: See pages - Siehe Seiten - Voir pages - Ver páginas 118-129
*) See graph - Siehe Abbildung - Voir image - Ver gráfica

4.9 <u>Relative depth doses of high-energy-electrons</u>
<u>Relative Tiefendosen schneller Elektronen</u>
<u>Rendements en profondeur pour des électrons accélérés</u>
<u>Dosis relativas para electrones de alta energía</u>

4.9.1 <u>1 - 10 MeV Energy - Energie - Énergie - Energía</u>

(40) - 60 - (80) cm SSD - QHA - DSP - DFP

(10) - 50 - (100) cm^2 Field - Feld - Champ - Campo

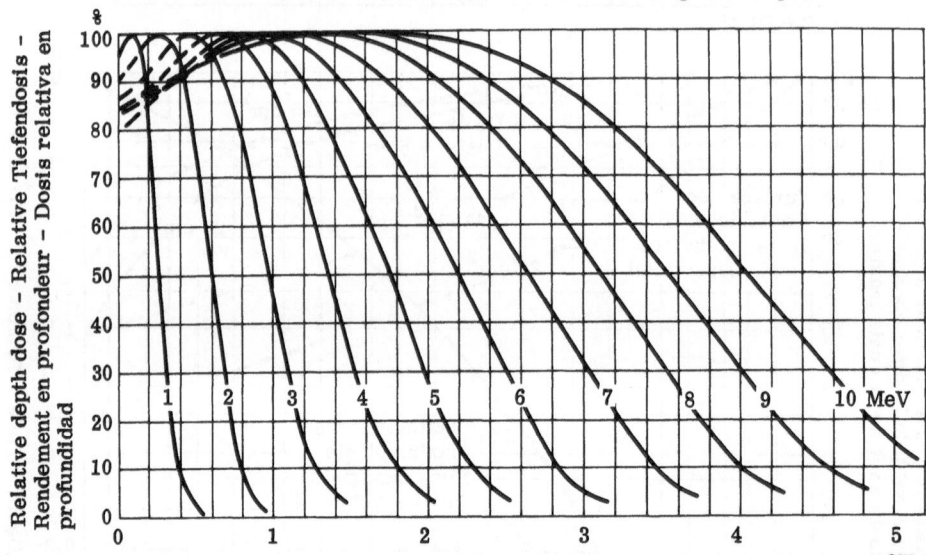

Depth - Tiefe - Profondeur - Profundidad (d)

d	Depth doses as % of the maximum dose - Tiefendosis in % der Maximaldosis - Rendement en profondeur en % de la dose maximum Dosis en profundidad en % de la dosis máxima									
	Energy - Energie - Énergie - Energía:									MeV
cm	1	2	3	4	5	6	7	8	9	10
O	(96)	(90)	(87)	(83)	(80)	(82)	(83)	(84)	(85)	(86)
0.1	100	(95)	(83)	(87)	(82)	(84)	(84)	(85)	(86)	(87)
0.2	83	(98)	(91)	(88)	(86)	(86)	(86)	(87)	(89)	(90)
0.3	34	100	(96)	(91)	(88)	(89)	(88)	(89)	(91)	(91)
0.4	8	94	(99)	(94)	(92)	(91)	(90)	(92)	(94)	(93)
0.6	(1)	50	97	(99)	(98)	(94)	(93)	(96)	(95)	(94)
0.8	–	10	80	98	100	(99)	(98)	(99)	(96)	(96)
1.0	–	(1)	47	89	98	100	100	100	(98)	(97)
1.2	–	–	17	69	94	98	100	100	(99)	(98)
1.4	–	–	4.5	4.5	82	92	98	100	100	(99)
1.6	–	–	(2)	22	66	84	94	98	100	100
1.8	–	–	–	10	46	74	88	96	99	100
2.0	–	–	–	4	26	62	81	92	96	99
2.5	–	–	–	(2)	4	30	58	76	87	93
3.0	–	–	–	–	(2)	4	32	55	72	80
3.5	–	–	–	–	–	(2)	9	31	51	68
4.0	–	–	–	–	–	–	(3)	10	30	48
5.0	–	–	–	–	–	–	–	–	(4)	12

4.9.2 10 - 100 MeV Energy - Energie - Energie - Energía

(40) - 60 - (100) cm SSD - QHA - DSP - DFP

(15) - 100 - (200) cm^2 Field area - Feld - Champ - Campo

Relative depth dose - Relative Tiefendosis
Rendement en profondeur - Dosis relativa
en profundidad

Depth - Tiefe - Profondeur - Profundidad (d)

d	Depth doses as % of the maximum dose - Tiefendosis in % der Maximaldosis - Rendement en profondeur en % de la dose maximum - Dosis en profundidad en % de la dosis máxima									
	Energy - Energie - Énergie - Energía									MeV
cm	10	15	20	25	30	40	50	60	70	100
0	(86)	(87)	(88)	(88)	(88)	(89)	(88)	(88)	(87)	(85)
1	(97)	(96)	(95)	(94)	(93)	(93)	(92)	(91)	(90)	(88)
2	99	100	100	(99)	(99)	(97)	(96)	(95)	(94)	(92)
3	80	97	99	100	100	(98)	(98)	(98)	(96)	(94)
4	48	88	97	99	100	(99)	(99)	(99)	(98)	(96)
5	12	70	90	96	97	100	100	100	99	(99)
6	2	50	79	88	94	98	99	100	100	(100)
7	-	28	63	78	88	95	99	98	99	(100)
8	-	7	44	68	81	91	96	97	97	(99)
9	-	3	26	55	72	85	93	94	96	(99)
10	-	-	9	40	61	78	88	92	94	(98)
12	-	-	3	12	39	64	77	83	87	(96)
14	-	-	-	4	17	50	66	74	81	(90)
16	-	-	-	6	5	34	54	64	73	(84)
18	-	-	-	-	-	18	42	53	63	(78)
20	-	-	-	-	-	7	29	42	53	(72)
22	-	-	-	-	-	-	18	31	42	(64)
24	-	-	-	-	-	-	10	21	32	(57)
26	-	-	-	-	-	-	8	13	22	(52)

Lit.: 1. GUND, K., WACHSMANN, F.: Strahlenther. 7, 573 (1948)
2. LAUGHLIN, J.S. et al.: Radiology 60, 165 (1953)
3. WEBSTER, E.W., TSIEN, K.C.: Atlas of Radiation Dose Distributions, IAEA, Vienna 1965
4. COHEN, M., JONES, D.E.A., GREENE, D.: Brit.J.Radiol., Suppl. 11 (1972)

4.10 Relative depth doses for heavy particles
Relative Tiefendosen schwerer Teilchen
Rendements en profondeur pour des particules lourdes
Dosis relativas en profundidad de particulas pesadas

4.10.1 Neutrons - Neutronen - Neutrons - Neutrones

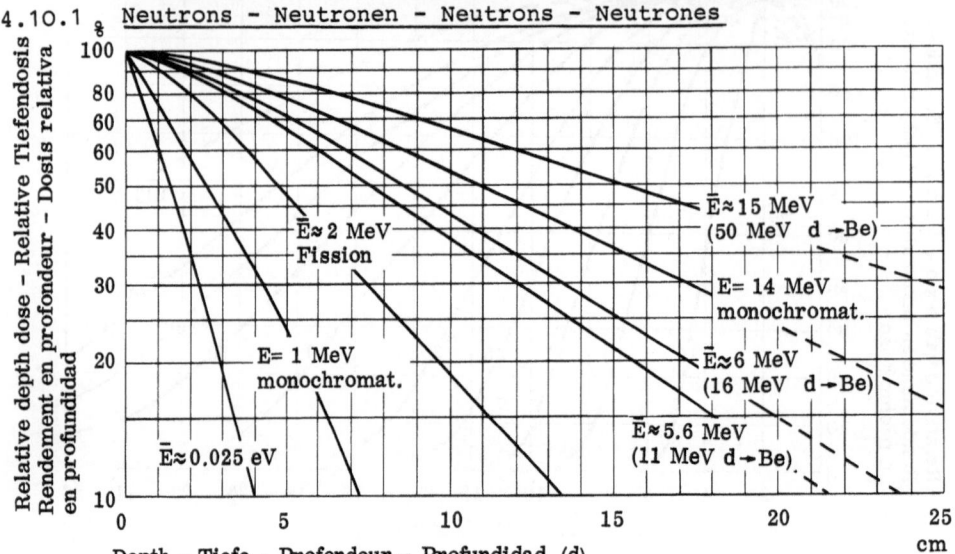

Depth - Tiefe - Profondeur - Profundidad (d)

d	Relative depth dose - Relative Tiefendosis - Rendement en profondeur - Dosis relativas en profundidad						
	Energy - Energie - Energie - Energía						
cm	$\overline{E}\approx$ 0.025 eV	E= 1 MeV	$\overline{E}\approx$ 2 MeV	$\overline{E}\approx$ 5.6 MeV	$\overline{E}\approx$ 6 MeV	E= 14 MeV	$\overline{E}\approx$ 15 MeV
0.5	76	87	97	98	98	99	100
1	60	76	91	94	96	98	99
1.5	45	66	86	92	94	96	98
2	30	57	80	88	90	94	97
3	19	43	68	81	83	88	93
4	10	32	57	73	77	83	89
5	-	24	47	66	71	78	85
6	-	16	40	60	65	73	82
7	-	11	33	53	59	67	78
8	-	-	27	48	53	63	74
10	-	-	18	38	43	53	66
12	-	-	13	30	35	46	60
14	-	-	-	24	28	39	54
16	-	-	-	19	23	33	48
18	-	-	-	15	18	28	43
20	-	-	-	(12)	(15)	(23)	(38)
22	-	-	-	-	(12)	(20)	(35)
24	-	-	-	-	-	(17)	(30)

Lit.: 1. BEWLEY, D.K.: Current Topics in Rad.Res., Amsterdam: North-Holland Publ.Co. (1970)
2. SNYDER, W.S.: NCRP Report No. 38, Washington (1971)
3. BROERSE, J.J. et al. in: Proc. First Symp. on Neutron Dosimetry, München (1972) (EUR 4896 dfe)
4. Brit.J.Radiol., Suppl. 11 (1972)

4.10.2 Protons, α-particles and mesons
        Protonen, α-Teilchen und Mesonen
        Protons, particules α et mésons
        Protones, particulas α y mesones

   1. 140 MeV Protons - Protonen - Protons - Protones
      1 - (12) cm Ø Field size - Feld - Champ - Campo 3)

   2. 570-605 MeV α-Particles-Teilchen-Particules-Particulas
      1- (2) cm Ø Field size - Feld - Champ - Campo 4)

   3. 84 MeV π- Mesons - Mesonen - Mésons - Mesones
      1- (2) cm Ø Field size - Feld - Champ - Campo 2)

   4. 58 - 77 MeV π- Mesons - Mesonen - Mésons - Mesones
      (1) - 5 cm Ø Field size - Feld - Champ - Campo 5)

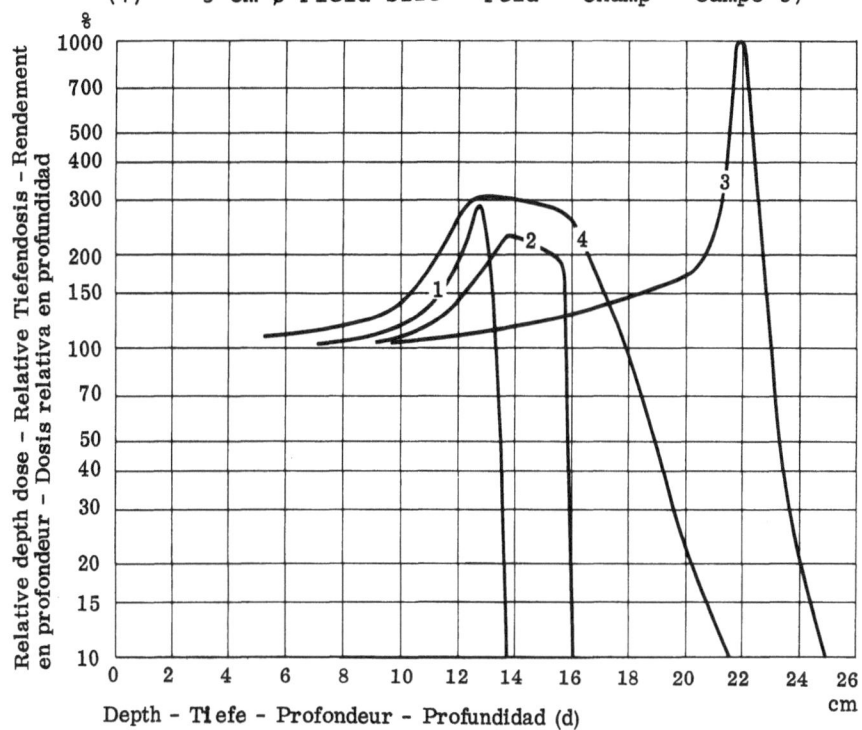

Depth - Tiefe - Profondeur - Profundidad (d)

Note - Bemerkung - Remarque - Nota:

The "biologic depth dose curves" have a different shape because the RBE of these radiations changes considerably with depth.

Die "biologischen Tiefendosiskurven" haben der sich mit der Tiefe stark ändernden RBW dieser Strahlungen wegen einen anderen Verlauf.

Les "courbes d'effet biologique en profondeur" ont une forme très différente car l'EBR de ces particules varie beaucoup en profondeur.

Las "curvas de dosis profundas biológicas" son distintas porque la EBR varia considerablemente con la profundidad.

Lit.: 1. CURTIS, S.C., RAJU, M.R.: Rad.Res. 34, 239 (1968)
      2. ALSMILLER, R.G. et al.: Nucl.Sci.Eng. 43, 257 (1971)
      3. KOEHLER, A.M., PRESTON, W.M.: Rad.Phys. 104, 191 (1972)
      4. ALSMILLER, R.G. et al.: ORNL-TM-4369 (1974)
      5. ARMSTRONG, T.W., CHANDLER, K.C.: Rad.Res. 58, 293 (1974)

4.11   Relative depth dose at different depths in tissue (water)
        Relative Tiefendosen in verschiedenen Gewebe-(Wasser-)Tiefen
        Rendements à différentes profondeurs de tissu (eau)
        Dosis relativas a diferentes profundidades de tejido (agua)

50 cm FSD - FHA - DFP - DFP

100 cm^2 Field size - Feldgröße - Champ - Campo

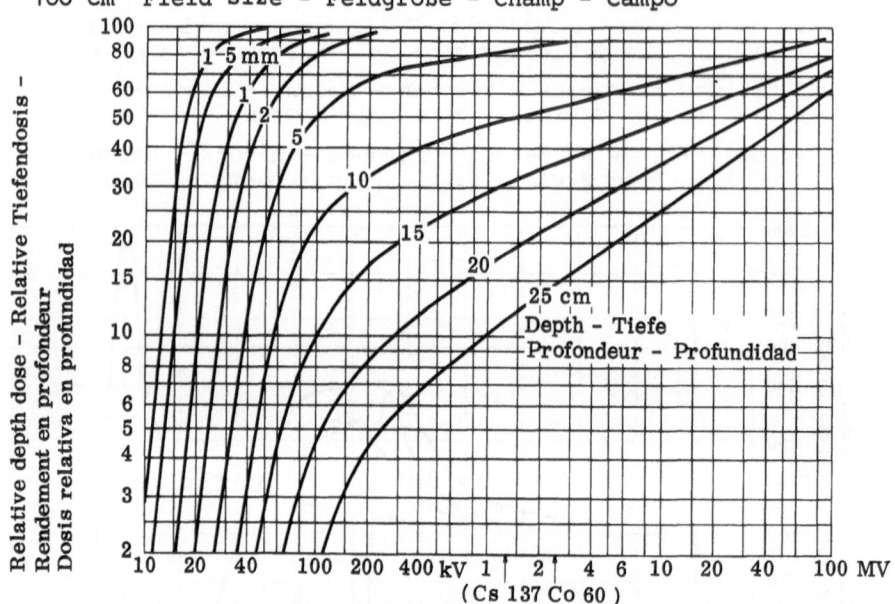

Tube voltage - Röhrenspannung - Tension d'alimentation - Voltaje del tubo

0,01 0,1   1   5 10 mm Al HVL-HWSD-CDA-CHR

0,3 1 2 4 6 8 10 mm Cu

Tube voltage Röhrenspannung Tension du tube Voltaje del tubo	Relative depth dose - Rel. Tiefendosis - Rendement en profondeur - Dosis relativa en profundidad %								
	Depth - Tiefe - Profondeur - Profundidad								
	1	5 mm	1	2	5	10	15	20	25 cm
10 kV	2.8	–	–	–	–	–	–	–	–
20 kV	70	44	10	–	–	–	–	–	–
30 kV	90	75	41	17	3.6	–	–	–	–
50 kV	99	91	76	53	23	7.5	2.8	–	–
100 kV	~100	(98)	92	81	51	23	11	4.5	–
200 kV	~100	~100	(99)	95	68	33	17	8.4	4.3
300 kV	~100	~100	~100	(98)	73	37	20	10	5.8
500 kV	~100	~100	~100	(99)	76	42	24	13	7.6
1 MV	~100	~100	~100	~100	83	49	29	16	10
2 MV	~100	~100	~100	~100	87	52	35	22	12
4 MV	~100	~100	~100	~100	(92)	58	40	27	17
10 MV	~100	~100	~100	~100	~100	67	48	36	25
20 MV	~100	~100	~100	~100	~100	74	57	44	33
50 MV	~100	~100	~100	~100	~100	83	70	59	48
100 MV	~100	~100	~100	~100	~100	90	80	73	62

Lit.: See pages - Siehe Seiten - Voir pages - Ver paginas 87 - 99,
      104 - 111, 118 - 122, 126 - 129

Table of contents - Inhaltsverzeichnis
Table des matières - Tabla de materias

137

5.1   <u>Back scatter of X- and gamma rays</u>
<u>Rückstreuung von Röntgen- und Gammastrahlung</u>
<u>Rétrodiffusion de rayons X et gamma</u>
<u>Retrodispersión de rayos X y gamma</u>

10 kV - Co 60

20 - 400 cm^2 Field size - Feld - Champ - Campo

5.1.1   <u>Quadratic or circular fields - Quadratische oder kreisrunde</u>
<u>Felder - Champs carrés ou circulaires - Campos cuadrados o</u>
<u>circulares</u>

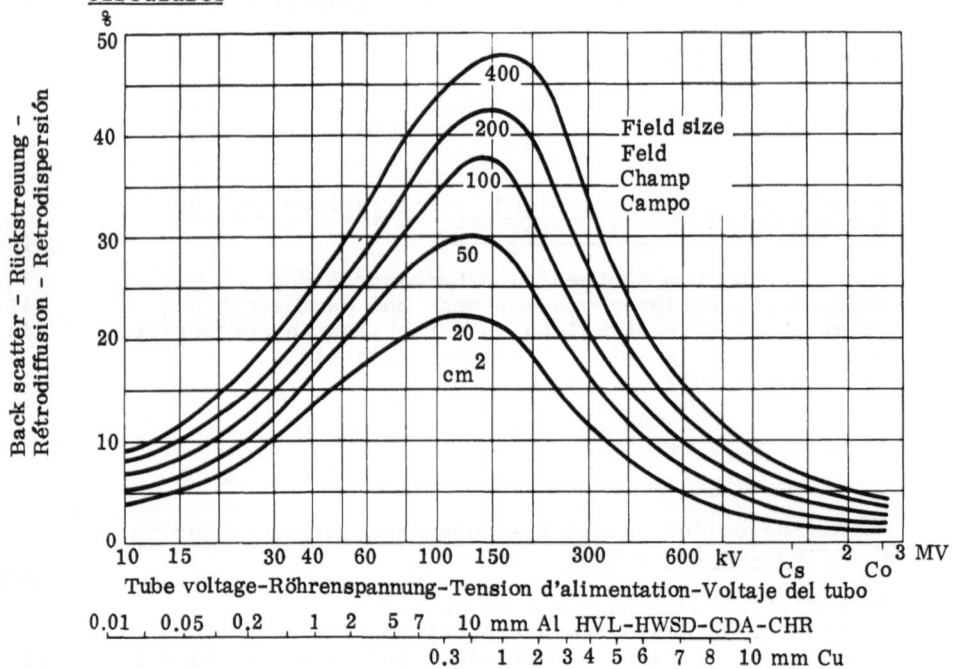

Radiation quality Strahlenqualität Qualité du rayonnement Calidad de la radiación		Back scatter - Rückstreuung - Rétrodiffusion - Retrodispersión % Field area - Feld - Champ - Campo cm^2				
kV-MV	HVL-HWSD-CDA-CHR	20	50	100	200	400
10 kV	0.013 mm Al	3.8	5.3	6.8	8.0	9.0
15 kV	0.045 " "	5.3	6.7	8.2	10.0	11.5
20 kV	0.10 " "	6.6	8.4	10.4	12.5	14.5
30 kV	0.35 " "	10.0	12.0	15.0	17.0	20
50 kV	1.7 " "	15.5	20	23	26	29
70 kV	4.0 " "	19.0	24	28	31	36
100 kV	8 mm Al 0.3 mm Cu	22	29	34	39	44
150 kV	0.8 mm Cu	22	29	37	42	48
200 kV	1.8 " "	18.0	25	32	40	46
300 kV	3.8 " "	11.5	16.0	20	26	34
400 kV	5.5 " "	8.0	11.5	15.0	18.0	24
600 kV	7.7 " "	5.0	7.0	9.5	12.5	15.5
1 MV	10 " "	2.2	4.0	5.8	7.4	9.3
Cs 137	–	1.7	2.9	4.4	5.9	7.2
2 MV	–	1.3	2.2	3.2	4.3	5.3
Co 60	–	1.2	1.8	2.6	3.5	4.3

5.1.2 Back scatter in the case of non-square fields
Rückstreuung bei nicht quadratischen Feldern
Rétrodiffusion par champs non-carrés
Retrodispersión con campos no cuadrados

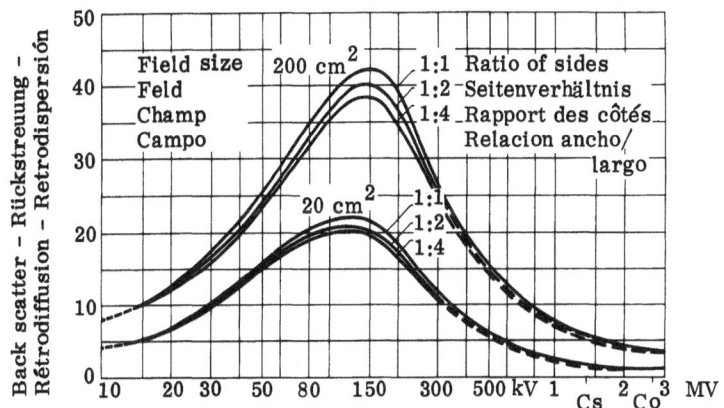

Tube voltage-Röhrenspannung-Tension d'alimentation-Voltaje del tubo

0.01 0.1 | 1 2 5 8 mm Al HVL-HWSD-CDA-CHR

0.3 1 2 3 5 6 8 10 mm Cu

Radiation quality Strahlenqualität Qualité du rayonnement Calidad de la radiación			Back scatter - Rückstreuung - Rétrodiffusion - Retrodispersión %					
Tube Röhre Ampoule Tubo	HVL - HWSD CDA - CHR		Field size and ratio of sides - Feldgröße und Seitenverhältnis - Dimensions du champ et rapport des côtés - Tamaño del campo y relación ancho/largo					
			$20\ cm^2$			$200\ cm^2$		
kV	mm Al	mm Cu	1:1	1:2	1:4	1:1	1:2	1:4
15	0.045	-	5.3	5.2	5.0	10.5	10.2	10.0
20	0.11	-	6.7	6.5	6.4	12.8	12.4	12.0
30	0.36	-	10.3	10.0	9.6	17.5	16.8	16.0
40	0.8	-	13.5	12.8	12.5	22	20.8	19.5
60	2.7	0.07	18.0	16.5	17.0	29	28	27
80	5.5	0.16	21	19.5	19.0	35	33	32
100	8	0.3	22	21	20	39	37	36
150	-	0.9	22	21	20	42	40	38
200	-	1.5	18.5	17.2	16.5	39	37	35
300	-	3.8	11.5	11.0	10.6	27	25	24
400	-	5.5	8.3	7.8	7.4	19.6	18.4	17.8
600	-	7.8	4.8	4.6	4.4	13.0	12.2	11.5
800	-	9	3.3	3.1	2.8	9.6	9.1	8.6
1000	-	10	2.5	2.3	2.1	7.8	7.4	7.0
Cs 137	-	-	1.7	1.5	1.3	6.0	5.5	5.3
2000	-	-	1.2	1.2	1.1	4.5	4.2	3.8
Co 60	-	-	1.1	1.1	1.1	3.9	3.8	3.4
3000	-	-	1.0	1.0	1.0	3.7	3.5	3.3

Lit.: 1. MAYNEORD, W.V., LAMERTON, L.F.: Brit.Radiol. **14**, 255 (1941)
2. JOHNS, H.E.: Brit.J.Radiol. **25**, 369 (1952)
3. JOHNS, H.E.: Physics of Radiation Therapy, Springfield: C.C. Thomas 1971
4. COHEN, M., JONES, D.E.A.: Brit.J.Radiol., Suppl. 11 (1972)

5.1.3 Variation of back scatter with body thickness (d)
Rückstreuung bei verschiedener Dicke des Streukörpers (d)
Variation de la rétrodiffusion en fonction de l'épaisseur (d)
Retrodispersión para diferentes espesores del fantoma (d)

100 cm^2 Field size - Feld - Champ - Campo

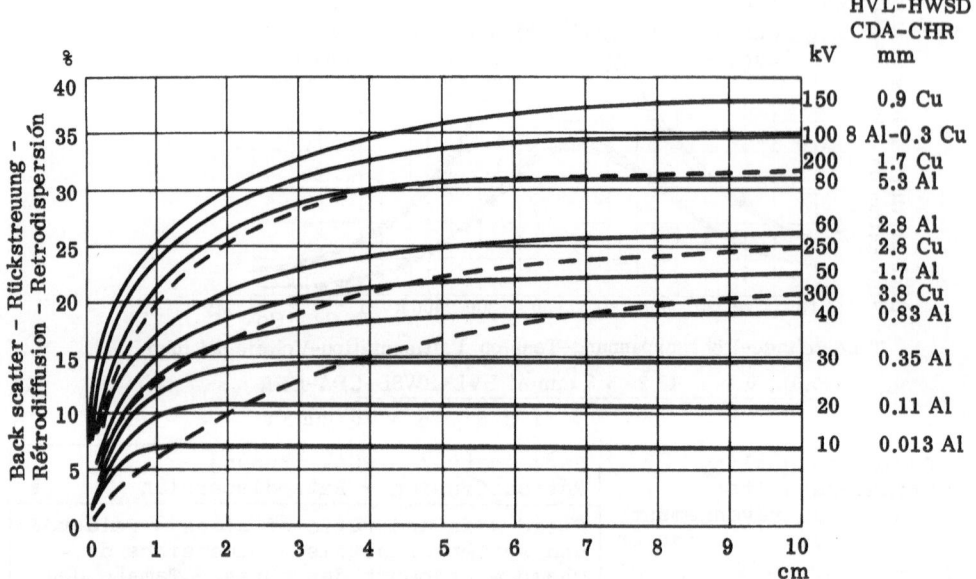

Body thickness - Körperdicke - Epaisseur du milieu - Espesor del cuerpo

d	Back scatter - Rückstreuung - Rétrodiffusion - Retrodispersión											%
	Radiation quality (normal radiation) - Strahlenqualität (Normalstrahlung) - Qualité du rayonnement (rayonnement normal) - Calidad de la radiación (radiación normal)											kV
cm	10	20	30	40	50	60	80	100	150	200	250	300
0.5	5.7	7.2	8.6	10	12	13	16	19	21	15	9.4	3.3
1	7.0	9.7	12	13	16	17	21	23	25	20	12	6.0
1.5	7.0	10	13	15	18	21	24	26	28	23	15	8.0
2	7.0	11	14	17	19	21	26	28	30	25	17	10
3	7.0	11	15	18	20	23	29	31	33	28	19	13
4	7.0	11	15	18	21	24	30	33	35	30	21	15
5	7.0	11	15	19	22	25	31	34	36	30	23	17
6	7.0	11	15	19	22	25	31	35	37	31	23	18
7	7.0	11	15	20	22	26	31	35	38	31	24	19
8	7.0	11	15	20	22	26	31	35	38	32	24	20
9	7.0	11	15	20	22	26	31	35	38	32	24	21
10	7.0	11	15	20	22	26	31	35	38	32	25	21

Lit.: 1. WACHSMANN, F., HECKEL, K., SCHIRREN, C.G.: Strahlenther. 94, 161 (1954)

5.2   Half-value depth (HVD) of X- and gamma rays in tissue
Gewebehalbwerttiefen (GHWT) von Röntgen- und Gammastrahlen
Profondeur demi attenuation (PDA 50 %) dans les tissus pour
des rayonnements X et γ
Profundidades hemireductoras (PHR) para rayos X y γ
expresadas en espesor de tejido

5.2.1   Low energy X-rays - Weiche Röntgenstrahlen - Rayons X mous -
Rayos X blandos

0.1 - 8 mm Al HVL - HWSD - CDA - CHR

100 cm^2 Field size - Feldgröße - Champ - Campo

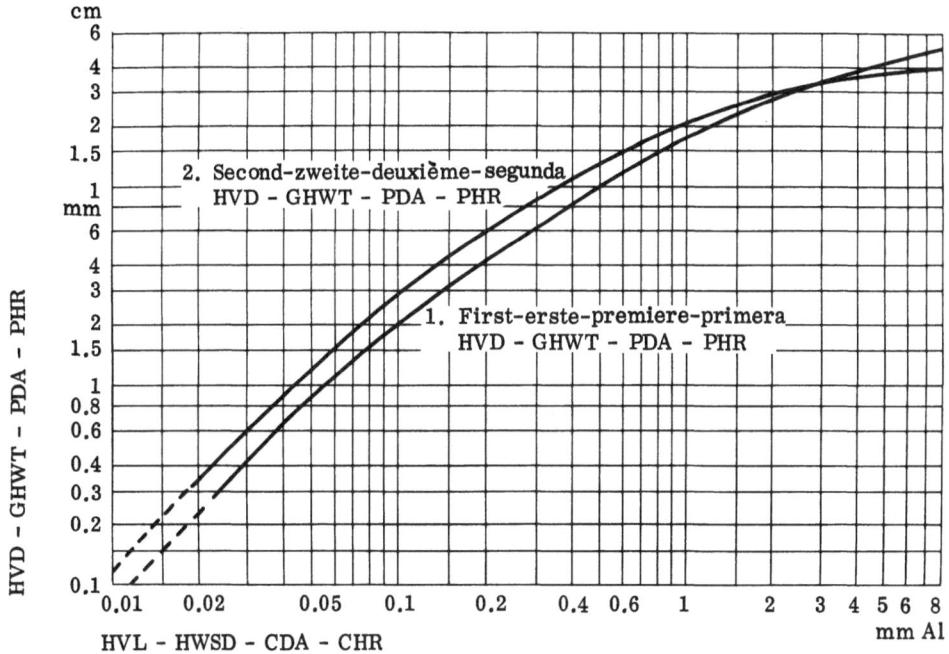

HVL - HWSD - CDA - CHR

HVL–HWSD CDA–CHR	HVD – GHWT PDA – PHR		HVL–HWSD CDA–CHR	HVD – GHWT PDA – PHR		HVL–HWSD CDA–CHR	HVD – GHWT PDA – PHR	
	1.	2.		1.	2.		1.	2.
mm Al	mm	mm	mm Al	mm	mm	mm Al	cm	cm
0.01	–	(0.12)	0.1	2.0	2.9	1	1.8	2.1
0.015	(0.15)	(0.22)	0.15	3.2	4.5	1.5	2.3	2.7
0.02	(0.23)	0.34	0.2	4.2	6.0	2	2.8	2.9
0.03	0.43	0.6	0.3	6.3	8.6	3	3.4	3.4
0.04	0.66	0.9	0.4	8.2	11	4	3.7	3.9
0.05	0.88	1.2	0.5	10	13	5	3.8	4.4
0.06	1.2	1.6	0.6	12	15	6	3.9	4.6
0.07	1.4	1.8	0.7	14	17	7	3.9	5.0
0.08	1.6	2.2	0.8	15	18	8	4.0	5.2
0.09	1.8	2.5	0.9	17	19			

Lit.: See pages - Siehe Seiten - Voir pages - Ver páginas 104 - 111

5.2.2 Orthovoltage X-rays - Harte Röntgenstrahlen - Rayons X classiques - Rayos X duros

0.5 - 8 mm Cu HVL - HWSD - CDA - CHR

50 cm FSD - FHA - DFP - DFP

25 - 100 - 200 cm^2 Field size - Feldgröße - Champ - Campo

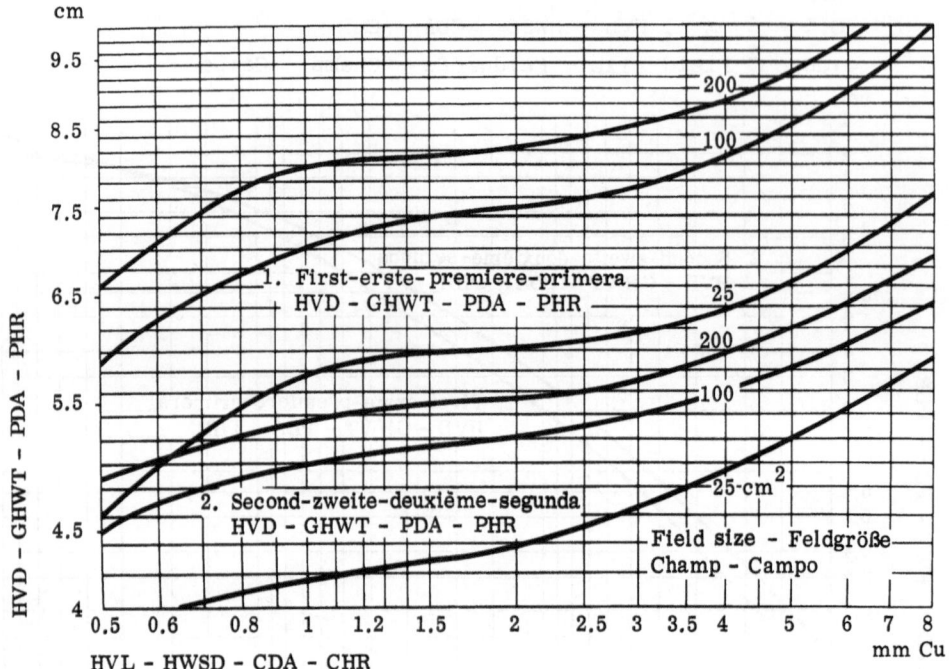

HVL-HWSD CDA-CHR	HVD - GHWT PDA - PHR (100 cm^2)		HVL-HWSD CDA-CHR	HVD - GHWT PDA - PHR (100 cm^2)	
	1.	2.		1.	2.
mm Cu	cm	cm	mm Cu	cm	cm
0.5	5.9	4.5	2	7.5	5.2
0.6	6.3	4.7	2.5	7.6	5.3
0.7	6.5	4.8	3	7.7	5.4
0.8	6.7	4.9	3.5	7.9	5.5
0.9	6.9	4.9	4	8.1	5.6
1	7.0	5.0	4.5	8.3	5.7
1.1	7.1	5.0	5	8.5	5.8
1.2	7.2	5.1	5.5	8.8	5.9
1.3	7.3	5.1	6	9.0	6.0
1.4	7.3	5.1	7	9.4	6.2
1.5	7.4	5.1	8	10	6.4

Lit.: See pages - Siehe Seiten - Voir pages - Ver paginas 87 - 99

5.2.3   Super- and megavoltage X- and gamma rays
        Sehr harte und ultraharte Röntgen- und Gammastrahlen
        Rayons X de haute et très haute énergie et rayons gamma
        Rayos X muy duros, ultraduros y gamma

0.5 - 100 MV

100 cm FSD - FHA - DFP - DFP

(50-) 100 (-200) cm^2 Field size - Feldgröße - Champ - Campo

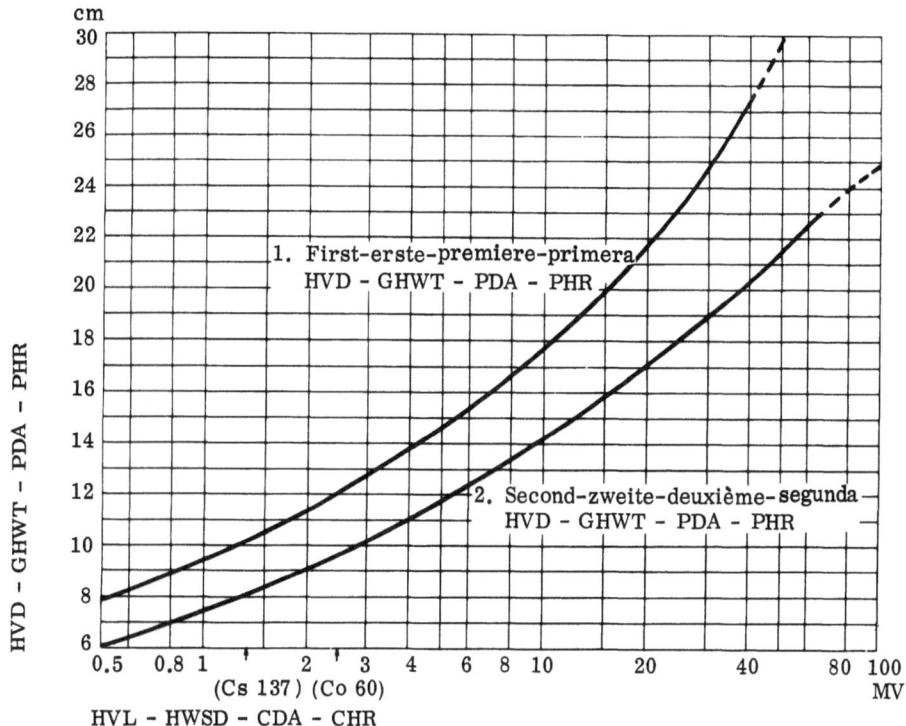

HVL–HWSD CDA–CHR	HVD – GHWT PDA – PHR (100 cm^2)		HVL–HWSD CDA–CHR	HVD – GHWT PDA – PHR (100 cm^2)	
	1.	2.		1.	2.
MeV	cm	cm	MeV	cm	cm
0.5	8.0	6.0	6	15.5	12.3
0.6	8.4	6.4	8	16.8	13.2
0.8	9.0	7.0	10	17.7	14.0
1	9.4	7.4	15	19.7	15.7
Cs 137	10.1	8.0	20	21.7	17.1
1.5	10.5	8.3	30	24.8	19.0
2	11.5	9.6	40	27.4	20.3
Co 60	12.1	9.7	50	(29.6)	21.4
3	12.5	10.3	60	-	22.4
4	13.8	11.1	80	-	(24.0)
5	14.5	11.7	100	-	(24.9)

Lit.: See pages-Siehe Seiten-Voir pages-Ver paginas 118-122, 126-129

5.3 <u>Primary and scattered radiation at different depths</u>
<u>Primär- und Streustrahlung in verschiedenen Tiefen</u>
<u>Rayonnement primaire et diffusé à diverses profondeurs</u>
<u>Radiación primaria y dispersa a distintas profundidades</u>

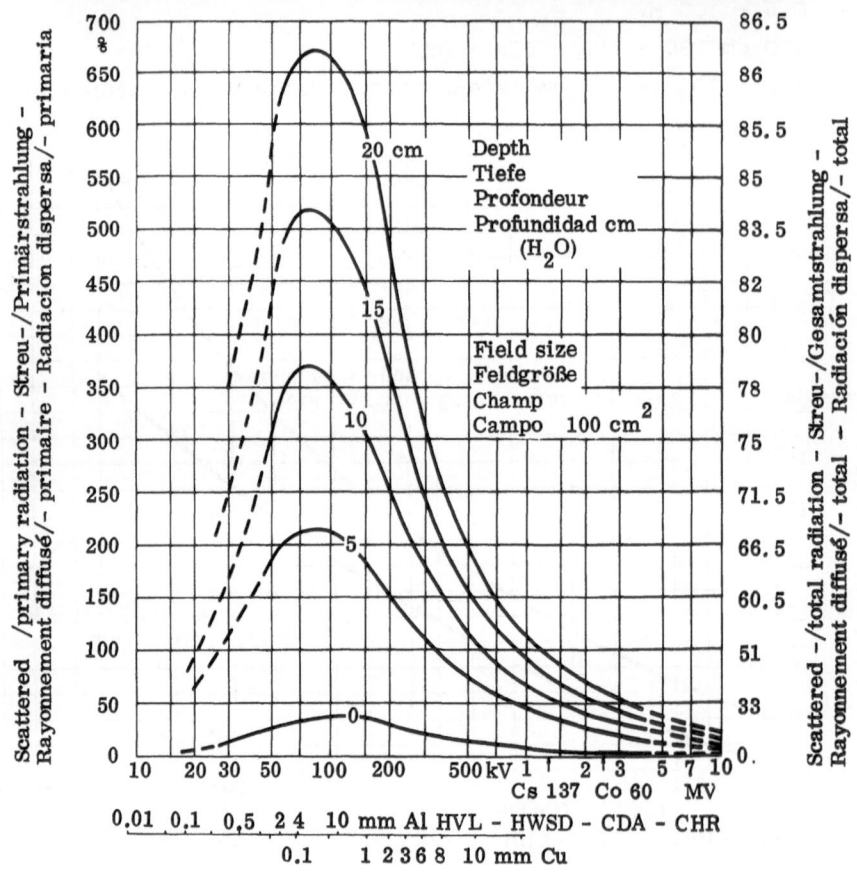

Tube voltage - Röhrenspannung - Tension d'alimentation
Tensión del tubo

In the case of larger or smaller fields the amount of scattered radiation increases or decreases, respectively, approximately with the square root of the field size.

Bei größeren bzw. kleineren Feldern wächst bzw. fällt der Streustrahlenanteil etwa mit der Quadratwurzel aus der Feldgröße.

Pour de plus grands ou de plus petits champs, la proportion du rayonnement diffusé augmente ou diminue à peu près avec la racine carrée de la dimension du champ.

En el caso de campos mayores o menores, la porción de radiación dispersada aumenta o disminuye aproximadamente con la raiz cuadrada de la magnitud del campo.

Lit.: 1. GAJEWSKI, H.: Fortschr. Röntgenstr. <u>80</u>, 642 (1954)

Radiation quality Strahlenqualität Qualité du rayonnement Calidad de la radiación		Scattered/primary radiation Streu-/Primärstrahlung Rayonnement diffusé/- primaire Radiación dispersa/- primaria %				
kV-MV	HVL - HWSD CDA - CHR mm	Depth-Tiefe-Profondeur-Profundidad cm				
		0	5	10	15	20
20 kV	0.11 Al	–	(52)	(95)	–	–
30 kV	0.35	12	(110)	(170)	(275)	(370)
40 kV	0.83	19	(150)	(240)	(360)	(480)
50 kV	1.7 0.045 Cu	25	190	300	(440)	(580)
60 kV	2.8 0.07	29	210	350	480	640
80 kV	5.3 0.16	34	215	370	520	670
100 kV	8.0 0.30	38	212	360	505	665
150 kV	0.9	35	180	305	440	590
200 kV	1.7	29	150	250	360	475
300 kV	3.8	21	110	175	240	315
400 kV	5.8	18	90	140	185	290
500 kV	7.1	14	75	115	158	200
600 kV	8.0	12	65	100	137	168
800 kV	9.0	9	55	80	110	135
1 MV	10	7	45	67	93	114
Cs 137	–	5	40	57	76	95
2 MV	–	4	28	42	55	70
Co 60	–	2	22	37	47	62
5 MV	–	(1)	(14)	(21)	(30)	(39)

Radiation quality Strahlenqualität Qualité du rayonnement Calidad de la raciación		Scattered /total radiation Streu-/Gesamtstrahlung Rayonnement diffusé/- total Radiación dispersa/- total %				
kV-MV	HVL - HWSD CDA - CHR mm	Depth-Tiefe-Profondeur-Profundidad cm				
		0	5	10	15	20
20 kV	0.11 Al	–	(34)	(49)	–	–
30 kV	0.35	10	(52)	(63)	(73)	(78)
40 kV	0.83	16	(60)	(70)	(79)	(83)
50 kV	1.7 0.045 Cu	20	66	75	(82)	(86)
60 kV	2.8 0.07	22	67	78	83	86
80 kV	5.3 0.16	25	68	79	84	87
100 kV	8.0 0.30	27	68	78	83	86
150 kV	0.9	26	64	75	82	84
200 kV	1.7	23	60	72	78	83
300 kV	3.8	18	52	63	71	77
400 kV	5.8	15	47	58	65	75
500 kV	7.1	12	43	54	61	67
600 kV	8.0	10	40	50	57	63
800 kV	9.0	8	35	44	52	58
1 MV	10	6.5	31	40	48	53
Cs 137	–	4.7	28	36	43	49
2 MV	–	4.0	22	30	35	41
Co 60	–	2	18	28	32	38
5 MV	–	(1)	(12)	(17)	(23)	(28)

5.4 Dose fall-off outside the beam axis (dose decrement)
Abfall der Dosis seitlich vom Zentralstrahl (Dosisdekrement)
Décroissance de la dose en traversée
Disminución de la dosis lateral del rayo central

Values measured in a water phantom 80 x 40 x 30 cm for 50 cm FSD -
In einem Wasserphantom von 80 x 40 x 30 cm gemessene Werte bei 50 cm
FHA - Valeurs mesurées dans un fantôme d'eau de 80 x 40 x 30 cm, DSP
50 cm - Valores medidos en un fantoma de agua de 80 x 40 x 30 cm a
50 cm DFP

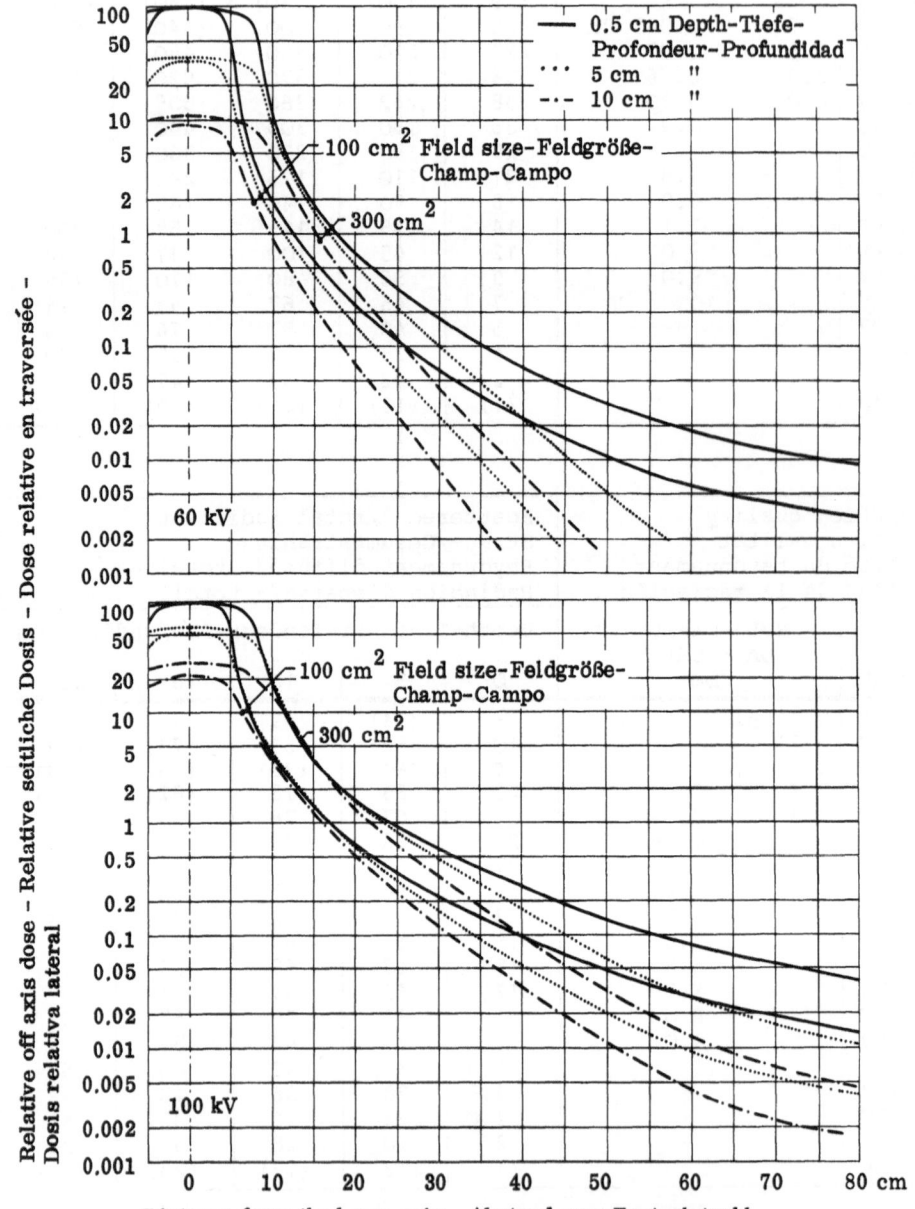

Distance from the beam axis - Abstand vom Zentralstrahl -
Distance de l'axe du faisceau - Distancia del rayo central

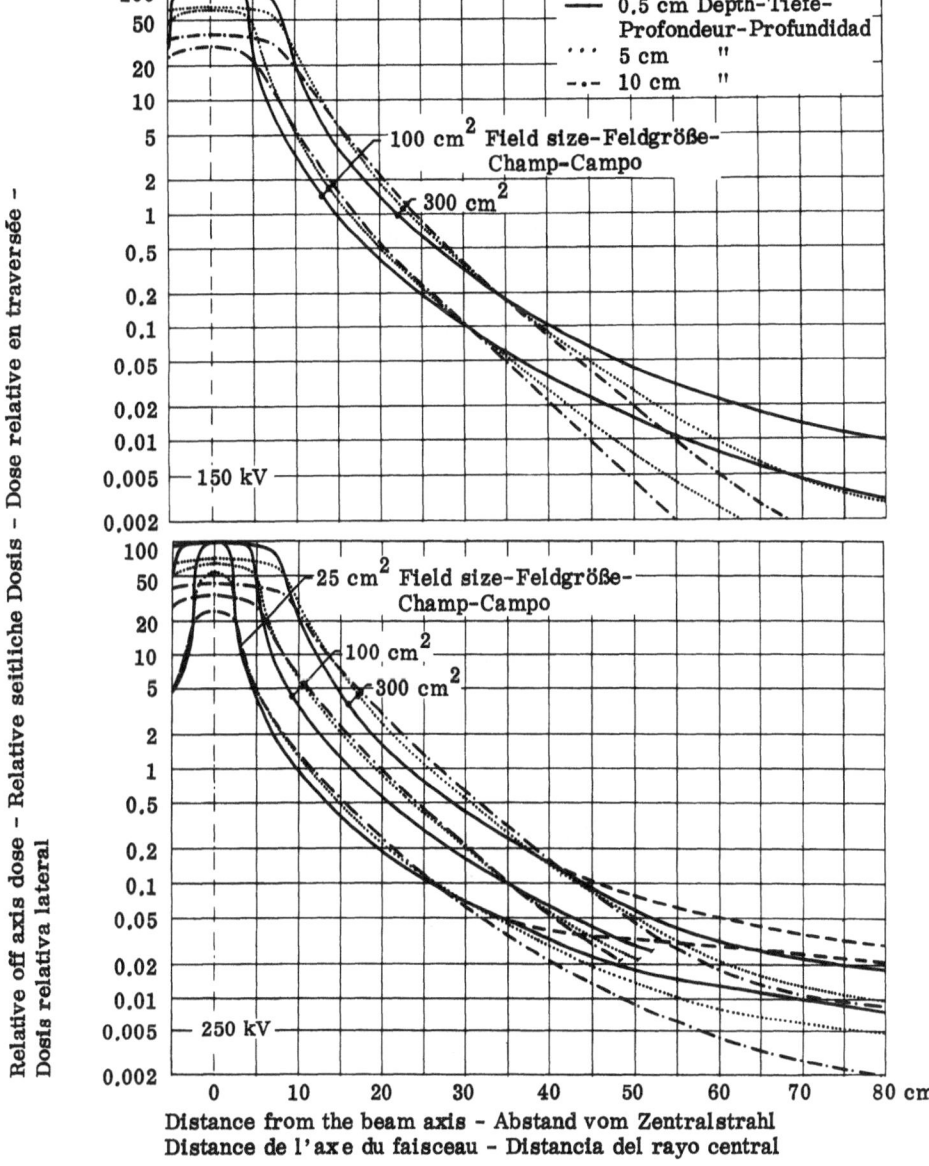

Distance from the beam axis - Abstand vom Zentralstrahl
Distance de l'axe du faisceau - Distancia del rayo central

--- Dose at 0.5 cm depth including the radiation passing through the
    tube housing (Siemens therapy tube housing Z Rhb 2, 250 kV)

--- Dosis in 0,5 cm Tiefe einschließlich der Gehäusedurchlaßstrahlung
    (Siemens Therapiehaube Z Rhb 2, 250 kV)

--- Dose à 0,5 cm de profondeur incluant la dose dûe au rayonnement
    de fuite à travers de la gaine du tube (gaine de thérapie Siemens
    Z Rhb 2, 250 kV)

--- Dosis a una profundidad de 0,5 cm incluida la radiación a través
    de la carcasa del tubo (carcasa para la terapia, Siemens Z Rhb 2,
    250 kV)

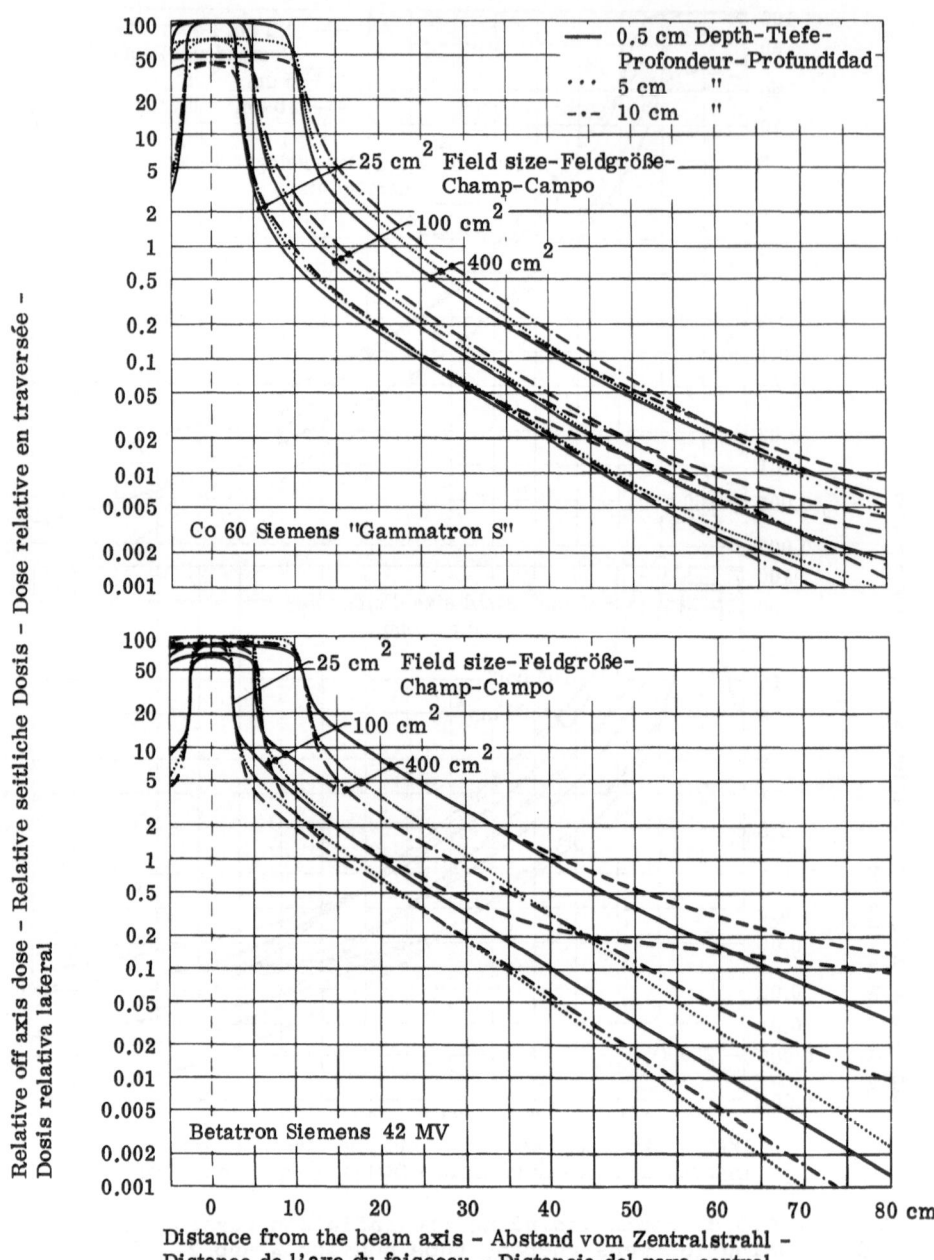

Relative off axis dose - Relative seitliche Dosis - Dose relative en traversée - Dosis relativa lateral

Distance from the beam axis - Abstand vom Zentralstrahl - Distance de l'axe du faisceau - Distancia del rayo central

--- See page - Siehe Seite - Voir page - Ver página 147

Lit.: 1. SEELENTAG, W., KLOTZ E.: Strahlenther. 108, 112 (1959)
      2. WACHSMANN, F., JASCHKE, R.: Biophysik 1, 108 (1963)
      3. TROUT, D.E., KELLEY, J.P.: Am.J.Roentgenol. 85, 546 (1965)
      4. CZEMPIEL, H., MÜHLE, P., REGULLA, D.F., WACHSMANN, F.:
         Fortschr.Röntgenstr. 124, (1976) im Druck

Table of contents - Inhaltsverzeichnis
Table des matières - Tabla de materias

6.1 Radionuclides used in nuclear medicine
In der Nuklearmedizin verwendete Radionuklide
Radionucleides utilisés en médecine nucléaire
Radionuclidos utilizados en medicina nuclear

Nuclide Nuklid Nucléide Nuclido	$T_{1/2}$	Decay Zerfall Décroissance Desintegr.	Energy-Energie Energie-Energía E_β max. MeV	E_γ max. MeV	P_γ %	Γ $\dfrac{R\ m^2}{Ci\ h}$	Appl.
^{3}H, T	12.3 a	β^-	0.0186	-	-	-	D,R,T
^{14}C	5700 a	β^-	0.156	-	-	-	D,R,T
^{13}N	10 min	β^+	1.2	0.511	200	0.59	D
^{18}F	110 min	β^+,EC	0.64	0.511	190	0.57	D,R
^{22}Na	2.6 a	β^+,EC	0.54 1.8	0.511 1.27	180 200	1.19	D
^{24}Na	15 h	β^-	1.39	1.37 2.75	100 100	1.82	D
^{32}P	14.3 d	β^-	1.71	-	-	-	D,Th
^{35}S	88 d	β^-	0.167	-	-	-	D
^{40}K	1.28·10^{9}a	β^-,EC	1.32	1.46	11	0.0803	R
^{42}K	12.4 h	β^-	3.52	1.52	18	0.137	D
^{45}Ca	165 d	β^-	0.252	-	-	-	D,R
^{47}Ca	4.53 d	β^-	0.67 1.98	0.5 0.81 1.3	5 5 74	- 0.54	D
^{51}Cr	27.8 d	E		0.32	9	0.018	D
^{52}Fe	8 h	β^+,EC	0.80	0.17 0.511	100 112	0.41	D
^{55}Fe	2.6 a	EC	-	0.006*)		-	D
^{59}Fe	45 d	β^-	0.48	0.19 1.1 1.29	3 56 44	0.62	D
^{57}Co	269 d	EC	-	0.006*) 0.014 0.12 0.14	9 87 11	0.093	D
^{58}Co	713 d	β^+,EC	0.47	0.006*) 0.511 0.81	30 99	0.54	D
^{60}Co	5.27 a	β^-	0.31	1.17 1.33	100 100	1.30	Th,T D,R
^{64}Cu	12.8 h	β^-,EC β^-	0.66 0.57	0.008*) 0.511 -	38 -	0.116 -	D
^{65}Zn	246 d	β^+	0.33	0.511 1.12	3 49	0.30	D

Nuclide Nuklid Nucléide Nuclido	$T_{1/2}$	Decay Zerfall Décroissance Desintegr.	Energy-Energie Energie-Energía E_β max. MeV	E_γ max. MeV	P_γ %	Γ $\dfrac{R\,m^2}{Ci\,h}$	Appl.
^{68}Ga	68 min	β^+,EC	1.9	0.009*) 0.511 1.08	176 4	0.54	D
^{72}Ga	14.2 h	β^-	3.1	0.60 0.63 0.84 0.89 2.2 2.5	8 27 96 10 26 20	1.31	D,R
^{68}Ge	275 d	EC	-	0.009*)		-	D,R
^{74}As	17.7 d	β^+,EC β^+ β^-	0.95 1.5 1.4	0.01*) 0.511 0.6 0.64	59 61 14	0.45	D
^{76}As	26.4 h	β^-	2.97	0.56 0.66 1.22	43 6 5	0.25	D,R
^{75}Se	122 d	EC	-	0.011*) 0.12 0.14 0.26 0.28 0.4	17 57 60 25 12	0.20	D,R
^{85}Kr	10.2 a	β^-	0.67	0.51	4	0.0012	D,T
^{86}Rb	18.7 d	β^-	1.78	1.08	9	0.051	D
^{87}Rb	$4.8 \cdot 10^{10}$ a	β^-	0.27	-		-	D
^{85}Sr	64.7 d	EC	-	0.014*) 0.511	100	0.30	D
^{87m}Sr	2.8 h	-	0.37 e 0.39 e	0.39	80	0.18	D
^{89}Sr	53 d	β^-	1.46	-	-	-	D,R
^{90}Sr	28 a	β^-	0.55	-	-	-	Th,T
^{90}Y	64 h	β^-	2.27	-	-	-	Th
^{99}Mo	66.5 h	β^-	1.23	0.04 0.18 0.37 0.74 0.78	2 7 1 12 4	0.83	D,R
^{99m}Tc	6.0 h		0.12 e	0.14	90	0.061	D
^{111}Ag	7.4 d	β^-	1.05	0.25 0.34	1 6	0.013	D
^{113m}In	102 min		0.36 e 0.39 e	0.39	64	0.145	D
^{113}Sn	120 d	EC	-	0.015*) 0.25	1.8	0.003	D,R

Nuclide Nuklid Nucléide Nuclido	$T_{1/2}$	Decay Zerfall Décroissance Desintegr.	Energy-Energie Energie-Energia E_β max. MeV	E_γ max. MeV	P_γ %	$\dfrac{\Gamma}{R\ \dfrac{m^2}{Ci\ h}}$	Appl.
^{132}Te	77.8 h	β^-	0.22	0.05 0.23	17 90	0.121	D,R
^{123}I^{123}J	13.1 h	EC	-	0.028*) 0.16	83	0.072	R
^{125}I^{125}J	59.2 d	EC	-	0.028*) 0.035	7	0.004	D
^{128}I^{128}J	25 min	β^-,EC	2.12	0.028*) 0.441	14	0.053	D
^{131}I^{131}J	8.07 d	β^-	0.61 0.81	0.08 0.28 0.36 0.64	3 5 82 7	0.21	D,Th
^{132}I^{132}J	2.35 h	β^-	2.1	0.52 0.67 0.77 0.96 1.14 1.28 1.4	20 144 89 22 6 7 14	1.13	D,Th
^{133}Xe	5.4 d	β^-	0.35	0.08	37	0.014	D
^{137}Cs	30 a	β^-	0.51 1.18	0.662	85	0.323	Th,T
^{170}Tm	129 d	β^-	0.97	0.084	3.3	0.001	D,R
^{182}Ta	115 d	β^-	0.52 1.71	0.07 0.1 0.15 0.22 1.12 1.19 1.22 1.23	42 14 7 8 34 16 27 13	0.68	Th
^{192}Ir	74.3 d	β^-,EC	0.67	0.3 0.31 0.32 0.47 0.59 0.6 0.61	29 30 81 49 4 9 6	0.51	Th,T
^{198}Au	2.7 d	β^-	0.96	0.41 0.68	95 1	0.233	D,Th
^{199}Au	3.15 d	β^-	0.3 0.46	0.16 0.21	37 8	0.078	R,Th
^{197}Hg	65 h	EC	-	0.071*) 0.08 0.19	18 2	0.009	D
^{203}Hg	47.1 d	β^-	0.21	0.28	77	0.175	D

Nuclide / Nuklid / Nucléide / Nuclido	$T_{1/2}$	Decay / Zerfall / Décroissance / Desintegr.	Energy-Energie Energie-Energía $E_{\beta,\alpha}$ MeV	E_γ max. MeV	P_γ %	Γ $\dfrac{R\ m^2}{Ci\ h}$	Appl.
^{206}Bi	6.24 d	EC		0.077*) 0.52 0.8 0.88 1.7	46 99 72 36	1.86	Th,D
^{222}Rn	3.82 d	α	5.49				R,Th
^{224}Ra	3.64 d	α	5.45	0.24	4	0.005	T,Th
^{226}Ra	1600 a	α	4.78	0.186	4	0.004 0.83**)	T,Th
^{228}Th	1.91 a	α	5.34 5.43	0.084	2	0.007	T
^{230}Th	$7.9\cdot10^4$a	α	4.62 4.68	0.068	0.6	0.0003	T,R
^{232}T	$1.4\cdot10^{10}$a	α	3.9 4.0				R,T
^{235}U	$7\cdot10^8$a	α	4.37 4.40 4.58	0.11 0.14 0.16 0.18 0.2	2.5 11 5 54 6	0.071	T
^{238}U	$4.5\cdot10^9$a	α	4.15 4.20				T
^{239}Pu	$2.4\cdot10^4$a	α	5.11 5.16	0.013 0.038 0.051	17	0.02	T
^{252}Cf	2.2 a	α	6.12 6.08	0.043 0.1 0.160			Th
^{252}Cf	85 a	n	2.13				

P_γ: Emission probability (% of disintegrations) - Emissionswahr-scheinlichkeit (% der Zerfälle) - Probabilité d'émission (% du nombre de desintégrations) - Probabilidad de emisión (% de desintegración)

Γ: Specific gamma-ray constant - Spezifische Gammastrahlenkon-stante - Constante de débit d'exposition - Constante especí-fica de radiación gamma

Appl.: Application - Anwendung - Utilisation - Aplicación

D: Diagnosis; Th: Therapy; R: Research; T: Technology

e: Conversion electrons - Konversionselektronen - Conversion interne - Electrones de conversión

EC: Electron capture - Elektroneneinfang - Capture électronique - Captura de electrones

*) K-radiation - K-Strahlung - Rayonnement K - Radiación K
**) Ra 226 + decay products - Ra 226 + Zerfallsprodukte - Ra 226 + produits de désintegration - Ra 226+ productos de desintegración

6.2 Desintegration schemes of radionuclides
Zerfallsschemen von Radionukliden
Schémas de désintégration des radionucléides
Esquemas de desintegración de radionúclidos

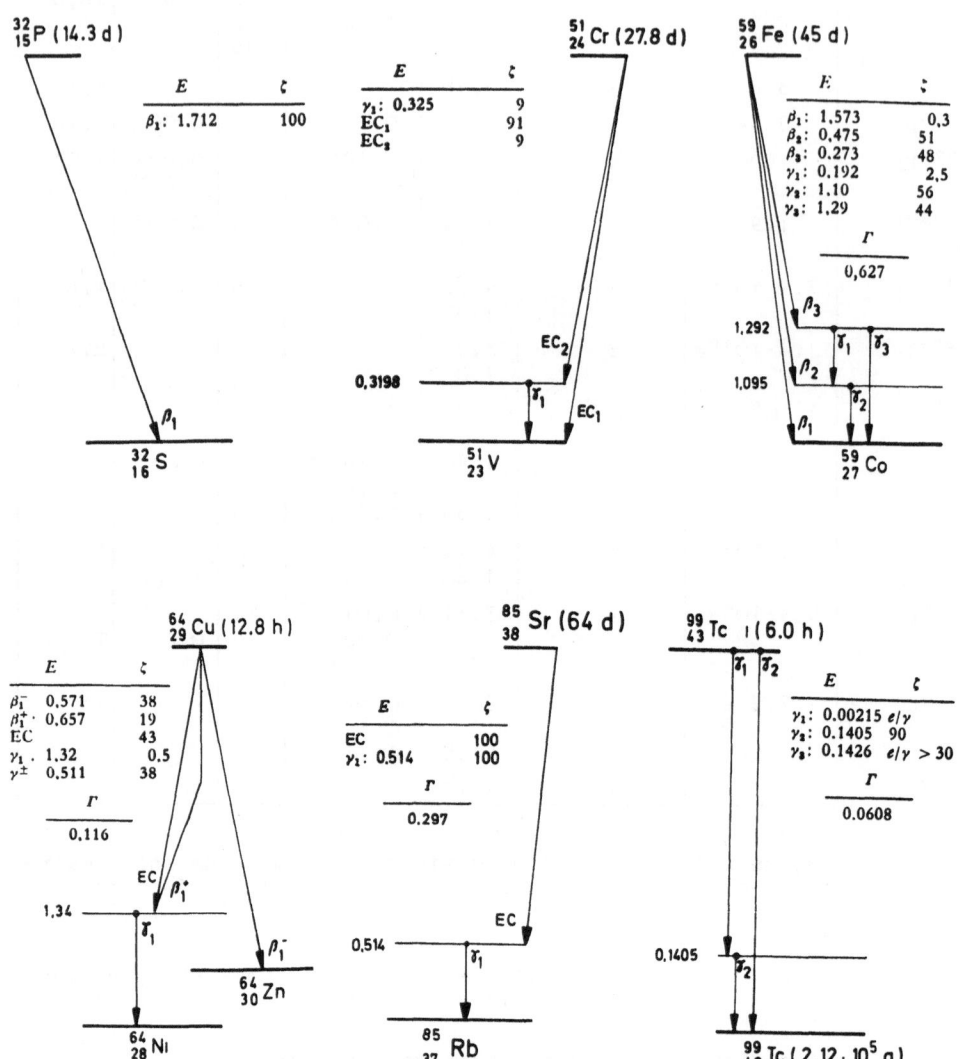

Lit.: 1. LEDERER, C.M., HOLLANDER, J.M., PERLMAN, J.: Table of Isotopes, New York: J. Wiley & Sons, Inc. 1967

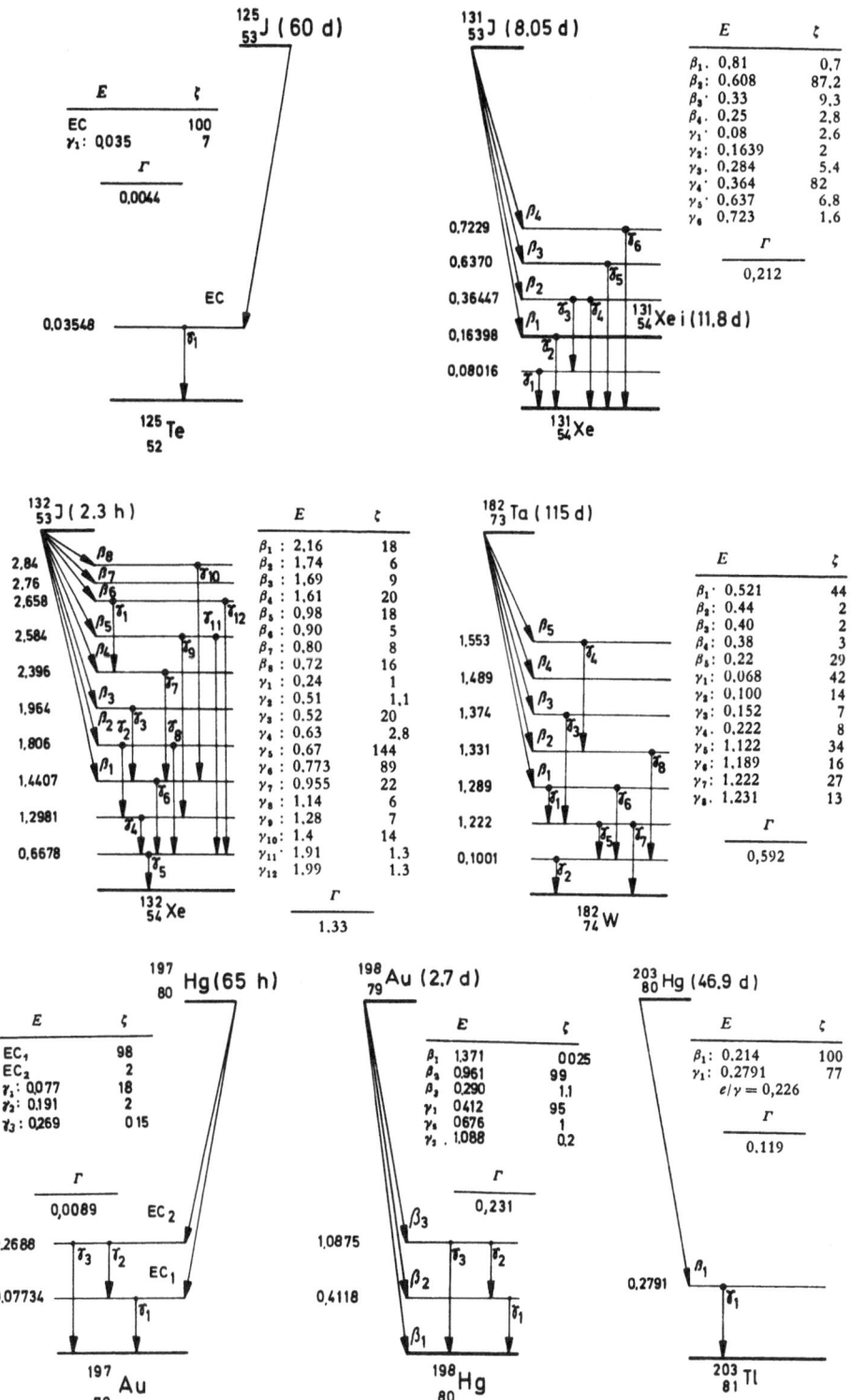

$^{125}_{53}J$ (60 d)

	E	ζ
EC		100
γ_1:	0,035	7

Γ

0,0044

EC

0,03548 γ_1

$^{125}_{52}Te$

$^{131}_{53}J$ (8,05 d)

	E	ζ
β_1.	0,81	0,7
β_2:	0,608	87,2
β_3:	0,33	9,3
β_4:	0,25	2,8
γ_1:	0,08	2,6
γ_2:	0,1639	2
γ_3:	0,284	5,4
γ_4.	0,364	82
γ_5:	0,637	6,8
γ_6:	0,723	1,6

Γ

0,212

0,7229 β_4 γ_6
0,6370 β_3 γ_5
0,36447 β_2 γ_3 γ_4 $^{131}_{54}Xe\ i$ (11,8 d)
0,16398 β_1
0,08016 γ_2
         γ_1

$^{131}_{54}Xe$

$^{132}_{53}J$ (2,3 h)

	E	ζ
β_1 :	2,16	18
β_2 :	1,74	6
β_3 :	1,69	9
β_4 :	1,61	20
β_5 :	0,98	18
β_6 :	0,90	5
β_7 :	0,80	8
β_8 :	0,72	16
γ_1 :	0,24	1
γ_2 :	0,51	1,1
γ_3 :	0,52	20
γ_4 :	0,63	2,8
γ_5 :	0,67	144
γ_6 :	0,773	89
γ_7 :	0,955	22
γ_8 :	1,14	6
γ_9 :	1,28	7
γ_{10} :	1,4	14
γ_{11} .	1,91	1,3
γ_{12}	1,99	1,3

Γ

1,33

2,84 β_8
2,76 β_7 γ_{10}
2,658 β_6
       γ_1 γ_{11} γ_{12}
2,584 β_5
       γ_9
2,396 β_4
       γ_7
1,964 β_3
1,806 β_2 γ_2 γ_3 γ_8
1,4407 β_1
       γ_6
1,2981 γ_4
0,6678 γ_5

$^{132}_{54}Xe$

$^{182}_{73}Ta$ (115 d)

	E	ζ
β_1.	0,521	44
β_2:	0,44	2
β_3:	0,40	2
β_4:	0,38	3
β_5:	0,22	29
γ_1:	0,068	42
γ_2:	0,100	14
γ_3:	0,152	7
γ_4:	0,222	8
γ_5:	1,122	34
γ_6:	1,189	16
γ_7:	1,222	27
γ_8:	1,231	13

Γ

0,592

1,553 β_5 γ_4
1,489 β_4
1,374 β_3 γ_3
1,331 β_2 γ_8
1,289 β_1 γ_1 γ_6
1,222 γ_5 γ_7
0,1001 γ_2

$^{182}_{74}W$

$^{197}_{80}Hg$ (65 h)

	E	ζ
EC_1		98
EC_2		2
γ_1:	0,077	18
γ_2:	0,191	2
γ_3:	0,269	0,15

Γ

0,0089 EC_2

0,2688 γ_3 γ_2 EC_1
0,07734 γ_1

$^{197}_{79}Au$

$^{198}_{79}Au$ (2,7 d)

	E	ζ
β_1	1,371	0,025
β_2	0,961	99
β_3	0,290	1,1
γ_1	0,412	95
γ_2	0,676	1
γ_3	1,088	0,2

Γ

0,231

1,0875 β_3
        γ_3 γ_2
0,4118 β_2
        γ_1
        β_1

$^{198}_{80}Hg$

$^{203}_{80}Hg$ (46,9 d)

	E	ζ
β_1:	0,214	100
γ_1:	0,2791	77
$e/\gamma = 0,226$		

Γ

0,119

0,2791 β_1
         γ_1

$^{203}_{81}Tl$

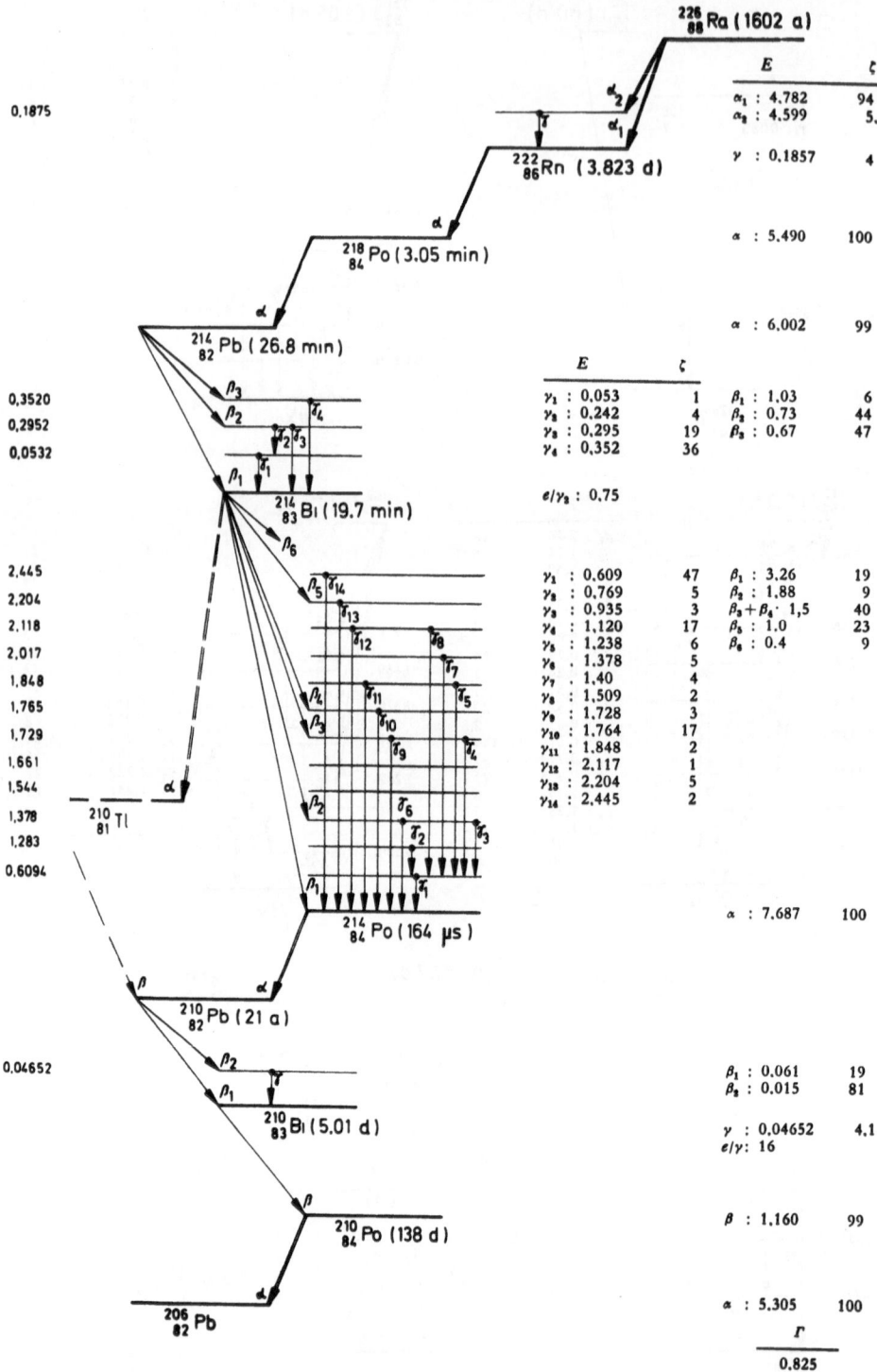

$^{226}_{88}$Ra (1602 a)

	E	ζ
α_1 :	4,782	94
α_2 :	4,599	5,4
γ :	0,1857	4

0,1875

$^{222}_{86}$Rn (3,823 d)

α : 5,490   100

$^{218}_{84}$Po (3,05 min)

α : 6,002   99

$^{214}_{82}$Pb (26,8 min)

0,3520
0,2952
0,0532

	E	ζ			
γ_1 :	0,053	1	β_1 :	1,03	6
γ_2 :	0,242	4	β_2 :	0,73	44
γ_3 :	0,295	19	β_3 :	0,67	47
γ_4 :	0,352	36			

e/γ_3 : 0,75

$^{214}_{83}$Bi (19,7 min)

2,445
2,204
2,118
2,017
1,848
1,765
1,729
1,661
1,544
1,378 $^{210}_{81}$Tl
1,283
0,6094

	E	ζ			
γ_1 :	0,609	47	β_1 :	3,26	19
γ_2 :	0,769	5	β_2 :	1,88	9
γ_3 :	0,935	3	$\beta_3 + \beta_4$:	1,5	40
γ_4 :	1,120	17	β_5 :	1,0	23
γ_5 :	1,238	6	β_6 :	0,4	9
γ_6 .	1,378	5			
γ_7 .	1,40	4			
γ_8 :	1,509	2			
γ_9 :	1,728	3			
γ_{10} :	1,764	17			
γ_{11} :	1,848	2			
γ_{12} :	2,117	1			
γ_{13} :	2,204	5			
γ_{14} :	2,445	2			

$^{214}_{84}$Po (164 μs)

α : 7,687   100

$^{210}_{82}$Pb (21 a)

0,04652

β_1 :	0,061	19
β_2 :	0,015	81

$^{210}_{83}$Bi (5,01 d)

γ : 0,04652   4,1
e/γ : 16

$^{210}_{84}$Po (138 d)

β : 1,160   99

$^{206}_{82}$Pb

α : 5,305   100

Γ

0,825

6.3   Exposure rates of radium and other radionuclides at dif-
       ferent distances from point sources given in Ci and Bq

       Dosisleistung von Radium und anderen Radionukliden in ver-
       schiedenen Abständen von punktförmigen Quellen in Ci und Bq

       Débit d'exposition pour le radium et autres radionucléides
       à diverses distances de sources ponctuelles en Ci et Bq

       Potencia de dosis del radio y otros radionúclidos a diferen-
       tes distancias de fuentes puntiformes expresado en Ci y Bq

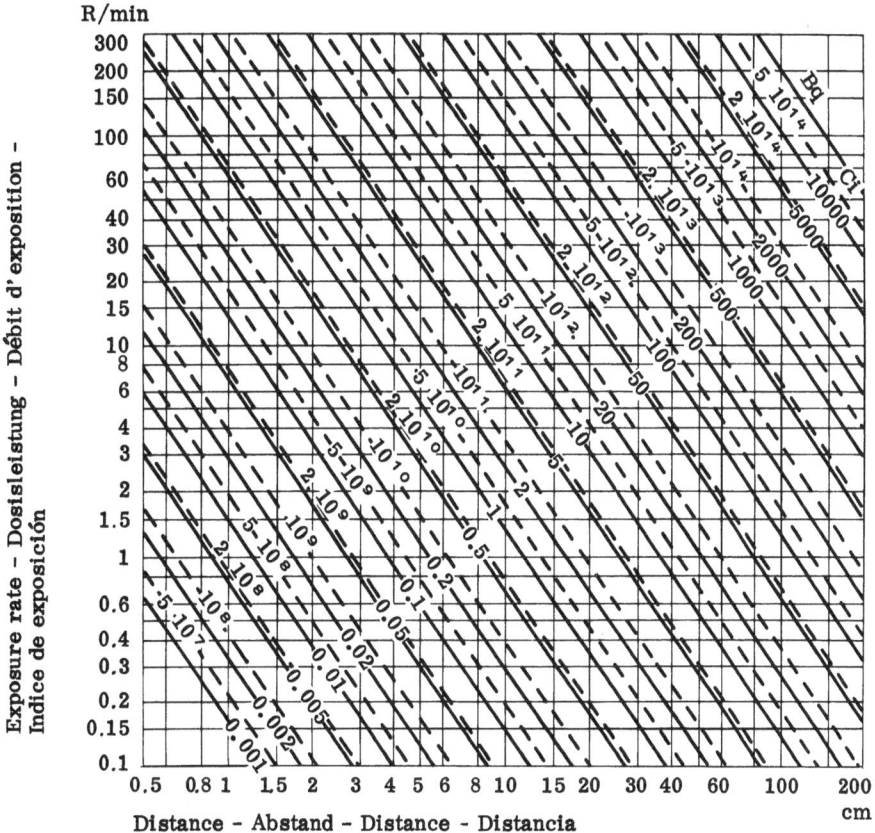

The exposure rates of radium sources filtered with 0.5 mm Pt; self-
absorption in the source is disregarded.

Dosisleistungen von Radium bei einer Filterung von 0,5 mm Pt ohne
Berücksichtigung der Selbstabsorption in der Quelle.

Les débits d'exposition sont donnés pour le radium filtré par
0.5 mm Pt; on n'a pas tenu compte de l'autoabsorption dans la source.

Las potencias de las dosis indicadas están referidas al radio fil-
trado con 0,5 mm Pt, despreciando la autoabsorción en la fuente.

Activity Aktivität Activité Actividad	Exposure rate of Ra 226 at various distances - Dosisleistung von Ra 226 in verschiedenen Abständen - Débit d'exposition de Ra 226 à diverses distances - Potencia de la dosis de Ra 226 a varias distancias R/min								
	Distance - Abstand - Distance - Distancia cm								
Ci	1	1.5	2	2.5	3	4	5	6	8
1	138	61.5	34.5	22.1	15.3	8.6	5.5	3.83	2.15
1.2	166	73.8	41.5	26.5	18.4	10.4	6.6	4.60	2.57
1.4	194	86.0	48.4	31.0	21.4	12.1	7.7	5.3	3.00
1.6	221	98.5	55.3	35.4	24.5	13.8	8.8	6.1	3.45
1.8	249	110	62.3	39.8	27.5	16.6	9.9	6.9	3.87
2	276	124	69	44.2	30.6	17.2	11.0	7.7	4.3
2.5	345	154	86.4	55.2	38.3	21.6	13.8	9.6	5.4
3	415	185	104	66.5	46.0	25.9	16.5	11.5	6.5
3.5	484	216	121	77.5	53.6	30.2	19.2	13.4	7.5
4	552	247	138	88.6	61.2	34.4	22.0	15.3	8.6
4.5	622	277	155	99.6	68.8	38.8	24.8	17.2	9.6
5	690	308	172	111	76.6	43.2	27.5	19.2	10.8
6	830	370	207	133	92.0	51.8	33.0	23.0	12.9
7	970	432	242	155	107	60.4	38.5	26.8	15.1
8	1104	493	276	177	122	68.8	44.0	30.6	17.2
9	2242	554	310	199	138	77.8	49.5	34.5	19.4
TBq	1	1.5	2	2.5	3	4	5	6	8
1	37.2	16.5	9.3	6.0	4.1	2.32	1.48	1.03	0.58
1.2	44.8	19.8	11.2	7.2	5.0	2.78	1.77	1.23	0.70
1.4	52.1	23.1	13.0	8.4	5.8	3.25	2.07	1.44	0.81
1.6	59.7	26.5	14.9	9.6	6.6	3.72	2.37	1.64	0.93
1.8	67.2	29.7	16.8	10.8	7.5	4.17	2.67	1.85	1.04
2	74.4	33.0	18.6	12.0	8.3	4.65	2.95	2.05	1.16
2.5	93.0	41.3	23.3	15.0	10.4	5.8	3.70	2.56	1.45
3	111	49.5	27.9	18.0	12.4	6.7	4.45	3.08	1.74
3.5	130	57.8	32.5	21.0	14.5	8.1	5.2	3.60	2.04
4	148	66.1	37.2	24.0	16.5	9.3	5.9	4.10	2.32
4.5	167	74.4	41.9	27.0	18.6	10.5	6.7	4.60	2.62
5	185	82.8	46.5	30.0	20.6	11.6	7.4	5.1	2.90
6	222	99.0	55.8	36.0	24.8	14.0	8.9	6.2	3.48
7	259	116	65.1	42.0	28.9	16.2	10.4	7.2	4.05
8	296	132	74.5	48.0	33.0	18.6	11.8	8.2	4.65
9	334	148	83.8	54.0	27.1	20.9	13.3	9.2	5.2

For activities other than those listed in the table, the exposure rates can easily be calculated in direct proportion to the activity and in inverse proportion to the square of the distance by means of decimal factors.

Für andere als in der Tabelle angegebene Aktivitäten lassen sich die Dosisleistungen proportional der Aktivität und umgekehrt proportional dem Quadrat des Abstandes unter Verwendung dekadischer Multiplikationsfaktoren leicht berechnen.

Pour des activités autres que celles figurant dans la table, les débits d'exposition peuvent facilement être calculés en proportion directe de l'activité et en proportion inverse du carré de la distance.

Actividades diferentes a las que aparecen en la tabla se pueden calcular facilmente mediante proporción directa de la actividad y proporción inversa del cuadrado de la distancia utilizando factores de multiplicación decimales.

The exposure rates for other radionuclides than Ra 226 can be calculated by multiplication of the values from the curve or the table by
the following values which correspond to the relationship of specific gamma ray constants ($\Gamma_x/\Gamma_{Ra\ 226}$).

Die Dosisleistungen anderer Radionuklide als Ra 226 ergeben sich
durch Multiplikation der aus den Kurven oder aus der Tabelle entnom-
menen Werten mit folgenden, dem Verhältnis der spezifischen Gamma-
strahlenkonstanten entsprechenden, Werten ($\Gamma_x/\Gamma_{Ra\ 226}$).

Les débits d'exposition pour d'autres radionucléides que Ra 226
peuvent être calculés en multipliant les valeurs des courbes où de
la table par les facteurs suivants de débit d'exposition
($\Gamma_x/\Gamma_{Ra\ 226}$).

La potencia de la dosis de otros radionúclidos del que Ra 226 se
puede calcular multiplicando los valores des las curvas o de la
tabla por los siguientes valores que corresponden a las relaciones
de las constantes específicas de rayos gamma ($\Gamma_x/\Gamma_{Ra\ 226}$).

Specific γ-ray constants - Spezifische γ-Strahlenkonstanten - Facteurs specifiques de rayons γ - Constantes especificas de rayos γ Γ					
^{46}Sc	^{60}Co	^{110}Ag	^{131}I	^{137}Cs	^{144}Ce
1.32	1.58	1.80	0.255	0.39	0.03
^{154}Eu	^{160}Tb	^{170}Tm	^{182}Ta	^{192}Ir	^{198}Au
0.78	0.98	0.0012	0.83	0.62	0.283

The self-absorption which, for Co 60, amounts to about 10 % per cm
of source height and for Cs 137, to about 15 % per g/cm^2, is diffi-
cult to calculate because the packing density of the radioactive
material is usually unknown. Therefore, the activity of large sources presently is expressed not in Ci, but directly in R/h at a 1 m
distance in free air, or preferably in water at 5 cm depth.

Die Selbstabsorption, die bei Co 60 etwa 10 % je cm Quellenhöhe und
bei Cs 137 etwa 15 % der g/cm^2 beträgt, läßt sich wegen der meist
unbekannten Packungsdichte des radioaktiven Materials schwer berechnen. Deshalb wird die Stärke von Großquellen heute nicht in Ci son-
dern direkt in R/h in 1 m Abstand frei in Luft oder besser in 5 cm
Wassertiefe angegeben.

L'auto-absorption qui s'élève à environ 10 % par cm de hauteur pour
les sources de Co 60 et à 15 % par g/cm^2 pour le Cs 137 est diffi-
cile à calculer car la densité réelle du matériau radioactif est
habituellement inconnue. C'est pourqoi l'activité des grandes sourses
est actuellement exprimée ne pas en Ci, mais directement en R/h à
une distance de 1 m, dans l'air, ou de préférence à une profondeur
de 5 cm dans l'eau.

La autoabsorción, que para el Co 60 supone aproximadamente el 10 %
por cm de altura de la fuente y para el Cs 137 aproximadamente el
15 % por g/cm^2, se puede calcular dificilmente debido a que generalmente no se conoce la densidad de empaquetamiento del material radioactivo. Por esta razón la intensidad de fuentes grandes no se mide
hoy en Ci sino en R/h a 1 m de distancia en aire o mejor a 5 cm de
profundidad de agua.

6.4 Decay of the activity of radionuclides with time
Abnahme der Aktivität von Radionukliden mit der Zeit
Décroissance de l'activité des radionucléides avec le temps
Disminución de la actividad de radionúclidos con el tiempo

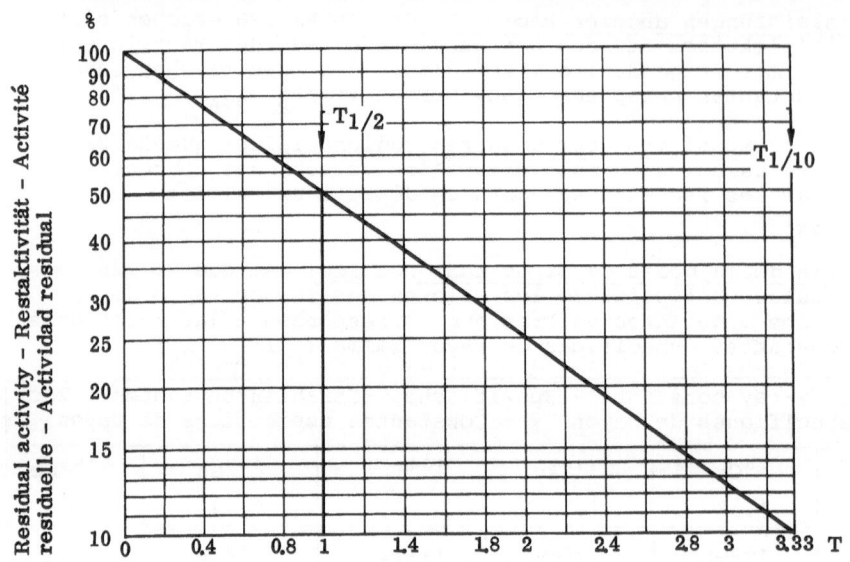

Time - Zeit - Temps - Tiempo

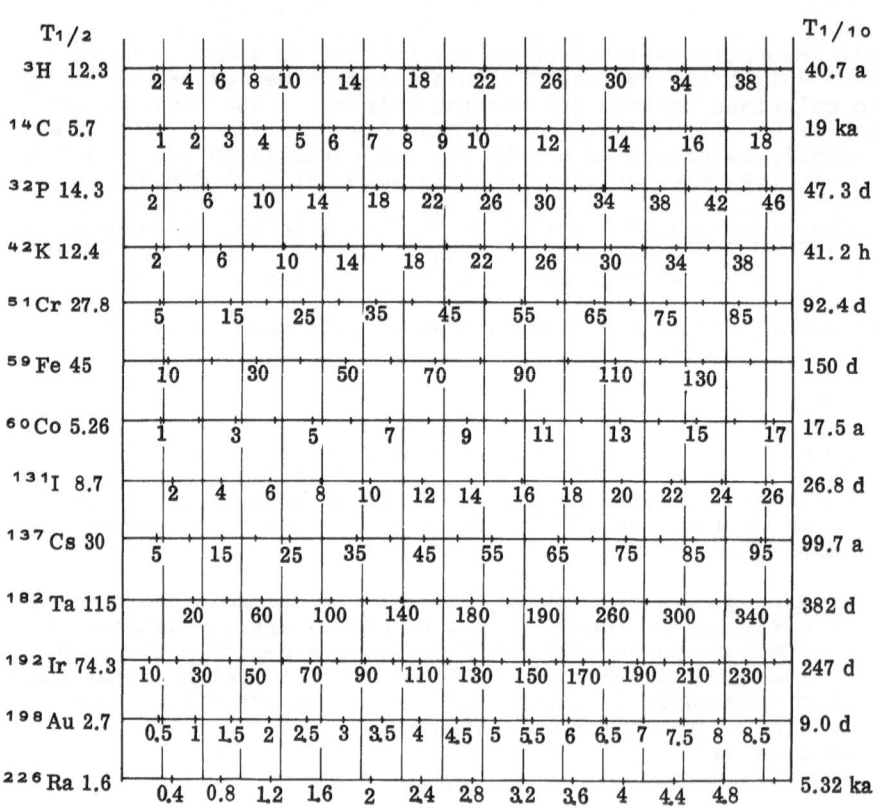

$T_{1/2}$		$T_{1/10}$
³H 12.3		40.7 a
¹⁴C 5.7		19 ka
³²P 14.3		47.3 d
⁴²K 12.4		41.2 h
⁵¹Cr 27.8		92.4 d
⁵⁹Fe 45		150 d
⁶⁰Co 5.26		17.5 a
¹³¹I 8.7		26.8 d
¹³⁷Cs 30		99.7 a
¹⁸²Ta 115		382 d
¹⁹²Ir 74.3		247 d
¹⁹⁸Au 2.7		9.0 d
²²⁶Ra 1.6		5.32 ka

6.4.1 Time required to reach a given residual activity
Zeit zum Erreichen einer bestimmten Restaktivität
Temps nécessaire pour atteindre une activité résiduelle
Tiempo necesario para alcanzar una actividad residual

Nuclide Nuklid Nucléide Nuclido	Time - Zeit - Temps - Tiempo h, d, a, ka									
	Residual activity - Restaktivität - Activité résiduelle - Actividad residual %									
	90	80	70	60	50	40	30	25	20	10
^{3}H	1.87	3.96	6.33	9.06	12.3	16.3	21.4	24.6	28.6	40.4 a
^{14}C	866	1.83	2.93	4.20	5.7	7.53	9.90	11.4	13.2	18.9 ka
^{32}P	2.17	4.60	7.36	10.5	14.3	18.9	24.8	28.6	33.2	47.5 d
^{42}K	1.88	3.99	6.38	9.14	12.4	16.4	21.5	24.8	28.8	41.2 h
^{51}Cr	4.23	8.95	14.3	20.5	27.8	36.7	48.3	55.6	64.6	92.4 d
^{59}Fe	6.84	14.5	23.2	33.2	45.0	59.5	78.2	90.0	104	150 d
^{60}Co	800	1.69	2.71	3.88	5.26	6.95	9.14	10.5	12.2	17.5 a
^{131}I	1.23	2.60	4.15	5.95	8.07	10.7	14.0	16.1	18.7	26.8 d
^{137}Cs	4.56	9.66	15.4	22.1	30.0	39.7	52.1	60.0	69.7	99.7 a
^{182}Ta	17.5	37.0	59.2	84.7	115	152	200	230	267	382 d
^{192}Ir	11.3	23.9	38.2	54.8	74.3	98.2	129	149	173	247 d
^{198}Au	410	869	1.39	1.99	2.70	3.57	4.69	5.40	6.27	8.97 d
^{226}Ra	243	515	823	1.18	1.60	2.12	2.78	3.20	3.72	5.32 ka

For half-lives of additional radionuclides see page 150
Die Halbwertzeiten weiterer Radionuklide siehe Seite 150
Pour les périodes des autres radionucléides, voir page 150
Periodo de vida media de otros radionúclidos, vease página 150

The residual activity of a radionuclide after a given time can be found in table 6.4.2. next page. For example I 131 after 18 days, it amounts to 21.3 % of the initial activity.

Die von einem Radionuklid nach einer bestimmten Zeit noch vorhandene Restaktivität läßt sich aus der Tabelle 6.4.2 herauslesen. Sie beträgt z.B. für J 131 nach 18 Tagen noch 21,3 % der Anfangsaktivität.

L'activité résiduelle d'un radionucléide peut être obtenue à partir de la table 6.4.2. Pour l'Iode 131, par ex. l'activité résiduelle après 18 jours est 21,3 % de l'activité initiale.

La actividad residual de un radionúclido que permanece después de un tiempo determinado se puede leer en la tabla 6.4.2. P. ej. para el I 131 después de 18 días, importa el 21,3 % de la actividad inicial.

6.4.2 Residual activity after different time intervals
Restaktivität nach verschieden langen Zeiten
Activité résiduelle après différents temps
Actividad residual después de diferentes periodos de tiempo

Residual activity in % of the initial activity – Restaktivität in % der Anfangsaktivität – Activité résiduelle en % de l'activité initiale – Actividad residual en % de la actividad inicial   Time – Zeit – Temps – Tiempo   %

Nuclide – Nuklid / Nucléide – Núclido $T_{1/2}$	col1	col2	col3	col4	col5	col6	col7	col8	col9	col10	unit
Time row A	0.5	1	2	3	4	5	6	7	8	9	
Time row B	10	12	14	16	18	20	22	24	26	28	
Time row C	30	35	40	45	50	55	60	65	70	75	
Time row D	80	90	100	110	120	130	140	150	160	170	
Time row E	200	230	260	290	320	350	380	410	440	470	
³H 12.3 a	97.2	94.5	89.3	84.4	79.8	75.4	71.3	67.4	63.7	60.2	a
	56.9	50.9	45.4	40.6	36.3	32.4	28.9	25.9	23.1	20.6	
¹⁴C 5.7 ka	94.1	88.6	78.4	69.4	61.5	54.4	48.2	42.7	37.8	33.5	ka
	29.6	23.2	18.2	14.3	11.2	8.79	6.89	5.40	4.24	3.32	
³²P 14.3 d	97.6	95.3	90.8	86.5	82.4	78.5	74.8	71.2	67.9	64.7	d
	61.6	55.9	50.7	46.1	41.8	37.9	34.4	31.2	28.4	25.7	
	23.4	18.3	14.4	11.3	8.86	6.95	5.46	4.28	3.36	2.64	
⁴²K 12.4 h	97.2	94.6	89.4	84.6	80.0	75.6	71.5	67.6	63.9	60.5	h
	57.2	51.1	45.7	40.9	36.6	32.7	29.2	26.1	23.4	20.9	
	18.7	14.1	10.7	8.08	6.11	4.62	3.49	2.64	2.0	1.51	
⁵¹Cr 27.8 d	98.8	97.5	95.1	92.8	90.5	88.3	86.1	84.0	81.9	79.9	d
	77.9	74.1	70.5	67.1	63.8	60.7	57.8	55.0	52.3	49.8	
	47.3	41.8	36.9	32.6	28.7	25.4	22.4	19.8	17.5	15.4	
⁵⁹Fe 45 d	99.2	98.5	97.0	95.5	94.0	92.6	91.2	89.8	88.4	87.1	d
	85.7	83.1	80.6	78.2	75.8	73.5	71.3	69.1	67.0	65.0	
	63.0	58.3	54.0	50.0	46.9	42.9	39.7	36.7	34.0	31.5	
	29.2	25.0	21.4	18.4	15.7	13.5	11.6	9.92	8.50	7.29	
⁶⁰Co 5.26 a	99.5	98.9	97.8	96.8	95.7	94.7	93.6	92.6	91.6	90.6	Mo *)
	89.6	87.7	85.7	83.9	82.1	80.3	78.5	76.8	75.2	73.5	
	71.9	68.1	64.5	61.0	57.7	54.7	51.7	49.0	46.4	43.9	
	41.5	37.2	33.3	29.9	26.8	24.0	21.5	19.3	17.3	15.5	
¹³¹I 8.07 d	95.8	91.8	84.2	77.3	70.9	65.1	59.7	54.8	50.3	46.2	d
	42.4	35.7	30.0	25.3	21.3	18.0	15.1	12.7	10.7	9.03	
¹³⁷Cs 30 a	98.9	97.7	95.5	93.3	91.2	89.1	87.1	85.1	83.1	81.2	a
	79.4	75.8	72.4	69.1	66.0	63.0	60.2	57.4	54.8	52.4	
¹⁸²Ta 115 d	94.2	93.0	91.9	90.8	89.7	88.6	87.6	86.5	85.5	84.5	d
	83.5	81.0	78.6	76.2	74.0	71.8	69.7	67.6	65.6	63.6	
	61.7	58.1	54.7	51.5	48.5	45.7	43.0	40.5	38.1	35.9	
	30.0	25.0	20.9	17.4	14.5	12.1	10.1	8.45	7.05	5.88	
¹⁹²Ir 74.3 d	99.5	99.1	98.2	97.2	96.3	95.4	94.6	93.7	92.8	92.0	d
	91.1	89.4	87.8	86.1	84.5	83.0	81.5	79.9	78.5	77.0	
	75.6	72.1	68.9	65.7	62.7	59.9	57.1	54.5	52.1	49.7	
	47.4	43.2	39.3	35.8	32.6	29.7	27.1	24.7	22.5	20.5	
¹⁹⁸Au 2.7 d	99.5	98.9	97.9	96.8	95.8	94.8	93.8	92.8	91.8	90.8	h
	89.9	88.0	86.1	84.3	82.5	80.7	79.0	77.4	75.7	74.1	h
	88.0	77.4	59.8	46.3	35.8	27.7	21.4	16.6	12.8	9.92	d

*) Months – Monate – Mois – Meses

6.5   Dosage of radium sources
       Dosierung von Radiumpräparaten
       Détermination de la dose des sources de radium
       Dosificación de fuentes de radio

6.5.1 Exposure rate of point sources
       Dosisleistung punktförmiger Präparate
       Débit d'exposition des sources ponctuelles
       Rendimiento de fuentes puntiformes

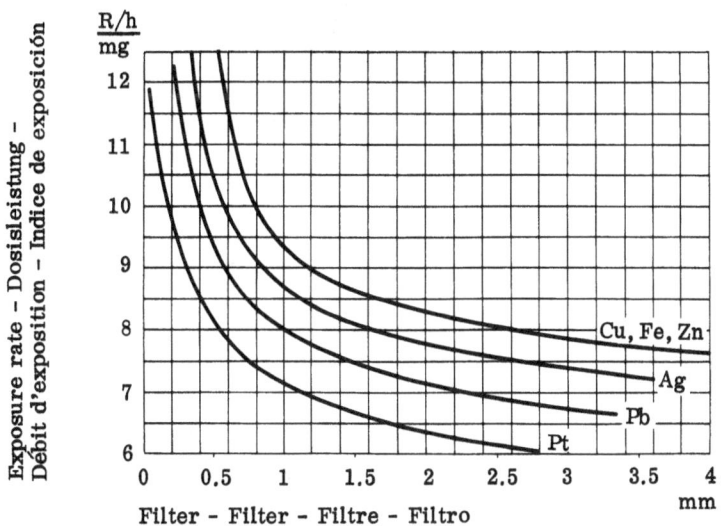

Filter - Filter - Filtre - Filtro

Filter Filter Filtre Filtro	Exposure rate at a distance of 1 cm from the source Dosisleistung in 1 cm Entfernung vom Präparat Débit d'exposition à 1 cm de distance de la source Indice d'exposición a 1 cm de distancia de la fuente			$\frac{R/h}{mg}$
	Filtration - Filterung - Filtration - Filtración			
mm	Pt	Pb	Ag	Cu,Fe,Zn
0.1	10.8	-	-	-
0.2	9.6	-	-	-
0.3	8.8	11.0	-	-
0.4	8.5	10.0	11.5	-
0.5	8.15	9.4	10.5	(13.0)
0.6	7.8	8.9	9.9	11.5
0.8	7.4	8.3	9.1	10.0
1.0	7.15	8.0	8.7	9.3
1.5	6.7	7.5	8.1	8.6
2.0	6.3	7.15	7.8	8.3
2.5	6.1	6.9	7.6	8.1
3.0	-	6.7	7.4	7.8
3.5	-	-	7.2	7.7
4.0	-	-	-	7.6

Lit.: 1. GLASSER, O. et al.: Physical Foundations of Radiol.,
         2. Edit., New York: Harper & Row 1952
      2. MITCHELL, R.G.: Brit.J.Radiol. 29, 631 (1956)
      3. MINDER, W.: Dosimetrie rad. Stoffe, Wien: Springer 1961

6.5.2 <u>Dosage of linear sources</u>
<u>Dosierung von linearen Präparaten</u>
<u>Doses pour des sources linéaires</u>
<u>Dosificación de fuentes lineales</u>

0.5 mm Pt Filtration - Filterung - Filtration - Filtración

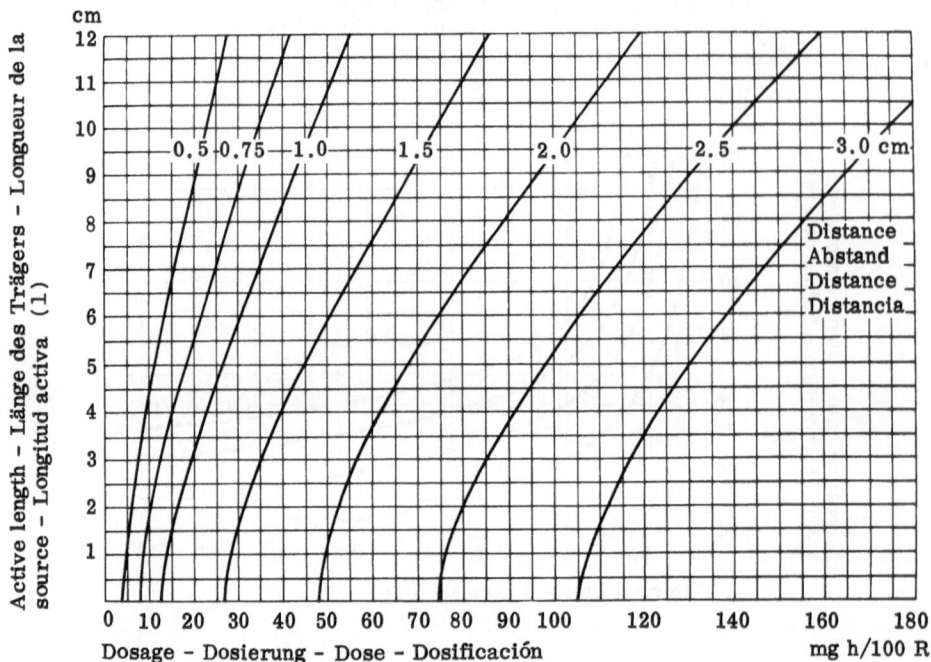

Active length - Länge des Trägers - Longueur de la source - Longitud activa (1)

Dosage - Dosierung - Dose - Dosificación   mg h/100 R

mg h required to give a dose of 100 R Zum Erreichen einer Dosis von 100 R erforderliche mg h mg h nécessaires pour obtenir une dose de 100 R mg h necesarios para alcanzar una dosis de 100 R							$\frac{\text{mg h}}{100\ \text{R}}$
l	Distance from source - Abstand vom Träger - Distance de la source - Distancia de la fuente						cm
cm	0.5	0.75	1.0	1.5	2.0	2.5	3.0
0.5	3.8	8.3	13	27	49	75	106
1	4.5	8.5	14	28	50	76	108
2	5.8	10	16	31	52	80	112
3	7.5	12	19	35	57	85	117
4	9.0	15	23	39	62	92	123
5	11	18	26	45	68	98	131
6	12	21	31	50	75	106	139
8	18	28	39	63	90	122	157
10	23	35	47	74	105	141	175
12	28	42	55	87	120	160	-

Lit.: 1. PATERSON, R., PARKER, H.M.: Brit.J.Radiol.<u>11</u>,252,313 (1938)
2. QUIMBY, E.H.: Radiology <u>43</u>, 572 (1944)
3. MEREDITH, W.J.: Radium Dosage, Edinburgh: Livingstone 1947
4. YOUNG, M.E.J., BATHO, H.F.: Brit.J.Radiol. 37, 38 (1964)
5. IAEA Atlas of Radiation Dose Distributions, IV, Vienna 1972

6.5.3 Dosage of planar sources
   Dosierung von flächigen Präparaten
   Doses pour des applicateurs plans
   Dosificación de fuentes planos

0.5 mm Pt Filtration - Filterung - Filtration - Filtración

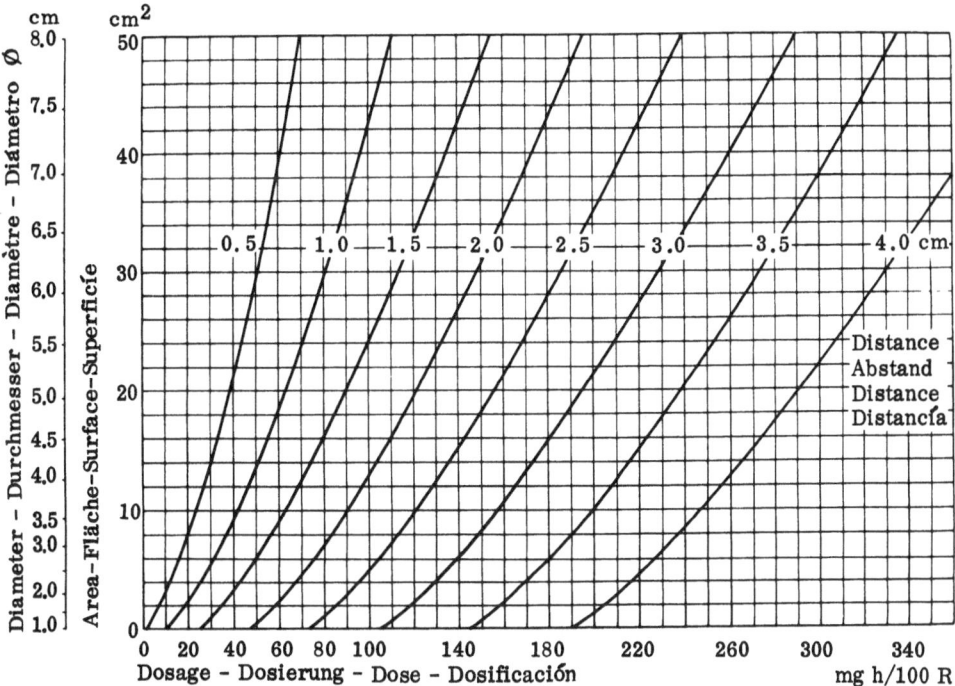

mg h/100 R

Dosage - Dosierung - Dose - Dosificación

mg h required to give a dose of 100 R Zum Erreichen einer Dosis von 100 R erforderliche mg h mg h nécessaires pour obtenir une dose de 100 R mg h necesarios para alcanzar una dosis de 100 R									$\frac{mg\ h}{100\ R}$

Ø cm	Area Fläche Surface Superficie cm²	Distance from source Abstand vom Träger Distance de la source Distancia de la fuente							cm
		0.5	1.0	1.5	2.0	2.5	3.0	3.5	4.0
1.6	2.0	7.2	18	35	58	85	119	159	204
2.3	4.0	12	25	43	67	96	130	170	217
2.8	6.0	16	32	50	75	105	140	181	228
3.2	8.0	20	36	56	83	113	150	190	238
3.6	10	23	42	63	90	121	158	200	247
4.4	15	31	53	77	107	139	177	220	270
5.0	20	38	63	90	122	156	196	239	292
5.7	25	45	73	102	135	172	213	257	312
6.2	30	51	81	114	148	187	230	274	331
6.7	35	56	89	124	161	200	246	291	350
7.1	40	61	96	135	173	214	261	307	(367)
7.6	45	64	104	145	185	227	276	323	-
8.0	50	70	111	154	196	240	290	336	-

Lit.: See pages - Siehe Seiten - Voir pages - Ver páginas 163/164

6.5.4   Evaluation of the minimum dose in interstitial therapy
        Ermittlung der Minimaldosis bei Spickung
        Evaluation de la dose minimale pour les applications inter-
        stitielles
        Evaluación de la dosis minima en el applicación intersticial

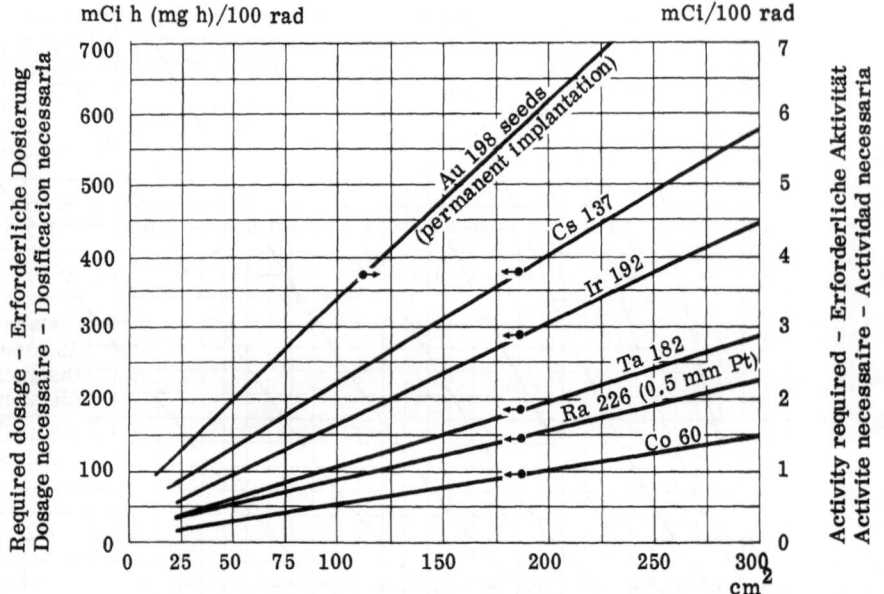

Surface of the target volume - Oberfläche des Zielvolumens
Surface du volume cible - Superficie de la volumen blanco

mg h (mCi h) required to obtain 100 rad in the target volume
Zum Erreichen von 100 rad im Zielvolumen erforderliche mg h (mCi h)
mg h (mCi h) nécéssaires pour obtenir 100 rad dans le volume-cible
mg h (mCi h) necessarios para obtener 100 rad dentro del volumen
blanco

Nuclide Nuklid Nucléide Nuclido	Surface area of the target volume - Oberfläche des Zielvolumens - Surface du volume cible - Superficie de la volumen blanco cm^2						
	25	50	100	150	200	250	300
Radium 226; 0.5 mm Pt (mg h/100 rad)	35	56	87	122	156	192	225
Co 60 (mCi h/100 rad)	16	28	52	74	102	125	150
Ta 182 "	38	61	105	151	195	240	280
Ir 192 "	62	95	165	235	305	375	445
Cs 137 "	90	133	220	310	406	490	570
Au 198 (mCi/100 rad)	1.30	2.00	3.35	4.75	6.20	7.60	8.90

Lit.: 1. LAUGHLIN, J.S., et al.: Am.J.Roentgenol. 89, 470 (1963)
      2. GOODWIN, P.N., QUIMBY, E.M., MORGAN, R.H.: Physical Founda-
         tions of Radiology, New York, London: Harper and Row 1970
      3. BUSCH, M.: Strahlenther., Sonderband 64 (1967)
      4. DIN 6809/2, Berlin: Beuth-Verlag 1975
See also - Siehe auch - Voir aussi - Ver tambien 163 - 164

6.6 <u>I 131 activity required for irradiation of the thyroid gland with a specified dose</u>

<u>Erforderliche J 131 Aktivität zur Bestrahlung der Schilddrüse mit einer bestimmten Dosis</u>

<u>Activité d'I 131 nécessaire pour obtenir une dose donnée dans la thyroide</u>

<u>Actividad necesaria del I 131 para obtener una dosis deseada en la glándula tiroidea</u>

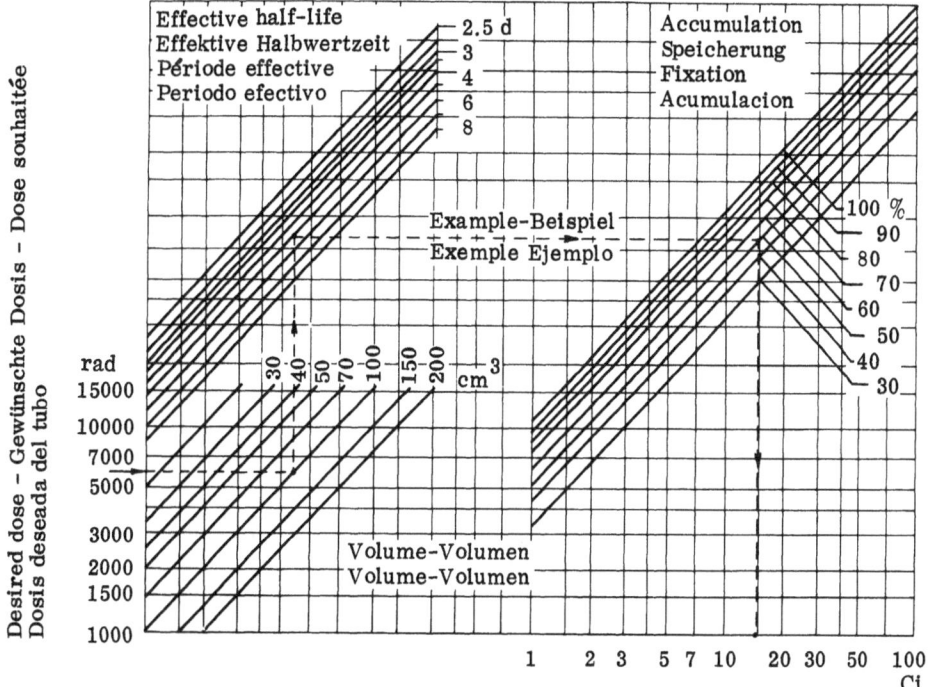

Activity required - Erforderliche Aktivität - Activite nécessaire - Actividad necesaria

Effective half-life and the accumulation must be determined in n each individual case by the iodine uptake test before administration of the therapeutic dose. The dotted line shows an example.

Die effektive Halbwertzeit und die Speicherung müssen in jedem Einzelfall vor der Verabreichung der therapeutischen Dosis durch den Jodtest bestimmt werden. Die gestrichelte Linie zeigt ein Beispiel.

La période effective et la fixation doivent êtra déterminées pour chaque cas particulier grâce aux tests à I 131 avant l'administration de la dose thérapeutique.

El valor del tiempo promedio efectivo y la acumulación se establecerán en cada caso individualmente antes de la administración de la dosis terapeútica por la prueba de compresión. La línea punteada muestra un ejemplo.

Lit.: 1. JOYET, G., MILLER, N.: Ann.Radiol. <u>5</u>, 21 (1962)

6.7 Exposure rate during handling of Tc 99m and I 131 sources
Dosisleistung beim Umgang mit Tc 99m und J 131
Débit d'exposition à distance de sources de Tc 99m et de I 131
Exposición en trato con fuentes de Tc 99m y I 131

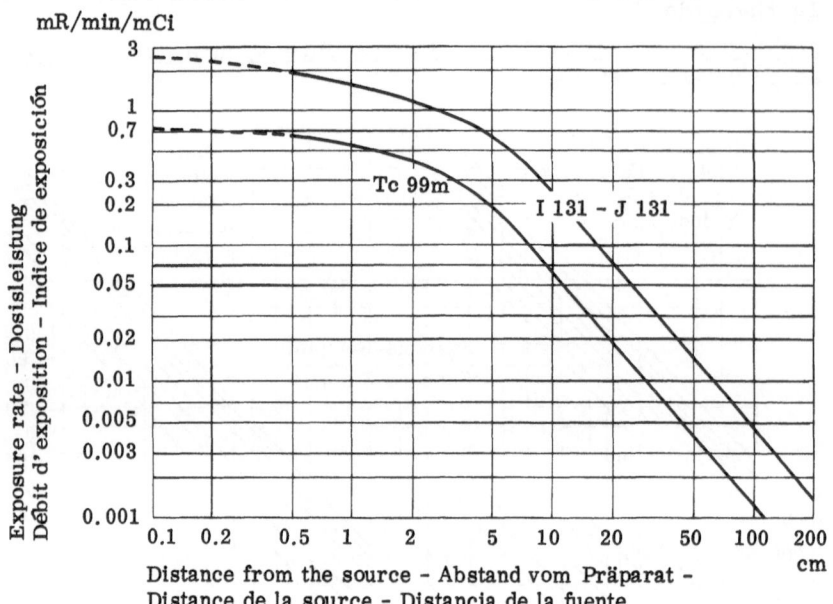

mR/min/mCi

Exposure rate – Dosisleistung – Indice de exposición
Débit d'exposition – Indice de exposición

Distance from the source – Abstand vom Präparat –
Distance de la source – Distancia de la fuente

Distance Abstand Distance Distancia	Exposure rate – Dosisleistung – Débit d'exposition – Indice de exposición						mR/min	
	For activity of – Bei einer Aktivität – Pour une activité – Con una actividad						mCi	
cm	1	2	5	10	20	50	100	150
Tc 99m								
0.1	(0.75)	(1.5)	(3.75)	(7.5)	(15)	(38)	(75)	(113)
0.2	(0.70)	(1.4)	(3.5)	(7.0)	(14)	(35)	(70)	(105)
0.5	0.65	1.3	3.25	6.5	13	32.5	65	98
1	0.55	1.1	2.75	5.5	11	27.5	55	83
2	0.42	0.84	2.10	4.2	8.4	21.0	42	63
5	0.19	0.38	0.95	1.9	3.8	9.5	19	29
10	0.052	0.104	0.26	0.52	1.04	2.6	5.2	7.8
20	0.019	0.038	0.095	0.19	0.38	0.95	1.9	2.9
50	0.004	0.008	0.020	0.040	0.08	0.20	0.40	0.60
100	0.0013	0.0026	0.007	0.013	0.26	0.07	0.13	0.20
150	0.0008	0.0016	0.004	0.008	0.016	0.04	0.08	0.12
I 131 – J 131								
0.1	(2.5)	(5.0)	(12.5)	(25)	(50)	(125)	(250)	(375)
0.2	(2.3)	(4.6)	(11.5)	(23)	(46)	(115)	(230)	(345)
0.5	1.9	3.8	9.5	19	38	95	190	285
1	1.6	3.2	8.0	16	32	80	160	240
2	1.2	2.4	6.0	12	24	60	120	180
5	0.65	1.3	3.2	6.5	13	32	65	98
10	0.25	0.5	1.25	2.5	5	12.5	25	38
20	0.075	0.15	0.37	0.75	1.5	3.7	7.5	11.2
50	0.015	0.03	0.075	0.15	0.3	0.75	1.5	2.25
100	0.0045	0.009	0.022	0.045	0.09	0.22	0.45	0.68
150	0.0027	0.0054	0.0135	0.027	0.054	0.135	0.27	0.40

6.8   Exposure rate in the vicinity of patients treated with I 131
Dosisleistung in der Umgebung von J 131-Patienten
Débit d'exposition au voisinage des malades traités par I 131
Exposición en la vecindad de pacientes tratados con I 131

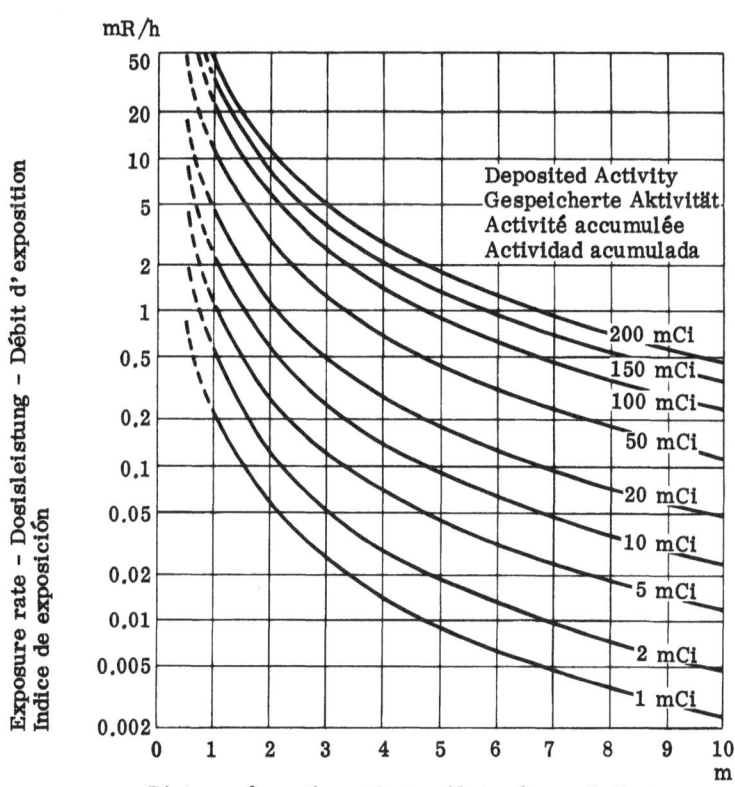

Distance from the patient - Abstand vom Patienten
Distance du malade - Distanica del paciente D

Distance Abstand Distance Distancia D m	Exposure rate - Dosisleistung - Débit d'exposition - Indice de exposición mR/h								
	When activity of ^{131}I deposited in the thyroid gland is - Bei einer in der Schilddrüse gespeicherten ^{131}J Aktivität von - Pour une activité d' ^{131}I fixée dans la thyroide de - Por una actividad de ^{131}I acumulada en la glandula tiroides de: mCi								
	1	2	5	10	20	50	100	150	200
0.5	(0.9)	(1.8)	(4.5)	(9.0)	(18)	(45)	(90)	(140)	(180)
1	0.23	0.46	1.15	2.3	4.6	11.5	23	35	46
1.5	0.10	0.20	0.50	1.0	2.0	5.0	10	15	20
2	0.06	0.12	0.29	0.58	1.2	2.9	5.8	8.6	11.5
3	0.026	0.05	0.13	0.26	0.51	1.28	2.56	3.8	5.1
4	0.014	0.028	0.072	0.14	0.29	0.72	1.44	2.16	2.88
5	0.009	0.018	0.046	0.092	0.18	0.46	0.92	1.38	1.84
6	0.006	0.012	0.032	0.064	0.13	0.32	0.64	0.96	1.28
7	0.005	0.010	0.024	0.047	0.094	0.24	0.47	0.70	0.94
8	0.004	0.007	0.018	0.036	0.072	0.18	0.36	0.54	0.72
10	0.002	0.005	0.012	0.023	0.046	0.12	0.23	0.35	0.46

6.9 Dose to critical organs in different scanning procedures - Strahlenbelastung der kritischen Organe bei verschiedenen szintigraphischen Untersuchungen - Doses aux organes critiques pour différents examens scintigraphiques - Dosis en órganos críticos en diferentes examenes scintigraficos

Organ Organ Organe Organo	1.	2.	3.	$T_{1/2}$	Chemical form Verbindung Forme chimique Especie química	Activity Aktivität Activité Actividad μCi	Critical organs Kritische Organe Organes critiques Organos críticos	Dose Dosis Dose Dosis rad
Brain Hirn Cerveau Cerebro	^{131}I ^{131}J	β⁻,γ	1-24 h	8.0 h	Serum albumin	350-500	Blood-Blut-Sang-Sangre Thyreoidea Whole body-Ganzkörper-Corps entier-Todo el cuerpo	2.5-3.5 7-25 0.7-1
	^{203}Hg	β⁻,γ	2-24 h	47 d	Neohydrin	750	Kidneys-Nieren-Reins-Rinones	315
	^{197}Hg	K,γ	2-4 h	27 d	Neohydrin	750	"	32
					HgCl₂	750	"	48
	^{99m}Tc	γ	30 min	6.0 h	Pertechnetat	5000-10000	Intestine-Darm-Intestin-Intestino	1
Heart Herz Coeur Corazón	^{131}I ^{131}J	β⁻,γ	5-10 min	8.0 d	Serum albumin	300-400	Blood-Blut-Sang-Sangre Thyreoidea Whole body-Ganzkörper-Corps entier-Todo el cuerpo	2-2.8 6-20 0.6-0.8
	^{99m}Tc	γ	5 min	6.0 h	Serum albumin	3000-4000	Blood-Blut-Sang-Sangre Whole body-Ganzkörper-Corps entier-Todo el cuerpo	0.5 0.2
	^{113m}In	γ	10 min	5 min	Serum albumin	1000-3000	"	0.015
Liver Leber Foie Higado	^{198}Au	β⁻,γ	30 min	2.7 d	Colloidal Au	150-400	Liver-Leber-Foie-Higado Spleen-Milz-Rate-Bazo	6-20 3.5-30
	^{131}I ^{131}J	β⁻,γ	10-20 min	8.0 d	Rose bengal	100-300	Liver-Leber-Foie-Higado Thyreoidea	0.1-0.3 5-15
	^{99m}Tc	γ	15-20 min	6.0 h	Colloidal Au	1000-3000	Liver-Leber-Foie-Higado Spleen-Milz-Rate-Bazo	0.3-1.6 0.2-1.3

1. Isotope - Isotope - Isotope - Isótopo   2. Type of decay - Zerfallsart - Type de décroissance - Tipo de desintegración   3. Time between application and examination - Zeit zwischen Verabreichung und Untersuchung - Temps entre l'administration et l'examen - Tiempo entre la administración y examen

Organ	Isotope	Radiation			Compound	Activity	Critical organ	Dose
Lungs / Lungen / Poumons / Pulmones	131I / 131J	β⁻,γ	5 min	8.0 h	Makroagg.HSA	300	Lungs-Lungen-Poumons-Pulmones Thyreoidea	∿5 local 20-30
	51Cr	K,γ	0.5-3 h	28 d	Makroagg.HSA	1000	Lungs-Lungen-Poumons-Pulmones	3-5
	90mTc	γ	0.5-3 h	6.0 h	Makroagg.HSA Colloid	1000-2000	"	0.6
Lymph nodes / Lymphknoten / Ganglions / Nud.linfát.	198Au	β⁻,γ	24 h	2.7 d	Colloidal Au	200	Site of injection / Injektionsstelle / Point d'injection / Lugar de la inyección	200-5000
Spleen / Milz / Rate / Bazo	51Cr	K	30 min	28 d	Erythrocytes	400-1000	Spleen-Milz-Rate-Bazo	12-20
	197Hg	K	1 h	2.7 d	BMPH incub. Blood,Blut	300-500	Kidneys-Nieren-Reins-Rinones	20-23
Kidneys / Nieren / Reins / Rinones	203Hg	β	1 h	47 d	Neotydrin	100-150	"	42-63
					Salyrgan	100-160	"	16-24
	197Hg	K	1 h	2.7 d	Neohydrin	100-200	"	6.3-8.4
					HgCl2	200-300	"	13-16
	99mTc	γ	1 h	6.0 h	Tc-Fe Komplex	2000	"	1.2
Thyreoidea	131I	β⁻	24-48 h	8.0 d	NaJ	25-100	Thyreoidea	25-50
	125I	K	24-48 h	60 d	NaJ	15-50	Thyreoidea	6-18
	99mTc	γ	20-30 min	6.0 h	Pertechnetat	500-1000	Thyreoidea Intestine-Darm-Intestin-Intestino	0.1-0.2 0.1-0.2
Bone / Knochen / Os / Huesos	85Sr	K	24 h	65 d	Sr(NO3)2 SrCL2	50-100	Bone-Knochen-Os-Huesos	2-4
	87mSr	IT	3-4 h	2.8 h	Sr(NO3)2	3000	Bone-Knochen-Os-Huesos	0.3
	99mTc	γ	2-4 h	6.0 h	Polyphosphat	5000-10000	Bladder-Blase-Vessie-Vejiga	1-2
	18F	β⁺,EC	1-3 h	1.8 h	Fluorid	2000-3000	Stomach-Magen-Estomac-Estómago / Bladder-Blase-Vessie-Vejiga	1-1.5 4-6
Tumor diagnosis	67Ga	K,EC	2-3 d	78 h	Citrat	2000-3000	Bone marrow-Knochenmark / Moelle-Médula / Liver-Leber-Foie-Higado	1-2

171

6.10 Radionuclide generators
Radionuklid Generatoren
Générateurs de radionucléide
Sistemas generadores de radionúclidos

Parent – Mutter – Père – Padre				Daughter – Tochter – Fils – Hijo			
Nuclide Nuklid Nucléide Núclido	*) $T_{1/2}$	**)	γ-Energy γ-Energie γ-Energie γ-Energía keV	Nuclide Nuklid Nucléide Núclido	*) $T_{1/2}$	**)	γ-Energy γ-Energie γ-Energie γ-Energía keV
^{99}Mo	2.8 d	β^-,γ	740 780	^{99m}Tc	6 h	γ	140
^{113}Sm	118 d	EC,γ	255	^{113m}In	1.7 h	γ	393
^{132}Te	3.2 d	β^-,γ	230	^{132}I	2.3 h	β^-,γ	670
^{87}Y	3.3 d	EC,β^+,γ	483	^{87m}Sr	2.8 h	γ	388
^{68}Ge	275 d	EC	–	^{68}Ga	68 min	β^+,γ	511
^{137}Cs	30 a	β^-	–	^{137m}Ba	2.6 min	γ	662
^{81}Rb	4.7 h	EC,β^+,γ	–	^{81m}Kr	13 s	γ	190
^{77}Br	58 h	β^-,γ	240 520	^{77m}Se	18 s	γ	161
^{191}Os	16 d	γ	130	^{191m}Ir	4.9 s	γ	129

*) $T_{1/2}$ = Time in which 1/2 of the radioactive atoms disintegrate (radioactive half-life)
Zeit, in der die Hälfte der radioaktiven Atome zerfallen sind
Temps au bout duquel la moitié des atomes radioactifs se sont désintégrés
Tiempo en el cual la mitad de los átomos radioactivos se desintegran

**) = Type of decay
Zerfallsart
Type de désintégration
Tipo de decaimiento

EC = Electron capture
Elektroneneinfang
Capture électronique
Captura de electrones

6.11 Some formulas used in counting statistics
Einige Formeln zur Zählstatistik
Quelques formules utilisées en statistiques
Algunas fórmulas para el tratamiento estadístico de datos

Arithmetic mean of a set of data $(x_1 \ldots x_i \ldots x_n)$
Arithmetischer Mittelwert eines Datensatzes $(x_1 \ldots x_i \ldots x_n)$
Moyenne arithmétique d'un ensemble de données $(x_1 \ldots x_i \ldots x_n)$
Media aritmética de un conjunto de valores $(x_1 \ldots x_i \ldots x_n)$

$$\bar{x} = \frac{1}{n} \sum_{i=1}^{n} x_i$$

Standard deviation of a set of data
Standardabweichung eines Datensatzes
Ecart type pour un ensemble de données
Desviación standard de un conjunto de datos

$$s_x^2 = \frac{1}{n-1} \left\{ \sum_{i=1}^{n} x_i^2 - \frac{\left(\sum_{i=1}^{n} x_i \right)^2}{n} \right\} ; \quad s_x = \sqrt{s_x^2}$$

Standard deviation of the mean
Standardabweichung des Mittelwertes
Ecart type de la moyenne
Desviación standard del valor medio

$$s_{\bar{x}} = \frac{s_x}{\sqrt{n}}$$

Covariance of two sets of data $(x_1 \ldots x_i \ldots x_n \ldots)$ and $(x_1 \ldots y_i \ldots y_n)$
Kovarianz zweier Datensätze $(x_1 \ldots x_i \ldots x_n)$ und $(y_1 \ldots y_i \ldots y_n)$
Covariance de deux ensembles de données $(x_1 \ldots x_i \ldots x_n)$ et $(y_1 \ldots y_i \ldots y_n)$
Covariancia de dos series de valores $(x_1 \ldots x_i \ldots x_n)$ y $(y_1 \ldots y_i \ldots y_n)$

$$s_{xy} = \frac{1}{n-1} \sum_{i=1}^{n} (x_i - \bar{x})(y_i - \bar{y}) = \frac{1}{n-1} \left\{ \sum x_i y_i - \frac{1}{n} \sum x_i \sum y_i \right\}$$

Correlation coefficient of two sets of data
Korrelationskoeffizient zweier Datensätze
Coefficient de correlation entre deux ensembles de données
Coeficiente de correlación de dos conjuntos de valores

$$r_{xy} = \frac{s_{xy}}{s_x s_y}$$

Poisson distribution - Poissonverteilung
Distribution de Poisson - Distribución de Poisson

$$P(x) = \frac{\bar{x}^x d^{-\bar{x}}}{x!}$$

173

Normal distribution - Normalverteilung
Distribution normale - Distribución normal

$$P(x) = \frac{1}{\sqrt{2\pi s_x}} \; e^{-\frac{(x-\bar{x})^2}{2s_x^2}}$$

Standard deviation of a Poisson or normal distribution
Standardabweichung einer Poisson oder Normalverteilung
Ecart type pour une distribution de Poisson ou pour une distribution normale
Desviación standard de una distribución de Poisson o normal

$$s_x = \sqrt{\bar{x}} \approx \sqrt{x}$$

Probability (W) that $\bar{x}$ lies in an interval $x \pm k \cdot s_x$
Wahrscheinlichkeit (W), daß $\bar{x}$ in einem Intervall $x \pm k \cdot s_x$ liegt
Probabilité (W) pour que $\bar{x}$ soit dans l'intervalle $x \pm k \cdot s_x$
Probabilidad (W) de que $\bar{x}$ este en un intervalo $x \pm k \cdot s_x$

k	0.675	1	1.65	2	2.58	3
W (%)	50	68.3	90	95.4	99	99.73

Standard deviation for difference of measured values
Standardabweichung für die Differenz von Meßwerten
Ecart type pour des différences de mesures
Desviación standard de la diferencia de valores experimentales

$$s_f = \sqrt{s_x^2 + x_y^2} \qquad f = x - y$$

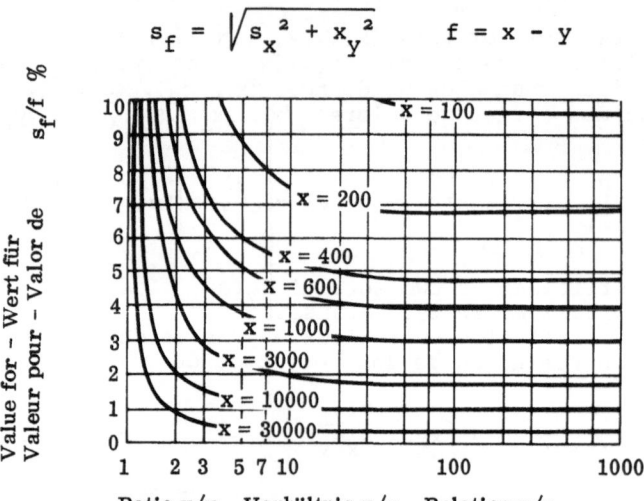

Ratio x/y - Verhältnis x/y - Relation x/y
Relación x/y

Lit.: 1. BURINGTON, R.: Handbook of Mathematical Tables and
          Formulas, New York, St.Louis, San Francisco, Toronto,
          London: Mc Graw-Hill 1965
       2. SACHS, L.: Statistische Auswertungsmethoden, Berlin,
          Heidelberg, New York: Springer Verlag 1969

Table of contents - Inhaltsverzeichnis
Table des matières - Tabla de materias

7.1　Factors affecting patient exposure
　　　Faktoren, die die Patientenexposition beeinflussen
　　　Facteurs intervenant sur l'exposition du malade
　　　Factores que influyen en la exposición de los pacientes

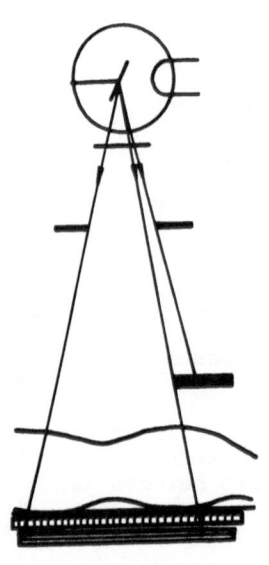

Kilovoltage - Spannung
Tension - Tensión

Tube current - Röhrenstrom
Courant du tube - Corriente del tubo

Filter - Filter - Filtre - Filtro

Collimator - Blende
Diaphragme - Colimador

Focus-film distance - Fokus-Film-Abstand
Distance foyer-film
Distancia foco-película

Shielding - Abdeckung
Écran de protection - Placa de protección

Grid - Streustrahlenraster
Grille antidiffusante - Parrilla antidifusora

Film/intensifying screens
Film/Verstärkerfolien
Film/écrans renforçateurs
Pelicula/cartulinas de refuerzo

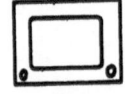

Image amplifier-TV - Bildverstärker-FS
Amplificateur de brillance-TV
Intensificador de imagen-TV

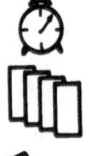

Fluoroscopic exposure time - Durchleuchtungs-
zeit - Durée de la radioscopie - Tiempo de la
radioscopia

Number of radiographs - Anzahl der Aufnahmen
Nombre de clichés - Cantidad de radiografias

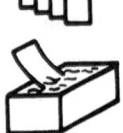

Development - Entwicklung
Développement - Revelado

Lit.: 1. SEELENTAG, W.: Dtsch.med.Wschr. 86, 2513 (1961)
　　　2. TER-POGOSSIAN, M.: The physical aspects of diagnosic radio-
　　　　 logy, New York, Evanston, London: Hoeber Medical Div. 1967
　　　3. DUTREIX, J., BISMUTH, V., LAVAL-JEANTET, M.: Traité de
　　　　 Radiodiagnostic, Vol. 1, Paris: Masson & Cie. 1969
　　　4. STIEVE, F.E.: Strahlenschutz in Forschung und Praxis 10,
　　　　 148 (1970)

7.2 Recommended kilovoltage ranges for radiography
Empfehlenswerte Spannungsbereiche für Röntgenaufnahmen
Domaines de tensions recommandés pour les radiographies
Márgenes de tensión recomendables para las radiografías

		kV	
Grid – Streustrahlenraster – grille antidiffusante – parilla antidifusora	Without-ohne-sans-sin	25 – 35	Mammography - Mammographie Mammographie - Mamografía
		40 – 50	Soft tissue (leg, neck) Weichteile (Bein, Hals) Parties molles (jambe, cou) Partes blandas (pierna, cuello)
	With – mit – avec – con	60 – 75	Petrous bone, cervical spine, shoulder, thorax, gall bladder, kidneys, knee, lower leg Felsenbein, Halswirbelsäule, Schulter, Thorax, Gallenblase, Nieren, Knie, Unterschenkel Rocher, colonne cervicale, épaule, thorax, vésicule biliaire, reins, genou partie inférieure de la jambe Hueso occipital, raquis cervical, hombro, thorax, vejiga biliar, rinon, rodilla, pierna
		75 – 90	Skull, thoracic and lumbar spine a.p., lung (children), trachea a.p., pelvis, femur Schädel, Brust- und Lendenwirbelsäule a.p., Lunge (Kinder), Trachea a.p., Becken, Oberschenkel Crâne, colonne dorsale et lombaire a.p., poumon (enfants), trachée-artère a.p., bassin, fémur Cráneo, raquis dorsal y lumbar a.p., pulmon (ninos), traquéa a.p., pelvis, femur
		90 – 125	Lung, lumbar spine lat., trachea lat., stomach, small intestine, colon, obstetric radiography Lunge, Lendenwirbelsäule und Trachea seitl., Magen, Dünndarm, Dickdarm, Schwangerschaftsaufnahmen Poumon, colonne lombaire lat., trachée-artère lat., estomac, intestin grêle, colon, radiographie obstétrique Pulmón, raquis lumbar lat., tráques lat., éstomago, intestino delgado, colon, radiografia obstetrica
		125 – 150	Lung lat. - Lunge seitl. Poumon lat. - Pulmón lat.

Lit.: 1. WIDENMANN, L.: Radiography 29, 81 (1963)
      2. ELEGEM van, P.: J. Belge Radiol. 55, 271 (1972)

7.3   Conversion factors for radiography
Umrechnungsfaktoren für Röntgenaufnahmen
Facteurs de conversion pour la radiographie
Factores de conversión para la radiografía

7.3.1   Variation of mAs with tube voltage
mAs-Produkt bei Änderung der Röhrenspannung
Variation du nombre de mAs avec la tension d'alimentation
Producto mAs con el cambio del voltaje del tubo

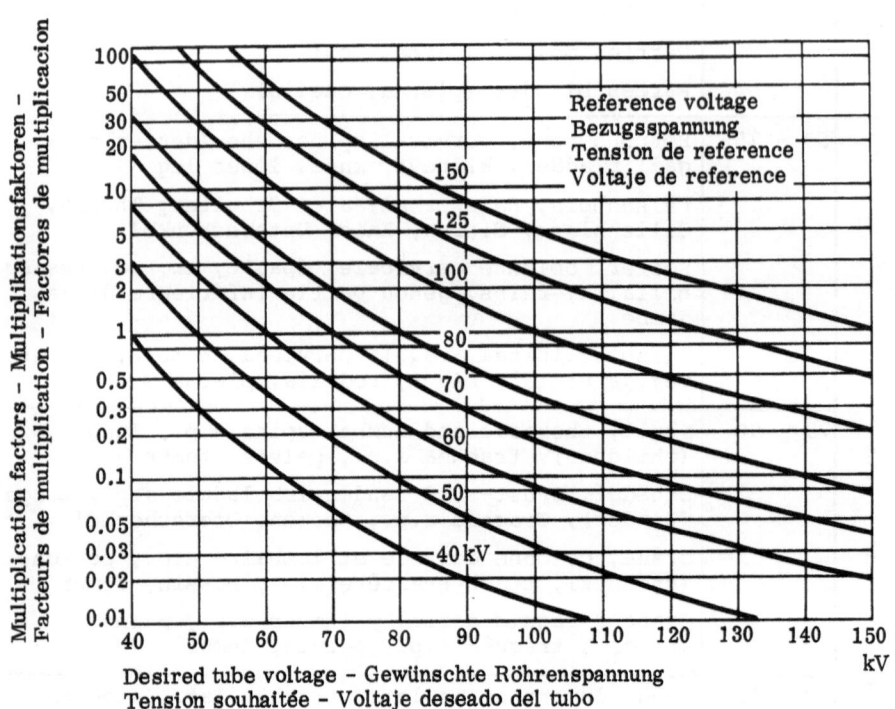

Desired tube voltage - Gewünschte Röhrenspannung
Tension souhaitée - Voltaje deseado del tubo

Reference voltage Bezugs-spannung Tension de réference Voltaje de reference	Multiplication factors - Multiplikationsfaktoren - Facteurs de multiplication - Factores de multiplicación f_{kV}								
	Desired tube voltage - Gewünschte Röhrenspannung - Tension souhaitée - Voltaje deseado del tubo kV								
	40	50	60	70	80	90	100	125	150
40 kV	1	0.3	0.13	0.06	0.03	0.016	0.014	0.0051	0.0021
50 kV	3.05	1	0.40	0.19	0.10	0.05	0.03	0.013	0.0051
60 kV	7.6	2.49	1	0.46	0.24	0.13	0.09	0.037	0.020
70 kV	16.4	5.4	2.2	1	0.53	0.28	0.19	0.077	0.037
80 kV	32	10.5	4.2	1.95	1	0.56	0.37	0.15	0.072
90 kV	57.6	19	7.6	3.51	1.80	1	0.66	0.27	0.13
100 kV	87.5	28.7	11.5	5.34	2.74	1.52	1	0.41	0.20
125 kV	214	70	28	13	6.7	3.7	2.44	1	0.48
150 kV	442	145	58	27	13.8	7.7	5.05	2.07	1

7.3.2 <u>Variation of mAs with changing focus-film-distance (FFD)</u>
       <u>mAs-Produkt bei Änderung des Fokus-Film-Abstandes (FFA)</u>
       <u>Variation du nombre de mAs avec la distance foyer-film (DFF)</u>
       <u>Cambio de la mAs con la distancia foco-película (DFP)</u>

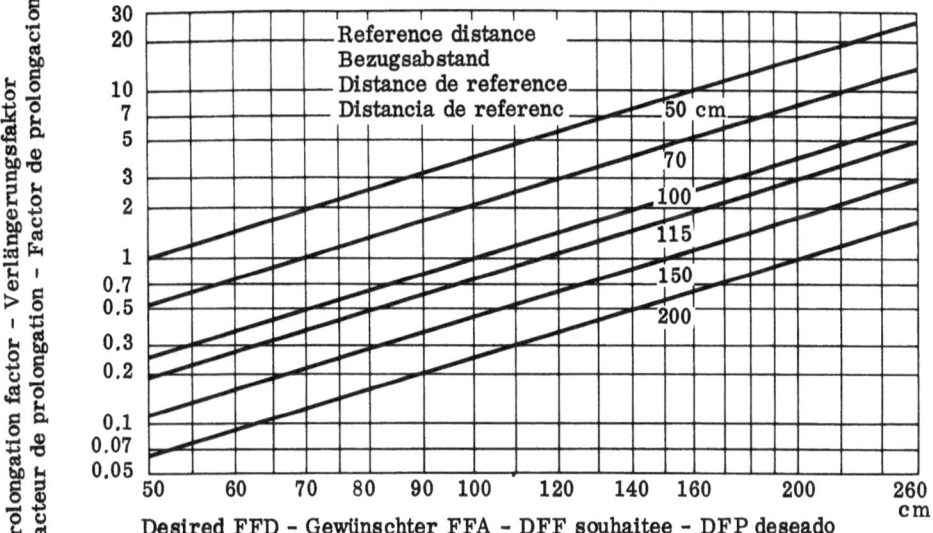

Desired FFD - Gewünschter FFA - DFF souhaitee - DFP deseado

7.3.3 <u>mAs when body thickness differs from a given value d</u>
       <u>mAs bei einer gegenüber dem Wert d abweichenden Körperdicke</u>
       <u>mAs quand l'épaisseur de corps diffère d'une valeur d donnée</u>
       <u>mAs cuando el espesor del cuerpo difiere de un valor d dado</u>

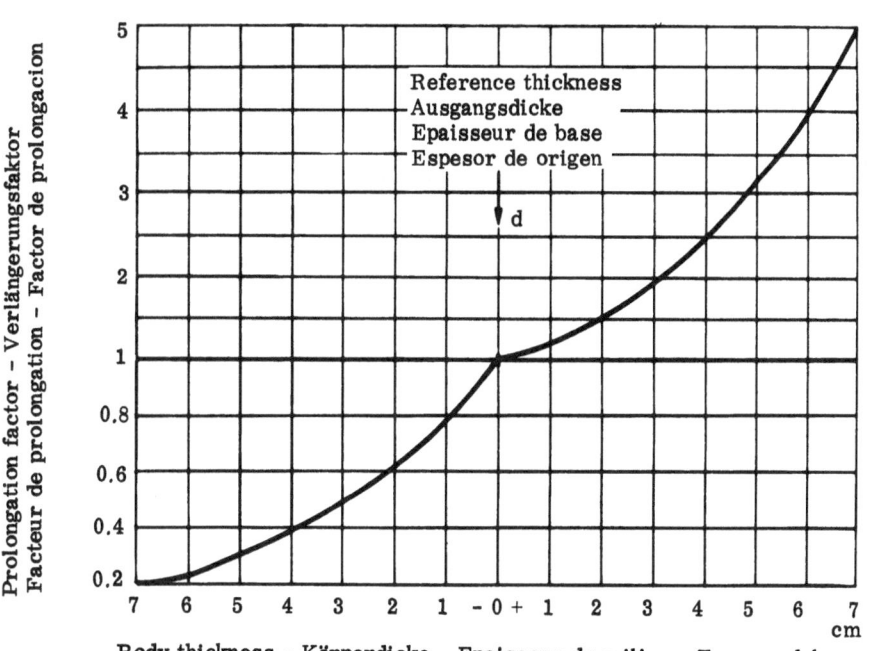

Body thickness - Körperdicke - Epaisseur du milieu - Expesor del cuerpo

7.4 Prolongation factors for exposure time in radiography with the use of antidiffusion grids (grid factors)

Verlängerungsfaktoren für die Belichtungszeit von Röntgenaufnahmen bei Verwendung von Streustrahlenrastern (Rasterfaktoren)

Facteurs pour l'accroissement du temps de pose en radiographie avec des grilles antidiffusantes (facteurs de grille)

Factores de prolongación para el tiempo de exposición usando rejillas antidifusoras (factores de rejilla)

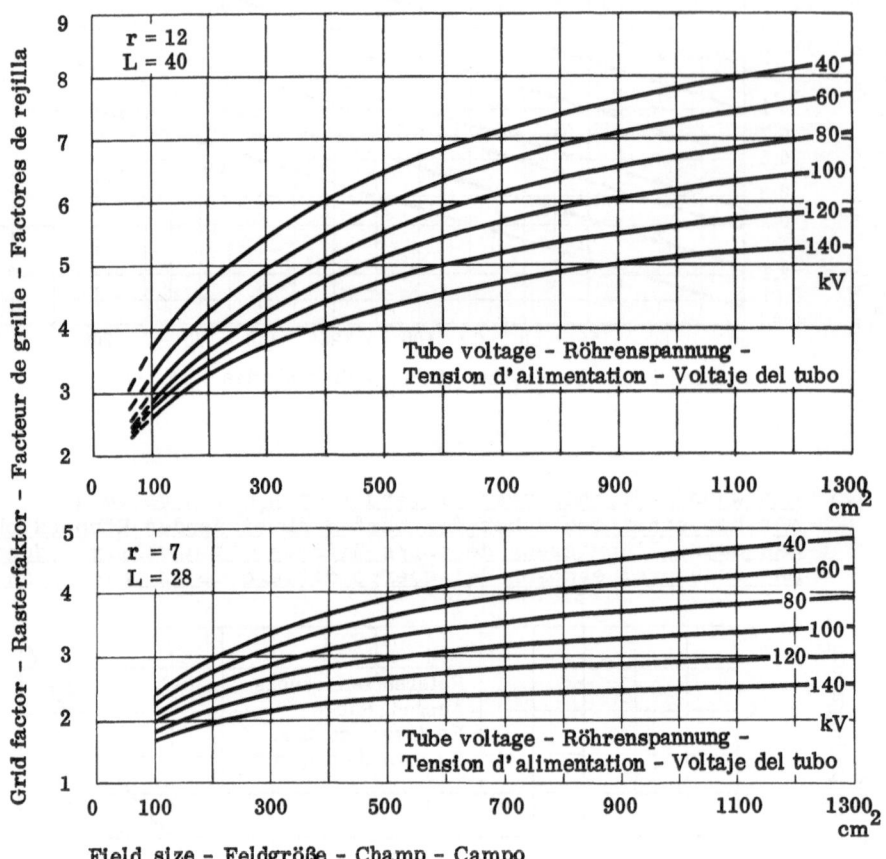

Field size - Feldgröße - Champ - Campo

r = Grid ratio - Schachtverhältnis - Rapport de grille - Razón de rejilla

L = Lines/cm - Linien/cm - Lames/cm - Lineas/cm

The values given in the graphs are valid for a 17 cm thick body (water phantom).

Die aus den graphischen Darstellungen zu entnehmenden Werte gelten für einen Körper (Wasserphantom) von 17 cm Dicke.

Les valeurs données dans les graphiques sont valables pour un corps (eau) de 17 cm d'épaisseur.

Los valores indicados en las gráficas son válidos para un cuerpo (muneco de agua) de un grosor de 17 cm.

7.5 <u>Nomogram for estimating the skin dose in diagnostic radiology</u>
<u>Nomogramm zur Abschätzung der Hautdosis in der Diagnostik</u>
<u>Nomogramme pour l'estimation de la dose à la peau en diagnostic</u>
<u>Nomograma para la estimacion de dosis en la piel en diagnóstico</u>

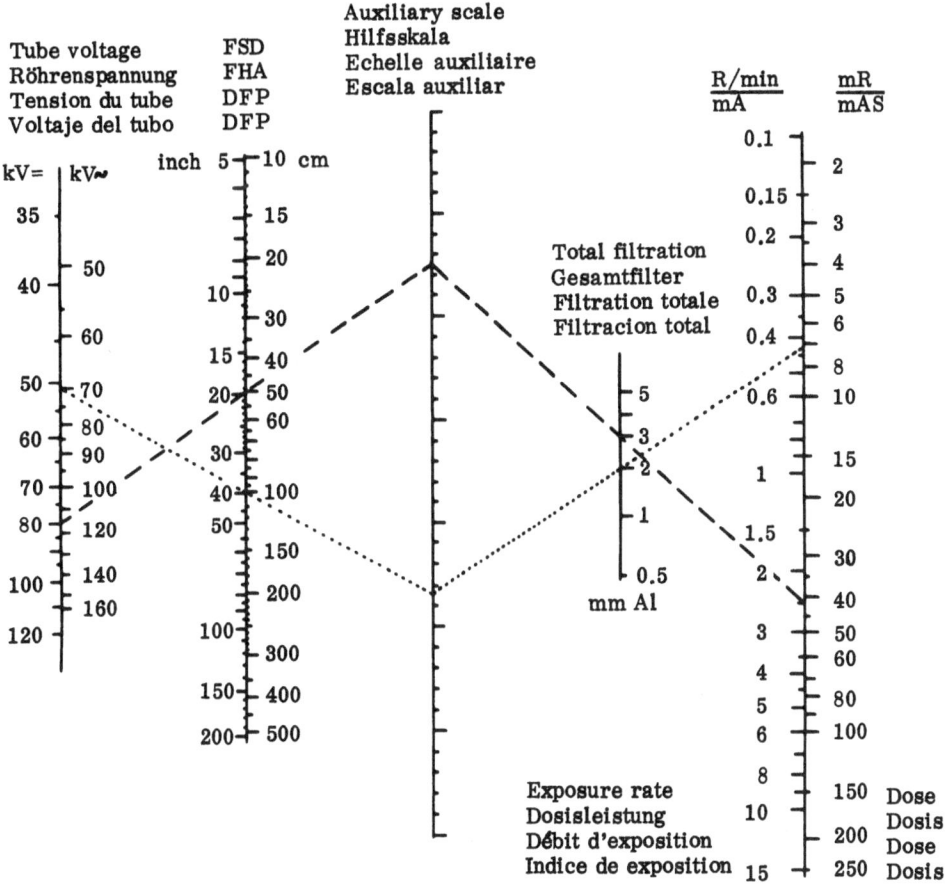

Examples - Beispiele - Exemples - Ejemplos:

(---) Fluoroscopy - Durchleuchtung - Radioscopie - Fluoroscopia
80 kV~; FSD - FHA - DFP - DFP 50 cm; Filter - Filter - Filtre -
Filtro 3 mm Al; Skin dose rate - Hautdosisleistung - Débit de
dose à la peau - Rendimiento de dosis en la piel ≅ 2.5 $\frac{R/min}{mA}$

(...) Radiography - Aufnahme - Radiographie - Radiografía 50 kV=;
FSD - FHA - DFP - DFP 100 cm; Filter - Filter - Filtre - Filtro
2 mm Al; Skin dose - Hautdosis - Dose à la peau - Dosis en la
piel ≅ 40 $\frac{mR}{mAs}$

Lit.: 1. WACHSMANN, F.: Fortschr. Röntgenstr. <u>6</u>, 728 (1951)

7.6 Depth dose curves for typical radiations used in diagnosis, and ratio of dose at entrance field/film dose (average values)

Dosisabfall der in der Diagnostik verwendeten typischen Strahlungen und Verhältnis Dosis-Strahleneintrittsfeld/Filmdosis

Rendements en profondeur pour des rayonnements typiques de radiodiagnostic; rapport de la dose à l'entrée du milieu à la dose au film (valeurs moyennes)

Disminución de la dosis de las radiaciones típicas usadas en el diagnóstico, y relaciones dosis en el campo de entrada/dosis película (valores aproximados)

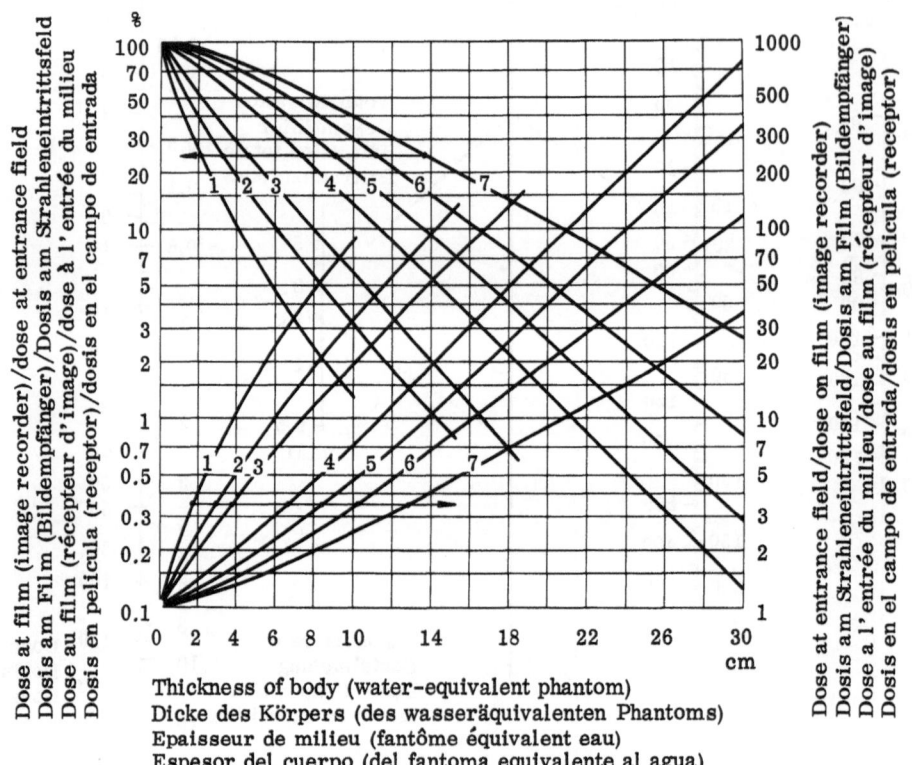

Thickness of body (water-equivalent phantom)
Dicke des Körpers (des wasseräquivalenten Phantoms)
Epaisseur de milieu (fantôme équivalent eau)
Espesor del cuerpo (del fantoma equivalente al agua)

Radiations used - Benützte Strahlungen - Rayonnements utilisés - Radiaciones utilizadas

Curve Kurve Courbe Curva	Application Anwendung Examen Aplicación	Tube voltage Röhrenspannung Tension du tube Voltaje del tubo	FSD FHA DFP DFP	Filtration Filterung Filtration Filtración	Field Feld Champ Campo	HVL HWSD CDA CHR
		kV	cm	mm	cm	mm
1	Mammography	Mo (17.7 keV)	45	0.1 Mo	15 x 15	∿1 Al
2	Dental X-rays	45 kV∿	15	1.5 Al	5 ∅	1.1 Al
3	Extremities	50 kV∿	50	1.5 Al	20 x 20	1.3 Al
4	General	60 kV∿	120	2 Al	30 x 30	1.6 Al
5	General	80 kV=	120	2 Al	30 x 30	2.4 Al
6	General	120 kV=	120	2 Al	30 x 30	3.4 Al
7	General	150 kV=	120	5 Al	30 x 30	0.3 Cu

7.7 Exposure (D) at the detector and resolution for radiographs
Dosis (D) am Detektor und Auflösung für Röntgenaufnahmen
Exposition (D) sur le détecteur et résolution pour radiographies
Exposición (D) en el detector y resolución para radiografías

Type of radiography - Aufnahmeart - Type de radiographie - Tipo de radiografía		Exposure Dosis (D)	Resolution *)
Non-screen radiography - Folienlose Aufnahme - Radiographie sans écran - Radiografía sin pantalla		10 - 100 mR	10 - 40
Photofluorography-Schirmbildfotographie Radiophotographie-Fluorografía		3 - 5 mR	1.5 - 3
Radiography with screens Aufnahmen mit Folien Radiographie avec écrans Radiografía con pantallas	High definition Feinzeichnend Haute définition Grano fino	0.7 - 2 mR	8 - 12
	Universal-Standard	300 - 800 µR	7 - 9
	High speed Hochverstärkend Rapide - Rápida	200 - 300 µR	5 - 7
	Rare earths Seltene Erden Terres rares Tierras raras	100 - 25 µR	4 - 7
Photographic recording from image intensifier Fotographische Aufzeichnung vom Bildverstärkerschirm Enregistrement photographique dè amplificateur de luminance Registro fotografico de intensificador de imagen		<u>70 - 100 mm:</u> 50 - 100 µR	1.5 - 4
		<u>Cine:</u> 2 - 20 µR	1.0 - 3.5
Photographic recording from TV monitor Fotographische Aufzeichnung vom FS-Schirm En registrement photographique de TV moniteur Registro fotografico de TV pantalla		0.5 - 2.0 µR	0.8 - 1.2
Xeroradiography - Xeroradiographie Xeroradiographie - Xeroradiografía		10 - 100 mR	**)

*) Periods/mm - Perioden/mm - Périodes/mm - Periodos/mm
**) Incomparable - Unvergleichbar - Incomparable - Incomparable

Lit.: 1. ROSSMANN, K.: Phys.Med.Biol., 9, 551 (1964)
2. DUTREIX, J., BISMUTH, V., LAVAL-JEANTET, M.: Traité de radiodiagnostic, Vol. I, Paris: Masson 1969
3. WIDENMANN, L.: Rö.Praxis 26, 85 (1973)
4. PUPPE, D.: Grundlagen u. Anwendungsmöglichkeiten, Ergebn. med. Radiologie, Bd. III, Stuttgart: Thieme 1971

7.8

Sensitivity of X-ray films (average values) – Empfindlichkeit von Röntgenfilmen (Richtwerte) –
Sensibilité des films radiographiques (valeurs moyennes) – Sensibilidad de películas para
rayos X (valores aproximados)

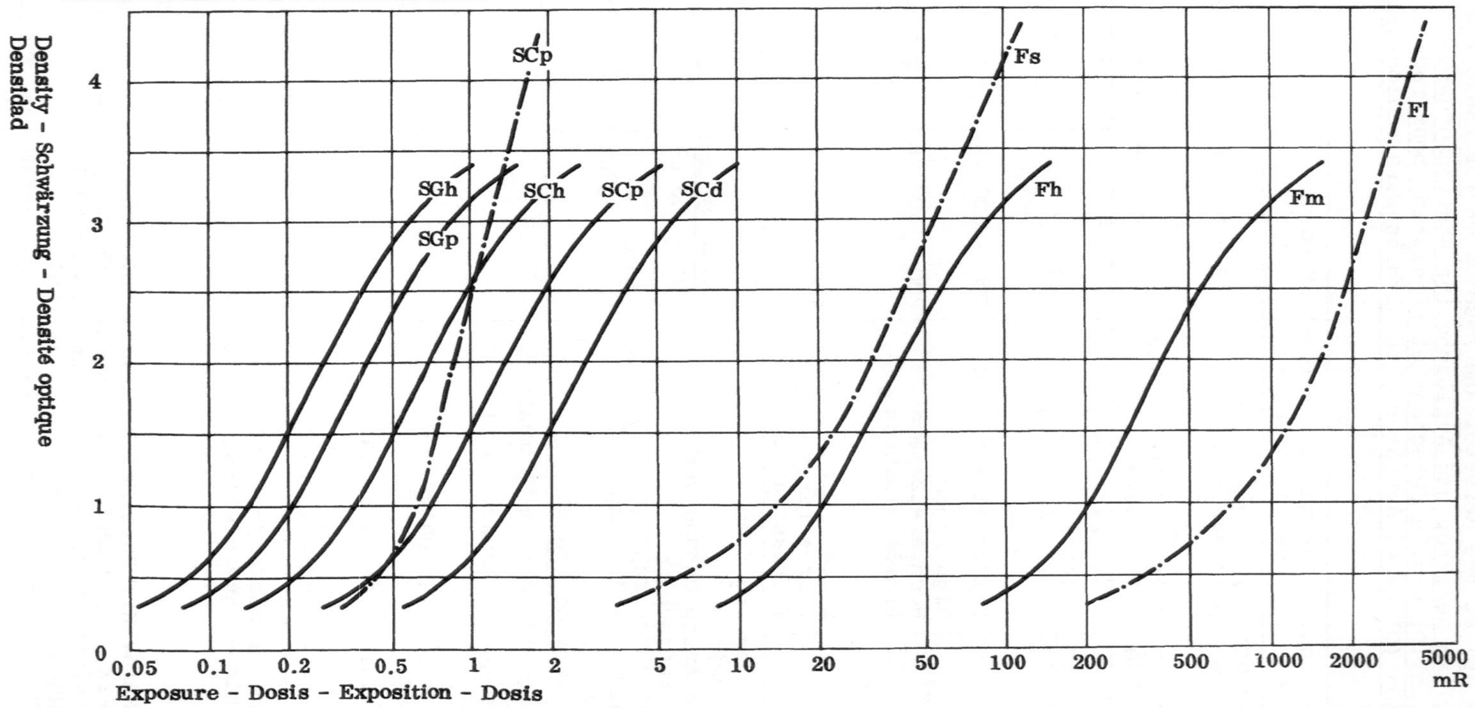

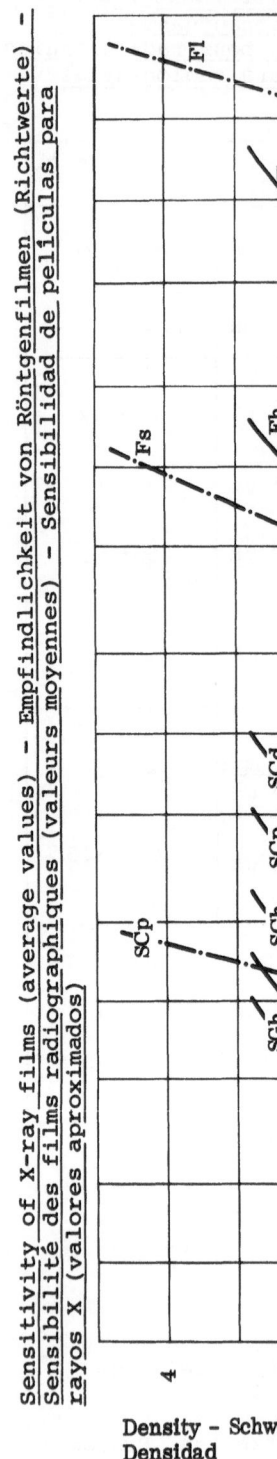

Density – Schwärzung – Densité optique
Densidad

Exposure – Dosis – Exposition – Dosis

For abbreviations see right page – Abkürzungen siehe rechte Seite – Pour les abréviations voir page de
droite – Para abreviaciones, ver página derecha

Lit.: 1. Brochures – Firmenprospekte – Prospekte – Prospectur des divers fabricants – Prospectos de casas de
       comercio
      2. BORCKE, E.: Röntgenpraxis 12, 277 (1970)
      3. KRAFT, A., NAHRSTEDT, U., WIDENMANN, L.: Röntgenpraxis 28, 264 (1975)
      4. Authors' measurements – Eigene Messungen – Mesures personelles – Medidas propias

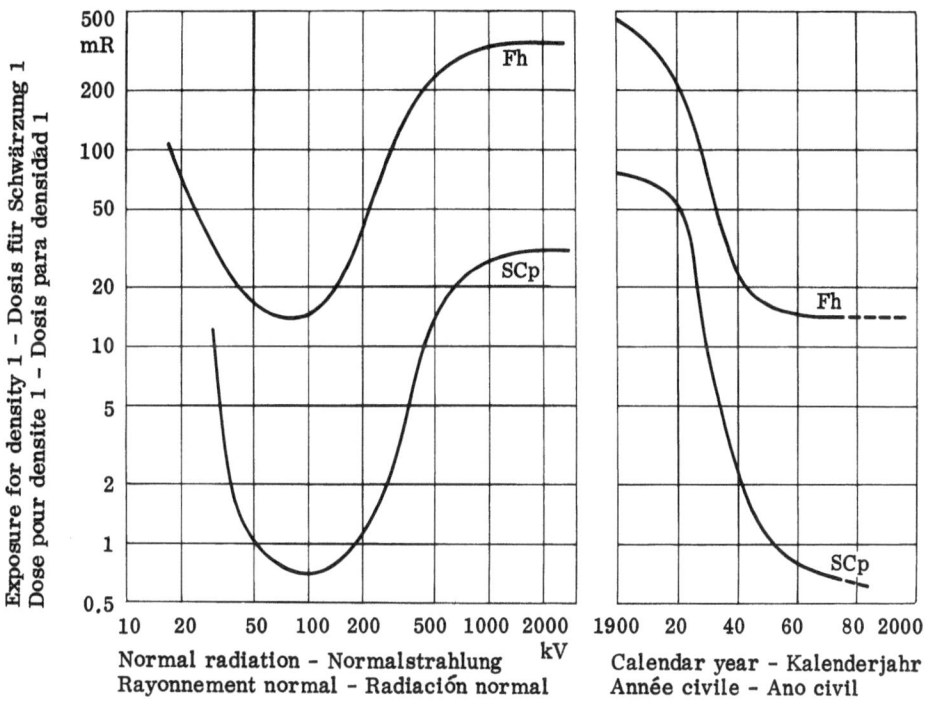

Exposure for density 1 - Dosis für Schwärzung 1
Dose pour densite 1 - Dosis para densidad 1

Normal radiation - Normalstrahlung kV
Rayonnement normal - Radiación normal

Calendar year - Kalenderjahr
Année civile - Ano civil

Intensifying screens - Verstärkerfolien - Ecrans renforçateurs - -
Pantallas reforzadoras:

S = Screen/film-combination - Film/Folien-Kombination - Combinai-
    son film/écran - Combinación-pantalla/película

F = Non screen films - Folienlose Filme - Films sans écrans -
    Películas sin pantalla

C = Ca WO$_4$

G = Gd$_2$ O$_2$ S: Tb

h = High-speed - Hochverstärkend - Rapides - Amplificación elevada

p = Parspeed - Universal - Standard - Universal

d = High definition - Feinzeichnend - Haute définition - Resolu-
    ción fina

X-ray films - Röntgenfilme - Films radiologiques - Películas radiolo-
gicas

s = High sensitivity-Hochempfindlich-Grande sensibilité-Alta
    sensibilidad (diagnostic, industrial, personal monitoring)

l = Low sensitivity-Wenig empfindlich-Faible sensibilité-Baja
    sensibilidad (industrial, personnel monitoring)

m = Mamography - Mammographie - Mammographie - Mamografía

Processing - Entwicklung - Développement - Relevado

—— = Automatic processing - Maschinenentwicklung - Développement
    automatique - Procesado automático

-•- = Manual processing - Handentwicklung - Développement manuel -
    Relevado manual

7.9   Effect of developer temperature (t) and developing time (T)
       on the doses needed for equal film density

       Einfluß von Entwicklertemperatur (t) und -zeit (T) auf die
       zur Erzielung gleicher Schwärzungen erforderlichen Dosen

       Influence de la température du révélateur (t) et du temps de
       développement (T) sur les doses nécessaires pour obtenir un
       noircissement donné

       Influencia de la temperatura (t) y tiempo (T) de revelado
       sobre las dosis necesarias para alcanzar densidades iguales

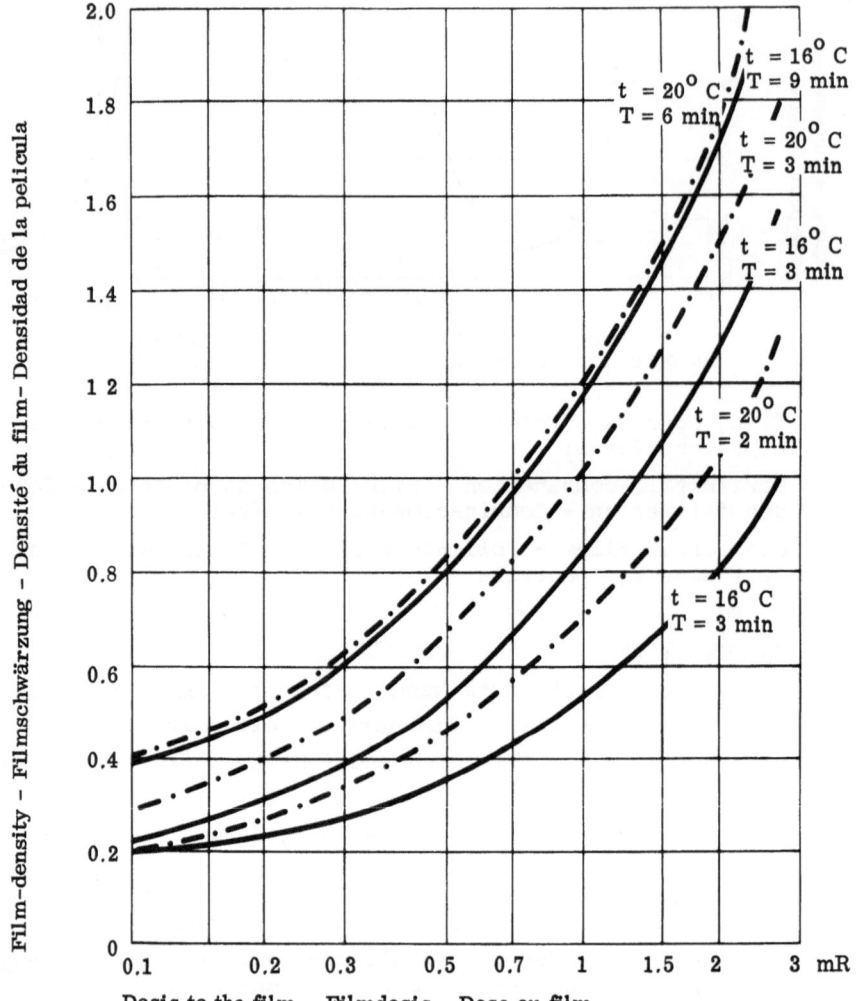

Dosis to the film - Filmdosis - Dose au film-
Exposición de la pelicula

Lit.: 1. STIEVE, F.E.: Strahlenschutz in Forschung und Praxis,
       7, 71, Freiburg: Rombach-Verlag 1967

Table of contents - Inhaltsverzeichnis
Table des matières - Tabla de materias

Type Bezeichnung Désignation Nombre	Frequency or energy Frequenz bzw. Energie Fréquence ou énergie Frecuencia o energía	Wavelength Wellenlänge Longueur d'onde Longitud de onda
Electromagnetic waves of low frequency - Elektromagnetische Oscillations électromagnétiques de basse fréquence -		
Short waves Kurzwellen Ondes courtes Ondas cortas	27.1 Mc/s - MHz [2]) 433.92 " " 2450 " "	11.06 m 69.14 cm 12.24 cm
Infrared Infrarot Infrarouge Rayos infrarrojos	0.2-1.5 eV	5-0.7 µm
Visible light Sichtbares Licht Lumière visible Luz visible	1.5-3 eV	760-400 nm
Ultraviolet Ultraviolett Ultra-violet Radiación ultravioleta	3-12 eV	400-230 nm
X-Rays - Röntgenstrahlen -		
Very soft X-rays Sehr weiche Strahlen Rayons X tres mous Rayos X may blandos	< 6-12 keV	> 6 nm
Low energy X-rays Weiche Strahlen Rayons X mous Rayos blandos	20-60 keV	6-2 nm
Medium-energy X-rays Mittelharte Strahlen Rayons X semi-durs Rayos semiduros	60-150 keV	2-0.8 nm
Orthovoltage X-rays Harte Strahlen Rayons durs (classiques) Rayos duros	150-400 keV	0.8-0.3 nm
High voltage X rays Sehr harte u. γ-Strahlen Rayons extra durs et γ Rayos muy duros y γ	400-3000 keV	0.3-0.04 nm

HVD [1]) GHWT PDA PHR H_2O	Applications Anwendungen Applicátions Aplicaciones	Mechanism of action Wirkungsmechanismus Mécanisme d'action Mecanismo de acción
	Schwingungen niederer Frequenz - Oscilaciónes electromagnéticas de frecuencia baja	
0.5-1 cm 2-9 cm 0.5-2 cm	Heat therapy Wärmetherapie Thermothérapie Termoterapia	Increase in blood circulation Durchblutungssteigerung Amélioration de la circulation sanguine Aumento de la circulación
1 mm	Light therapy Lichttherapie Photothérapie Fototerapia	Superficial heating Oberflächige Erwärmung Augmentation superficielle de la température Calentamiento superficial
0.5 mm	Light therapy Lichttherapie Photothérapie Fototerapia	Heat and photochemical effects Wärme und photochemische Wirkungen Chaleur et action photochimique Calor y efectos fotoquimicos
	Ultraviolet therapy Ultraviolett-Therapie Thérapie par UV Fototerapia con UV	Photochemical effects Photochemische Wirkungen Action photochimique Efectos fotoquímicos
	Rayons X - Rayos X	
0.2 mm	Skin therapy [4]) Hauttherapie Radiothérapie des lésions cutanées Terapia dermatologica	Cell damage by ionization Zellschädigungen durch Ionisation Lésions cellulaires par ionisation Lesión tisular por ionización LET [3]) 6-3 keV/µm ID [3])150-100/µm
2-30 mm	Skin and subcutaneous therapy [5]) Haut- u.Unterhautther. Radiothérapie cutanée et souscutanée Terapia cutánea y subcutánea	" LET $\sim$ 2.6 keV/µm ID $\sim$ 70/µm
30-70 mm	Intermediate therapy [5]) Halbtiefentherapie Thérapie semi- profonde Terapia semiprofunda	" LET 2.5-1.5 keV/µm ID 90-50/µm
7-8 cm	Deep therapy [6]) Tiefentherapie Radiothérapie profonde Terapia profunda	" LET 1.5-0.5 keV/µm ID $\sim$ 50-15/µm
8-12 cm	" " [7])	" LET 0.5-0.25 keV/µm ID $\sim$ 15-8/µm

Type Bezeichnung Désignation Nombre	Frequency or energy Frequenz bzw. Energie Fréquence ou énergie Frecuencia o energîa	Wavelength Wellenlänge Longueur d'onde Longitud de onda
Megavoltage rays [8]) Ultraharte Strahlen Rayons X de très haute énergie Rayos X ultraduros	3-50 MeV	< 0.04 nm
Corpuscular radiations - Korpuskularstrahlen -		
Alpha rays Alphastrahlen Rayons alpha Rayos alfa	1-10 MeV	-
Beta rays Betastrahlen Rayons beta Rayos beta	1-3 MeV	-
Fast electrons [9]) Schnelle Elektronen Electrons accélérés Electrones rápidos	5-50 MeV	-
Neutrons [10]) Neutronen Neutrons Neutrones	0.02 eV - 60 MeV	-
Protons [11]) Protonen Protons Protones	50-200 MeV	-

Definitons - Definitionen - Définitions - Definiciônes

[1]) HVD = Half-value depth (tissue)
    GHWT = Gewebe-Halbwerttiefe
    PDA = Profondeur demi atténuation tissulaire
    PHR = Profundidad hemi reductora en tejido

[2]) Mc/s = M cycle/s   = Megahertz/s
           = 10^6 Schwingungen/s
           = M oscillations/s
           = M oscilaciônes/s

HVD [1]) GHWT PDA PHR H₂O	Applications Anwendung Applications Aplicaciones	Mechanism of action Wirkungsmechanismus Mécanisme d'action Mecanismo de acción
∿ 15 cm	Deep therapy Tiefentherapie Thérapie des lésions profondes Terapía profunda	Cell damage Zellschädigung Lésion cellulaire Lesión tisular LET ∿ 0.25 keV/μm ID ∿ 7/μm

Rayonnements corpusculaires - Radiación corpuscular

5 μm	Contact therapy Kontaktbestrahlung Thérapie de contact Terapía de contacto	" LET keV/μm ID μm⁻¹ ∿ 150-30 ∿ 5000-1000
5 mm	Skin therapy Hauttherapie Thérapie cutanée Terapía dermatológica	" ∿ 0.3-0.2 ∿ 10-6
2-10 cm	Intermediate therapy Halbtiefentherapie Thérapie semiprofonde Terapía semiprofunda	" LET ∿ 0.2 keV/μm ID ∿ 7/μm
2-15 cm	In experimental stage Im Versuchsstadium Stade expérimental Fase experimental	" LET 1.5 keV/μm ID ∿ 50/μm
5-20 cm	"	" LET 0.3-0.15 ID ∿ 10-5/ m

[3]) LET - ID   See page - Siehe Seite - Voir page - Ver pagina 37-39

[4]) See page - Siehe Seite - Voir page - Ver pagina 87, 100 - 103
[5]) "   "   "   "   87 - 103
[6]) "   "   "   "   104 - 111
[7]) "   "   "   "   118 - 127
[8]) "   "   "   "   126 - 129
[9]) "   "   "   "   132 - 133
[10]) "   "   "   "   134
[11]) "   "   "   "   135

8.2 Data for the "reference man" (adult) – Angaben über den "Referenz-Menschen" (Erwachsener) – Données sur "l'homme référence" (adulte) – Datos sobre el "hombre-referencia" (adulto)

8.2.1 Organ weights – Organgewichte – Poids des organes – Peso del órgano

	Male Mann Homme Hombre g	Female Frau Femme Mujer g	Average value Mittelwert Valeur moyenne Valor medio g
Total body – Ganzkörper – Corps entier – Cuerpo total	70000	58000	
Skeletal muscles – Skelettmuskulatur – Muscles du squelette – Esqueleto muscularlos	28000	17000	
Skeleton (with bone marrow etc.) – Skelett (mit Knochenmark usw.) – Squelette (y compris la moelle etc.) – Esqueleto (incluida médula, etc.)	10000	6800	
Skin – Haut – Peau – Piel	2600	1790	
Subcutaneus tissue – Unterhautgewebe – Tissus souscutanés – Tejido subcutáneo	7500	13000	
Fat – Fett – Graisse – Grasa	16000	13500	
Red bone marrow – Rotes Knochenmark – Moelle rouge – Médula roja	1500	1300	
Yellow bone marrow – Weißes Knochenmark – Moelle jaune – Médula blanca	1500	1300	
Blood – Blut – Sang – Sangre	5500	4100	4800
Gastrointestinal tract (without contents) – Magen-Darm-Kanal (ohne Inhalt) – Tractus gastrointestinal (sans contenu) – Tubo digestivo (vacío)	1200	1200	
Gastrointestinal tract (content) – Magen-Darm-Kanal (Inhalt) – Tractus gastrointestinal (contenu) – Tubo digestivo (contenido)	1000	1000	
Liver – Leber – Foie – Hígado	1800	1400	1600
Brain – Hirn – Cerveau – Cerebro	1400	1200	1300
Lungs – Lungen – Poumons – Pulmones	1150	880	
Lymphoid tissue – Lymphatisches Gewebe – Tissu lymphoïde – Tejido linfático	700	580	
Heart – Herz – Coeur – Corazón	330	240	
Kidneys – Nieren – Reins – Riñones	310	275	
Spleen – Milz – Rate – Bazo	180	150	
Pancreas – Bauchspeicheldrüse – Pancréas – Páncreas	100	85	
Salivary glands – Speicheldrüsen – Glandes salivaires – Glándulas salivales	85	70	
Thyroid gland – Schilddrüse – Thyroïde – Tiroides	20	17	
Thymus – Thymus – Thymus – Timo			10
Testicles – Hoden – Testicules – Testículos	35	–	
Prostate gland – Prostata – Prostate – Prostata	16	–	

8.2.2 Daily food intake – Tägliche Nahrungsaufnahme
Quantités ingérées quotidiennement – Dieta alimenticia diaria

	Male Mann Homme Hombre	Female Frau Femme Mujer	Child 10 a Kind 10 a Enfant 10 a Nino 10 a
Water balance – Wasserhaushalt – Bilan en eau – Balance de agua	g/24 h		
Ingestion – Aufnahme – Ingestion – Ingestión			
In fluids – In Getränken – Dans les boissons – En bebidas	1950	1400	1400
In food – In der Nahrung – Dans l'alimentation – En comidas	700	450	400
By oxidation – Durch Verbrennung – Par oxydation – Por oxidación	350	250	200
Total – Zusammen – Total – Total	3000	2100	2000
Excretion – Ausscheidung – Sécrétion – Secreción			
Urine – Urin – Urine – Orina	1400	1000	1000
Feces – Stuhl – Fèces – Deposiciones	100	90	70
Insensible loss – Unmerkbar – Perte inapparente – Pérdidas imperceptibles	850	600	580
Sweat – Schweiß – Sueur – Transpiración	650	420	350
Total – Zusammen – Total – Total	3000	2100	2000

8.2.3 Breathed air – Atemluft – Air inhalé – Aire inhalado

	Male Mann Homme Hombre	Female Frau Femme Mujer	Child 10 a Kind 10 a Enfant 10 a Nino 10 a
	ℓ/8 h		
Light activity – Leichte Arbeit – Travail facile – Actividad moderada	9600	9100	6240
Nonoccupational activity – Freizeit – Activité non professionnelle – Tiempo libre	9600	9100	6240
Resting – Schlaf – Sommeil – Durante el sueño	3600	2900	2300
Total – Zusammen – Total – Total: Liters–Liter–Litres–Litros/24 h	22800	~21000	~15000

Lit.: 1. ICRP Publ. 23, Oxford: Pergamon Press (1975)

8.3 Dose/effect relationships of ionising radiations
Dosis/Wirkung Beziehungen ionisierender Strahlungen
Relations dose/effet pour les rayonnements ionisants
Relación dosis/efecto de radiaciones ionizantes

8.3.1 Target theory (based on mathematical considerations)
Treffertheorie (auf mathematischen Überlegungen basierend)
Théorie de la cible (basée sur des considérations mathematiques)
Teoría del blanco (basada en consideraciones matemáticas)

The term "hit" refers to an elementary physical event (e.g., formation of an ion pair) within a "sensitive volume" (e.g., cell nucleus or chromosome). Single hits (n = 1), plotted logarithmically, give linear dose-effect curves; curves for multiple hits (n = 2...n) are sigmoidal.

"Treffer" nennt man ein physikalisches Elementarereignis (z.B. Auslösung eines Ionenpaares) innerhalb eines "empfindlichen Volumens" (z.B. Zellkern oder Chromosom). Eintreffervorgänge (n = 1) ergeben logarithmisch dargestellt geradlinige Mehrtreffervorgänge (n = 2...n) sigmatoide Dosiswirkungskurven.

Le terme "coup" se rapporte à un évènement physique élémentaire (par exemple: formation d'une paire d'ions) à l'intérieur d'un volume sensible (par exemple: noyau cellulaire ou chromosome). Le modèle à un coup (n = 1) représenté avec des ordonnées logarithmiques, conduit à une courbe dose-effet linéaire; les modèles à plusieurs coups (n = 2...n) conduisent à des sigmoides.

El término "pegar en el blanco" o "impacto" se refiere a un evento fisico elemental (por ejemplo formación de pares de iones) en un "volumen sensible" (por ejemplo núcleos celulares o cromosomas). Procesos de impacto unitarios (n = 1) ofrecen perfiles lineales en representaciones logaritmicas de las relaciones de dosis/efecto, mientras que para procesos de impacto múltiple (n = 2...n) son sigmoidales.

Effect - Effekt - Effet - Efecto

n = Number of hits / Trefferzahl / Nombre de coups / Numero de blancos

D 1/2

Dose-Dosis-Dose-Dosis D 1/2

Object	Effect	n
Drosophila	Mutation	1
Viruses - Viren	Inactivation	1
B.coli, prodigiosus, etc.	Killing-Abtötung-Mort Muerta	1
Yeast - Hefe - Levures-Levadura	Damage-Schädigung-Dommage-Daño	3-5
Seeds-Keimlinge-Germes-Semillas	"	5-28
" depending on age " je nach Alter	"	
" and-und-et-y kV	"	1-18
Mammalian cells	"	15-20

Lit.: 1. TIMOFEEFF-RESSOWSKY, N.W., ZIMMER, K.G.: Das Trefferprinzip in der Biologie, Leipzig: Hirzel 1947
2. KELLERER, A.M.: Handbuch der Radiologie, Bd. II/3, Berlin, Heidelberg, New York: Springer 1972

8.3.2   Survival rate in cell cultures
         Überlebensrate in Zellkulturen
         Taux de survie de cultures de cellules
         Relación de supervivencia en cultivos celulares

         Note - Bemerkungen - Remarque - Nota

D_0 = Dose which reduces the number of surviving cells to the fraction
       1/e;

n   = "extrapolation number", i.e., the number of survivors, deter-
      mined by continuation of the linear portion of the damage curve
      to its intersection with the ordinate.

D_0 = Dosis, durch die die Zahl der jeweils überlebenden Zellen auf
       den 1/e-ten Teil vermindert wird;

n   = "Extrapolationsnummer", d.h. die Zahl der Überlebenden, gefunden
      durch Verlängerung des geradlinigen Teils der Schädigungskurve
      bis zum Schnittpunkt mit der Ordinate.

D_0 = Dose qui réduit le nombre de cellules survivantes à une fraction
       1/e;

n   = "nombre d'extrapolation", c'est à dire le nombre de survivants
      déterminé par extrapolation de la partie linéaire de la courbe
      de survie jusqu'à son intersection avec l'axe des ordonnées.

D_0 = Dosis mediante la cual el número de células que sobreviven dis-
       minuye a la porción 1/e;

n   = "número de extrapolación", es decir el número de sobrevivientes,
      que se obtiene prolongando la parte recta de la curva de dañados
      hasta que corta el eje de ordenadas.

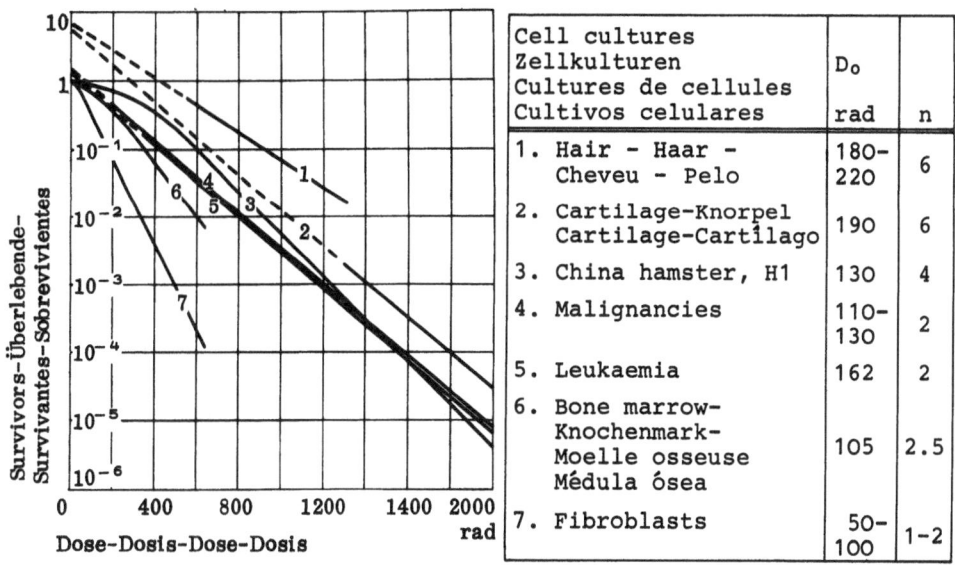

Cell cultures Zellkulturen Cultures de cellules Cultivos celulares	D_0 rad	n
1. Hair - Haar - Cheveu - Pelo	180-220	6
2. Cartilage-Knorpel Cartilage-Cartílago	190	6
3. China hamster, H1	130	4
4. Malignancies	110-130	2
5. Leukaemia	162	2
6. Bone marrow- Knochenmark- Moelle osseuse Médula ósea	105	2.5
7. Fibroblasts	50-100	1-2

Survivors-Überlebende-
Survivantes-Sobrevivientes

Dose-Dosis-Dose-Dosis

Lit.: 1.-3. PUCK, T.T., MARCUS, P.I. et al.: J.Exp.Med. 103, 273,
            485 (1956) and 106, 485 (1957)
         4. TROTT, K.R.: Hdb. der Radiologie, Bd. II/3, Berlin,
            Heidelberg, New York: Springer 1972

8.4.1 Relative biological effectivness (RBE) - Relative biologische Wirksamkeit (RBW) - Efficacité biologique relative (EBR) - Efectividad biológica relativa (EBR)

Since the RBE is strongly dependent on the object and its condition, the reaction under consideration, the temporal dose distribution, and extraneous circumstances, only examples can be given here. - Da die RBW stark von dem Objekt und seinem Zustand, der betrachteten Reaktion, der zeitlichen Dosisverabreichung und Nebenumständen abhängig ist, können hier nur Beispiele gegeben werden. - Etant donnée la dépendance marquée de l'EBR suivant le matériel et ses conditions, suivant le test biologique considéré, suivant la distribution de la dose dans le temps et suivant les conditions extérieures, seuls quelques exemples sont presentés. - Dado que la EBR depende en gran medida del objeto y su estado, reacción considerada, suministro de dosis temporal y circunstancias accesorias, solamente se pueden indicar aquí ejemplos.

Group / Gruppe / Groupe / Grupo	Object / Objekt / Matériel / Objeto	Observed reaction / Beobachtete Reaktion / Réaction observé / Reacción observada	LET – LET – TEL – TEL – RBE – RBW – EBR – EBR keV/µm 0.2 0.5 1 2 5 10 20 50 100 200 500 1000 / 6 15 30 60 150 300 600 1500 3000 6000 15000 30000 Ionisation density – Ionisationsdichte Pairs/µm – Densité d'ionisation – Densidad de ionización
Primitive plants	Fungi Pilze	Mutations 2) Deletions	Reference radiation: 1; 2 — 5.5; 5.5; 74
Higher plants	Arabidopsis, zea, nigella	Somatic and germline mutations 2)	1; 9 16 18 11.5 →1.5; 51–49 22–66 29–89
Insects	Drosophila, silk worm	Various mutations 2)	1; 1–2 2–4; 1–2.5 4
Mammals Säugetiere Mammifère Mamiferos	Mice, rats Different tissues	Mutations, translocations, and lethal 2)	1; 1.1–1.2 2 3–6 6
	Fast-growing tissues	Haemopoetic syndrome 1) Damage – death 1)	1; 1.2 1.5 2; 1–3 2–4 5 6
	Lens of eye	Induction of cataracta 3)	1; (2–) 8 (–20)
	Different cells	"Biologic effect" of fractionation 3)	1; single dose 1–1.1; 5 fractions/5 days 0.9–1.7

Lit.: 1. ICRP Report No. 14, Oxford: Pergamon-Press 1969
2. ICRP Report No. 18, Oxford: Pergamon-Press 1972
3. BROERSE, J.J.: Europ.J.Cancer. 10, 225 (1974)

8.4.2 Erythema dose as a function of radiation energy
Erythemdosis bei Strahlungen verschiedener Energie
Doses d'érythème en fonction de l'énergie du rayonnement
Dosis eritematosa en función de la energía de la radiación

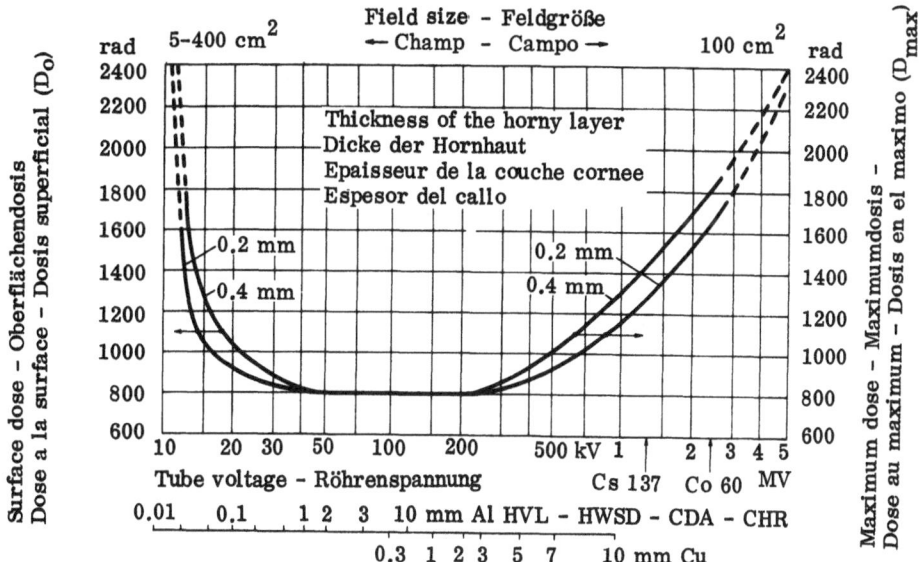

Note - Bemerkung - Remarque - Nota:

The absorption of soft X-rays in the horny layer of the skin and its steep dose decay respectively the significant build-up above 250 kV makes it possible to irradiate skin with higher surface doses (D_o) at low energies and with higher maximum doses (D_{max}) at high energies, without exceeding the erythema or tolerance threshold.

Die Schwächung in der Hornhaut und der steile Dosisabfall weicher Röntgenstrahlen bzw. der über 250 kV Bedeutung erlangende Aufbaueffekt bewirken, daß bei weichen Strahlungen höhere Oberflächendosen und bei sehr bis ultraharten Strahlungen höhere Maximumdosen (D_{max}) verabreicht werden können als im Bereich von 50 - 200 kV ohne die Erythem- oder Toleranzschwelle zu überschreiten.

L'absorption des rayons X mous dans la couche cornée de la peau et la décroissance rapide de la dose d'une part et d'autre part l'accroissement initial significatif de la dose au dessus de 250 kV permettent d'irradier la peau avec des doses à la surface (D_o) plus élevées pour les rayonnements de basse energie au pour les hautes énergies sans dépasser de seuil érythème où tolerance.

La atenuación en el callo y el escarpado descenso de la dosis de los rayos blandos o sea el efecto de build-up encima de 250 kV da lugar a que se puedan aplicar con rayos blandos dosis superficiales (D_o) y con rayos de alta energía dosis medidas en el máximo (D_{max}) más elevadas como en el intervalo 50 - 250 kV sin sobrepasar el límite eritematoso o de tolerancia.

Lit.: 1. REISNER, A.: Fortschr. Röntgenstr. 45, 293 (1932)
2. TRUMP, J.G.: Radiology 50, 645 (1948)
3. WACHSMANN, F.: Proceedings of the Congressus Int.Dermatologiae 1967, Vol. 2, Springer: Heidelberg 1968

8.5.1 Dependence of skin tolerance on field size
       Abhängigkeit der Hauttoleranz von der Feldgröße
       Variation de la tolérance cutanée avec la taille du champ
       Dependencia de la tolerancia de la piel con el campo

Conventional therapy; fractionation 20 single doses in 4 weeks
Konventionelle Therapie; Fraktionierung 20 Einzeldosen in
4 Wochen - Thérapie classique; fractionnement: 20 séances
en 4 semaines - Terapia convencional; fraccionamiento 20
dosis unitarias en 4 semanas

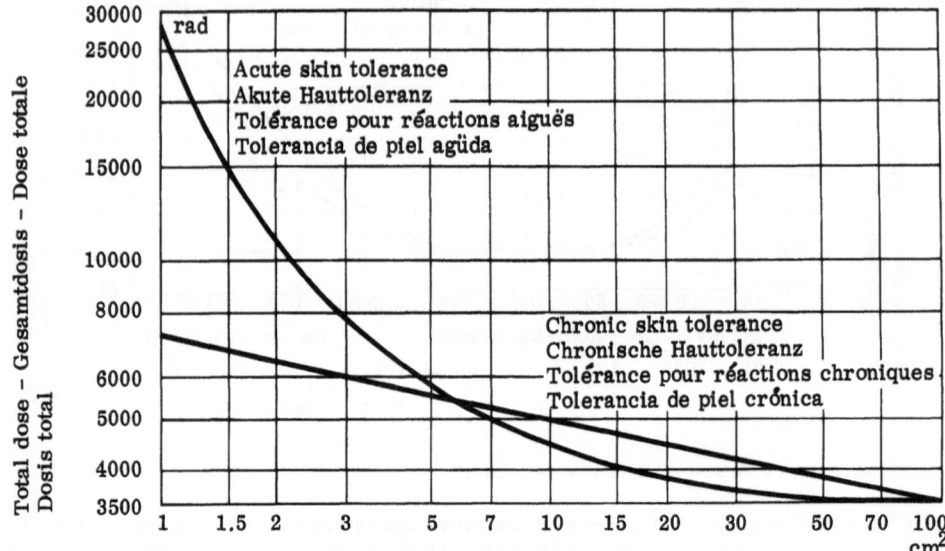

Field size - Feldgröße - Champ - Campo

Field size Feldgröße Champ Campo cm²	Skin tolerance - Hauttoleranz - Tolérance cutanée - Tolerancia de la piel rad	
	Acute - Akut Aiguë - Aguda	Chronic - Chronisch Chronique - Crónica
1	28 000 rad	7 300 rad
1.5	15 000	6 800
2	11 000	6 400
3	7 800	6 000
5	5 800	5 600
7	5 000	5 300
10	4 500	5 000
15	4 000	4 800
20	3 800	4 500
30	3 700	4 200
50	3 550	3 850
70	3 500	3 700
100	3 500	3 500

Lit.: 1. JOYET, G., HOHL, K.: Fortschr. Rö.Strl. 82, 387 (1955)
      2. von ESSEN, C.F.: in Frontiers of Radiation Therapy and
         Oncology, Vol. 6, Basel: S. Karger 1972

8.5.2 Skin reactions as a function of different fractionnation
Hautreaktionen bei verschiedener Fraktionierung
Réactions de la peau pour différents fractionnements
Reacciones de la piel según el fraccionamiento

Conventional therapy - Konventionelle Therapie - Thérapie classique — Terapía convencional ($\sim$ 200 kV)

100 cm^2 Field size - Feldgröße - Champ - Campo

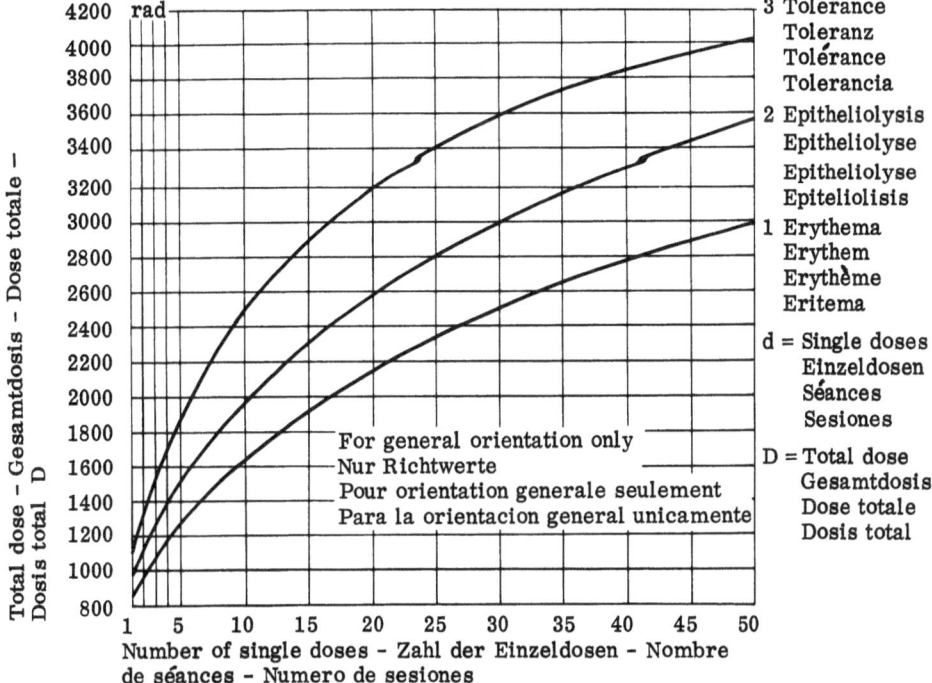

Total dose - Gesamtdosis - Dose totale - Dosis total D

3 Tolerance / Toleranz / Tolérance / Tolerancia

2 Epitheliolysis / Epitheliolyse / Epitheliolyse / Epiteliolisis

1 Erythema / Erythem / Erythème / Eritema

d = Single doses / Einzeldosen / Séances / Sesiones

D = Total dose / Gesamtdosis / Dose totale / Dosis total

For general orientation only
Nur Richtwerte
Pour orientation generale seulement
Para la orientacion general unicamente

Number of single doses - Zahl der Einzeldosen - Nombre de séances - Numero de sesiones

Number of single doses Zahl der Einzeldosen Nombre de séances Número de sesiones	Doses for various skin reactions - Dosen zur Erzeugung verschiedener Hautreaktionen - Expositions différentes pour reactions cutanées - Dosis para varias reacciones cutáneas rad					
	1		2		3	
	d	D	d	D	d	D
1	850	850	950	950	1100	1100
2	1000	425	1100	475	1350	550
3	1100	333	1300	366	1600	450
5	1300	260	1550	310	1900	380
7	1500	215	1750	250	2150	308
10	1650	165	1950	195	2500	250
15	1900	125	2300	153	2900	193
20	2150	110	2600	130	3200	160
25	2350	95	2800	112	3400	137
30	2500	85	3000	100	3600	120
35	2650	75	3150	90	3750	107
40	2800	70	3300	83	3850	97
45	2900	65	3450	77	3950	88
50	3000	60	3550	71	4000	80

Lit.: 1. WACHSMANN, F.: Strahlenther. 73, 636 (1943)
      2. STRANDQVIST, M.: Acta Radiol. Suppl. LV (1944)

8.6   "Nominal single doses" (NSD) in the fractionated radiotherapy
       "Nominale Einzel-Dosen" (NED) bei Fraktionierung
       Doses équivalentes en radiothérapie fractionnée (NSD)
       Dosis equivalente en la radioterapia fraccionada (NSD) 1-2)

Reference value 1000 rad; proportional transformation in other NSD
is possible. In certain tissues deviations may be occur.

Bezugswert 1000 rad; proportionale Umrechnung auf andere NED ist zu-
lässig. Bei gewissen Geweben sind Abweichungen möglich.

NSD équivalent de 1000 rad; une règle de proportionnalité est accep-
table pour d'autres NSD. Pour certains tissus des écarts sont possibles.

Valor de referencia 1000 rad; se puede realizar la conversión pro-
porcional a otras NSD. Para ciertos tejidos son posibles desviaciones.

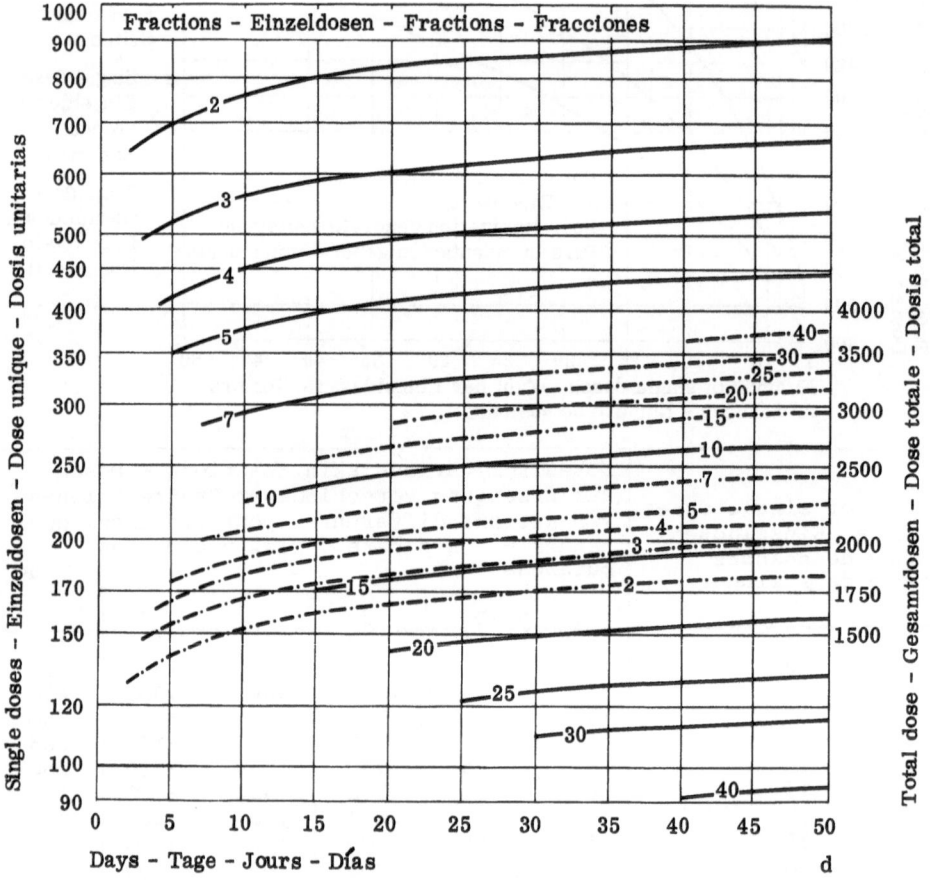

Days - Tage - Jours - Días   d

Lit.: 1. ELLIS, F.: Clin.Radiol. 20, 1 (1969)
      2. ELLIS, F. et al.: Brit.J.Radiol. 42, 715 (1969)
      3. KROENING, P.M. et al.: Am.J.Roentgenol. CXII, 803 (1971)

Equivalent single dose - Äquivalente Einzeldosen - Dose équivalente par séance - Dosis únitarias equivalentes											rad

Number of fractions - Zahl der Einzeldosen - Nombre de séances - Número de sesiones

d*)	2	3	4	5	7	10	15	20	25	30	40
2	635	-	-	-	-	-	-	-	-	-	-
3	670	490	-	-	-	-	-	-	-	-	-
4	690	505	405	-	-	-	-	-	-	-	-
5	705	520	415	350	-	-	-	-	-	-	-
7	720	535	430	365	280	-	-	-	-	-	-
10	760	560	450	380	295	225	-	-	-	-	-
15	795	585	470	395	310	235	172	-	-	-	-
20	825	600	485	410	315	240	177	143	-	-	-
25	840	620	500	420	325	250	182	146	123	-	-
30	860	630	510	430	330	255	186	150	126	110	-
40	890	650	520	445	340	260	192	154	130	113	91
50	910	665	535	455	350	270	196	158	133	115	93

Equivalent total doses - Äquivalente Gesamtdosen - Doses totales équivalentes - Dosis total equivalente

	2	3	4	5	7	10	15	20	25	30	40
2	1170	-	-	-	-	-	-	-	-	-	-
3	1340	1470	-	-	-	-	-	-	-	-	-
4	1580	1515	1620	-	-	-	-	-	-	-	-
5	1410	1560	1660	1750	-	-	-	-	-	-	-
7	1440	1605	1720	1825	1960	-	-	-	-	-	-
10	1520	1680	1800	1900	2065	2250	-	-	-	-	-
15	1590	1755	1880	1975	2170	2350	2580	-	-	-	-
20	1650	1800	1940	2050	2205	2400	2660	2860	-	-	-
25	1680	1860	2000	2100	2275	2500	2760	2920	3075	-	-
30	1720	1890	2040	2310	2550	2790	3000	3150	3300	-	-
40	1780	1950	2080	2225	2380	2600	2980	3080	3250	3390	3640
50	1820	1995	2140	2275	2450	2700	2940	3160	3325	3450	3720

Treatment time Behandlungszeit Durée du traitement Duración del tratamiento	Equivalent doses with 1 - 5 irradiations/week Äquivalente Dosen bei 1 - 5 Bestrahlungen/Woche Dose équivalente à 1 - 5 irradiations/semaine Dosis equivalentes con 1-5 irradiaciones/semana rad									
	Single doses-Einzeldosen Dose unique-Dosis únitarias rad					Weekly dose-Wochendosis Dose hebdomadaire Dosis semanales rad				
Weeks-Wochen Semaines-Semanas	1	2	3	4	5	1	2	3	4	5
1	1000	730	535	430	360	1000	1460	1615	1720	1800
2	780	465	345	280	235	780	930	1030	1120	1175
3	605	360	262	212	178	605	720	790	850	890
4	505	295	220	175	148	505	590	660	700	740
5	435	258	188	152	128	435	515	565	610	645
6	385	230	168	135	114	385	460	505	540	570
7	350	186	152	122	103	350	372	455	490	515

*) d = Duration of the treatment (days) - Behandlungsdauer (Tage) - Durée du traitement (jours) - Duración del tratamiento (dias)

(ret = $rad_{therapy}$)

8.7 Effect of dose protraction on various biological tissues and reactions (average values)

Einfluß der Protrahierung auf verschiedene Gewebe und Reaktionen (Richtwerte)

Influence de l'étalement de la dose sur différents tissus et différentes réactions biologiques (pour orientation seulement)

Efecto de la protracción de la dosis sobre diversos tejidos y reacciones biológicas (para orientación unicamente)

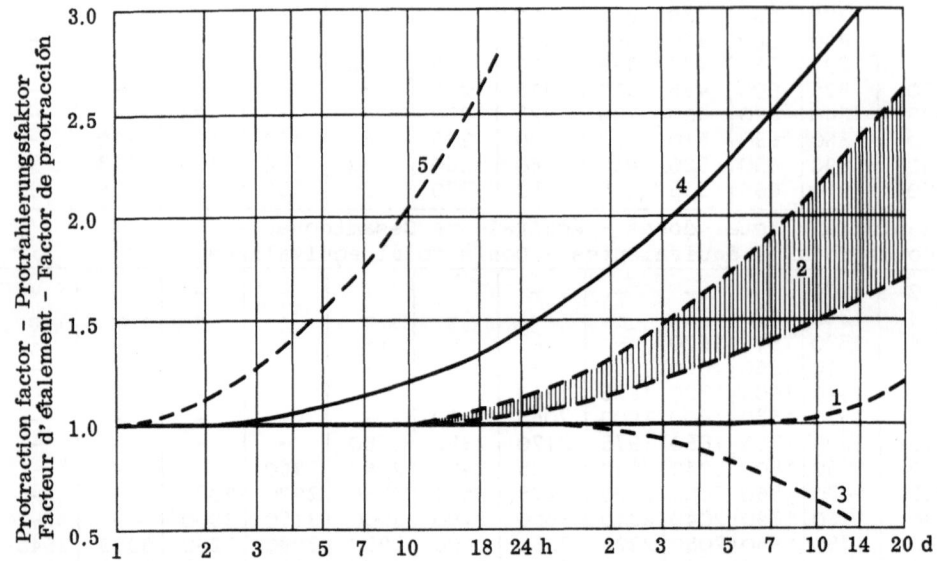

Irradiation time - Bestrahlungsdauer - Durée de l'irradiation
Duración de la radiación

1. Resting cells and mutations - Ruhende Zellen und Mutationen - Cellules au repos et mutations - Células en reposo y mutaciones

2. Tumour cells, killing - Tumorzellen, abtöten - Cellules tumorales, amortir - Destrucción de células tumorales

3. Germ cells - Samenepithel - Cellules germinales - Células seminales

4. Skin erythema - Hauterythem - Erythème cutané - Eritema cutáneo

5. Fast growing tissues - Schnell wachsende Gewebe - Tissus en croissance rapide - Tejidos de crecimiento rápido

Lit.: 1. QUIMBY, E.H., Mc COMB, W.S.: Radiology 29, 305 (1937)
      2. CHAOUL, H., WACHSMANN, F., ROSENBERGER, H.: Strahlenther. 76, 224 (1944)
      3. PATERSON, R.: Treatment of malignant disease by radium and X-rays, Baltimore: Williams and Wilkins 1948

Time Zeit Durée Tiempo	Protraction factors - Protrahierungsfaktoren*) Facteurs d'étalement - Factores de protracción					f_{ep} **)
	f_p1	f_p2	f_p3	f_p4	f_p5	1:2
1 h	1	1	1	1	1	1
2 h	1	1	1	1	1	1
3 h	1	1	1	1.02	1	>1
5 h	1	1	1	1.08	1	1.08
7 h	1	1	1	1.15	≫1	1.12
10 h	1	>1	1	1.20	≫1	1.20
15 h	1	>1	1	1.24	≫1	1.25
18 h	1	>1	1	1.33	≫1	1.30
24 h=1d	1	(1.05-1.1)	1	1.45	≫1	1.35
2 d	1	(1.1 -1.3)	1	1.75	≫1	1.55
3 d	1	(1.2 -1.45)	(>1)	1.95	≫1	1.65
4 d	1	(1.25-1.6)	(>1)	2.15	≫1	1.75
5 d	1	(1.35-1.7)	(>1)	2.25	≫1	1.75
7 d	1	(1.4 -1.9)	(>1)	2.5	≫1	1.8
10 d	(>1)	(1.5 -2.1)	(>1)	2.75	≫1	1.9
14 d	(>1)	(1.6 -2.4)	(>1)	3.05	≫1	2.0
20 d	(>1)	(1.7 -2.6)	(>1)	-	≫1	2.0

*) "Protraction factor " f_p = protracted dose/short-term dose, both of which produce the same biological effects; (1 - 5 see left page).

"Protrahierungsfaktor" f_p = Dosis protrahiert/Dosis kurzzeitig, bei beiden Verabreichungsarten gleiche biologische Wirkungen; (1 - 5 siehe linke Seite).

"Facteur d'étalement" f_p = dose avec irradiation étalée/dose avec irradiation aiguë qui produisent le même effet biologique; (1 - 5 voir page de gauche).

"Factor de protracción" f_p = dosis protraida/dosis aplicada en breve tiempo obteniéndose con ambas formas de tratamiento los mismos efectos biológicos (1 - 5 ver página izquierda).

**) "Therapeutic ratio" of dose protraction (e.g., tumor/skin: $f_{ep} = f_{p4}/f_{p2}$). The therapeutic ratio indicates how much the tumor dose can be increased while the reaction to healthy tissue (skin) remains unchanged.

"Elektivitätsfaktor" der Protrahierung (z.B. Tumor/Haut: $f_{ep} = f_{p4}/f_{p2}$). Der Elektivitätsfaktor gibt an, eine um wievielmal höhere Dosis dem Tumor bei gleichbleibender Belastung (Reaktion) des gesunden Gewebes (Haut) gegeben werden kann.

"Facteur de sélectivité" lié à l'étalement (par ex. tumeur/peau: $f_{ep} = f_{p4}/f_{p2}$). Il indique le facteur par lequel la dose à la tumeur peut être multipliée, pour que la réaction des tissus sains reste la même.

"Factor de electividad" de la protracción (p. ej. tumor/piel: $f_{ep} = f_{p4}/f_{p2}$). El factor de electividad indica en que proporción se puede suministrar al tumor una dosis superior, permaneciendo igual el daño (reacción) del tejido (piel) sano.

8.8   Growth of malignant tumours (average values)
       Wachstum bösartiger Geschwülste (Richtwerte)
       Croissance des tumeurs malignes (valeurs moyennes)
       Crecimiento de tumores malignos (valores promedios)

8.8.1 Theory of constant tumour doubling time (t_D)
       Theorie der gleichbleibenden Tumor-Verdopplungszeit (t_D)
       Théorie du temps de doublement constant de la tumeur (t_D)
       Teoría del tiempo constante de duplicación de los tumores (t_D)

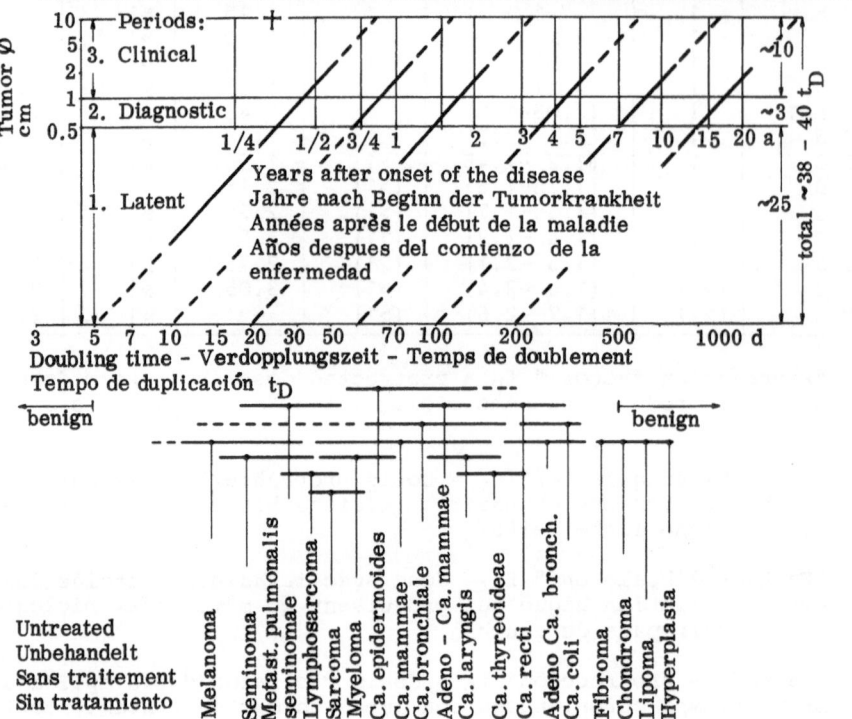

The graph indicates the approximate duration of the latent period, the period of
the possible diagnosis and the duration of the clinical phase. In practice many tumours grow faster in the initial phase and more slowly at the end of the clinical
phase, than corresponds to the doubling time.

Die Darstellung zeigt die ungefähre Dauer der Entstehungsphase, den frühestmög-
lichen Zeitpunkt der Diagnose und die Dauer der klinischen Phase. In der Praxis
wachsen Tumoren anfangs oft schneller und am Ende der klinischen Phase langsamer
als der Verdopplungszeit entspricht.

Le graphique indique la durée approximative de la periode de latence, le moment où
le diagnostic est possible et la durée de la phase clinique. En pratique de nombreuses tumeurs grossissent plus vite dans la phase initiale et plus lentement à la
fin de la phase clinique que ne le montre le temps de doublement.

La gráfica indica la duración aproximada de la fase de generación, el término de
la diagnosis y la duración de la fase clínica. En realidad los tumores crecen al
comienzo más rapidamente y al final de la fase clinica más lentamente de lo correspondiente al tiempo de duplicación.

Lit.: 1. COLLINS, V.P. et al.: Am.J.Roentgenol. 76, 988 (1956)
      2. CHARBIT, A. et al.: Europ.J.Cancer. 7, 307 (1971)
      3. OESER, H.: Krebsbekämpfung..., Stuttgart: Thieme 1974

8.8.2 Prognosis for malignant tumours following radiation therapy
Prognose maligner Tumoren nach Strahlentherapie
Prognose pour les tumeurs malignes après radiothérapie
Pronóstico de tumores malignos según la radioterapia

The average values given refer to patients who were treated between 1945 and 1965 - Die angegebenen groben Richtwerte beziehen sich auf Patienten, die etwa 1945 - 1965 behandelt wurden - Valeurs approchées se rapportant à des malades traites entre 1945 et 1965 - La cifras aproximadas se refieren a pacientes tratados entre 1945 y 1965

Tumour Tumor Tumeur Tumor	Frequency Häufigkeit Fréquence Frecuencia %	5-year survivors / 5-Jahre Überlebende / Survivants à 5 ans / 5 anos supervivencia Stage-Stadium-Stade-Fase					Remarks Bemerkungen Observations Observaciones
		1	2	3	4	total	
Bronchus	10					5	Inopérable
Collum uteri	9	60	60	30	7	55	Conventional
		75	75	45	10	70	Super voltage therapy
Mamma	8	80	40	-20-		50	Operable
		40	20	-10-		25	Inoperable
Rectum	4.3	40	40	-10-		30	(Intracavitary therapy 80 %)
Corpus uteri	3.4					55	Operable
		55	19			22	Inoperable
Ovarium	3.1	90	60	45	15		
Vulva	0.6	80	60	20	5	30	
Vagina	0.4	60	35	20	9	45	
Vesica urin.	1.7	65	30	15	8	30	
Oesophagus	1.0					3	
M. Hodgkin	0.9	55	40	14		30	(1972∿70 %)
Larynx	0.8	85	70	40	15	65	
Cutis	3	95	90	80		90	
Melanoma	0.7	70	30	12	∿0	60	
Lingua	0.2	65	30	15	5	60	
Labium oris	1.0					70	Contact therapy 90 %
Testis	0.3	85	70	25	5	70	

Lit.: 1. EICHHORN, H.J. et al.: Strahlenther. 131, 227 (1966)
2. BARTH, G., BECKER, J.: Klinische Radiologie, Stuttgart, New York: Schattauer-Verlag 1968
3. FLETCHER, G.H.: Textbook of Radiotherapy, Philadelphia: Lea and Febiger 1973
4. OESER, H.: Krebsbekämpfung..., Stuttgart: Thieme 1974

8.9   Typical dose values in biology and medicine
Typische Dosiswerte in Biologie und Medizin
Valeurs de dose typiques en biologie et en médecine
Valores típicos de dosis en biología y medicina

Average values - Richtwerte - Valeurs moyennes -
Valores aproximados

1. Smallest dose for which a biologic effect was observed [1]
   Kleinste Dosis, bei der ein biologischer Effekt be-
   obachtet wurde
   Plus petite dose pour laquelle un effet biologique a
   été observé
   Dosis mínima con la que se observa un efecto biológico   5 mrad

2. Dose which kills $1-1/e$ (= 63 %) of all cells (D_0) [2]
   Dosis, die $1-1/e$ (= 63 %) aller Zellen abtötet (D_0)
   Dose tuant $1-1/e$ (= 63 %) de toutes les cellules (D_0)
   Dosis que mata el $1-1/e$ (= 63 %) de todas las células (D_0)

   Ca cells in vitro - Ca-Zellen in vitro - Cellules
   cancereuses in vitro -Células cancerosas en vitro 100-200   rad

   Cells of root tips in beans - Wurzelspitzen-Zellen
   von Bohnen - Cellules de pointes de racines de fèves
   Células en las puntas de las raices en habas   1000   rad

   Escherichia coli bacteria   10 krad

   Yeast cells (Saccharomyces cerevisiae)   30 krad

   Viruses and bacteriophages   100 krad

3. D_0 for various cells of the living mouse
   D_0 für verschiedene Zellen der lebenden Maus
   D_0 pour différentes cellules de la souris in vivo
   D_0 de varias células de ratones, vivos

   Oocytes   5   rad

   Spermatogonia   180   rad

   Bone marrow stem cells   70   rad

   Intestinal crypt cells   200   rad

4. Suppression of germination in potatoes [3]
   Unterdrückung der Keimfähigkeit von Kartoffeln
   Arrèt de la germination des pommes de terre
   Supresión de la germinación en patatas   8-15 krad

5. Usual sterilising dose for medical products [4]
   Gebräuchliche Sterilisationsdosis für medizinische Erzeugnisse
   Dose stérilisante usuel pour des produits medicaux
   Dosis usual de esterilización, productos medicinales   1-3 Mrad

6. Human skin - Menschliche Haut - Peau humaine -
   Piel humana

   Epilation-transitory   >400   rad

   Epilation-irreversible   >800   rad

   Erythema (see page - siehe Seite - voir page -
   ver página 199)   800   rad

   Radiodermatitis exsudativa   1200   rad

Necrosis	2000	rad
Tolerance dose (field 100 cm^2)	1 x 1700	rad
Idem fractionated: 10 x /14 d =	3700	rad
Idem fractionated: 30 x /42 d =	5500	rad

7. Tolerance doses of different human organs (resulting damage) - Toleranzdosen verschiedener menschlicher Organe und (entstehende Schäden) - Dose de tolerance pour différents organes humains (l'esion résultante) - Dosis de tolerancia para diferentes órganos humanos (resultado del daño) 5)

Fractionated irradiation with 200 rad/d in the organ
Fraktionierte Bestrahlung mit 200 rad/d im Organ
Irradiation fractionnée avec 200 rads/d dans l'organe
Irradiación fraccionada con 200 rad/d en el órgano

Ren (Nephrosklerosis)	2300	rad
Hepar (Budd-Chiari)	3500	rad
Pulmones (Pneumonitis, Fibrosis)	4000	rad
Cerebrum (Necrosis)	5000	rad
Medulla spinalis (Myelitis)	5000	rad
Colon-rectum (Fistula, Stenosis)	5500	rad
Vesica uriniaris (Fistula, Fibrosis)	6000	rad
Os (Necrosis)	6000	rad
Cor (Myocarditis)	4000	rad
Lens (Cataracta)	500	rad
Testis (Azoospermia)	>500	rad
Ovarium (Menolysis)	>200	rad

8. Curative doses frequently used in therapy - in der Therapie zu kurativen Zwecken häufig verabreichte Herddosen Doses curatives fréquemment utilisées en radiothérapie Dosis frecuentemente utilizadas en terapía con fines curativos (Fractionated - Fraktioniert - Fractionnement Fraccionada 200 rad/d)

Seminoma	3000	rad
Lymphogranulomatosis (M. Hodgkin)	4000	rad
Carcinoma laryngis	> 6000	rad
Carcinoma mammae (post operationem)	4000-6000	rad
Osteosarcoma	> 7000	rad
Melanoma (fractionated: 300-1000 rad/d)	< 10-(20)	krad
Arthritis - Arthrosis etc. 5-10·10-20 rad (2/7 d)	50-200	rad

Lit.: 1. FORSSBERG, A.G.: Acta Radiol., Suppl. 49 (1943)
2. HOFMANN, E.G.: Rö.Prax. 23, 59 (1970)
3. CHADWICK, K.H.: Proc. IAEA Symp.Dos.Agriculture, Vienna 1973
4. HUG, O.: Med.Strahlenkunde, Berlin: Springer 1974
5. RUBIN, P., KELLER, B., QUICK, R. in: The Biological and Clinical Basis of Radiosensitivity, Springfield: Thomas 1974

8.10   <u>Grid or sieve therapy - Gitter- oder Siebbestrahlung -</u>
        <u>Radiothérapie à travers grilles - Irradiación con rejilla</u>

8.10.1 <u>Explanatory remarks - Erläuterungen - Explications -</u>
        <u>Explicaciones</u>

The <u>"grid factor"</u> f indicates how the surface dose administered
through a grid can be increased compared to that irradiating an open
field, while the skin tolerance remains unchanged. The factor increases as the relative aperture Ψ (Ψ = apertures/total field) and
the size of the grid holes decrease.

The <u>degree of homogeneity</u> Q is the ratio of the dose under the
shielded portions of the field to the dose under the exposed parts
of the field. To find the "effectiveness" η of the grid irradiation,
i.e., the possible increase in the mean depth dose, one multiplies
the grid factor by the relative aperture; i.e.:

$$\eta = f \cdot \Psi.$$

Der <u>"Gitterfaktor"</u> f gibt an, wie die über ein Gitter verabreichte
Oberflächendosis gegenüber der auf ein offenes Feld eingestrahlten
unter Einhaltung der Hauttoleranz erhöht werden kann. Er wächst mit
kleiner werdendem Öffnungsverhältnis Ψ (Ψ = Gitteröffnungen/Gesamt-
feld) und mit kleiner werdender Größe der Gitteröffnungen.

Der <u>Homogenitätsgrad</u> Q ist das Verhältnis der Dosis unter den abge-
deckten Feldpartien zur Dosis unter den offenen Feldteilen. Der
"Wirkungsgrad" η der Gitterbestrahlung, das ist die mögliche Erhöhung
der mittleren Tiefendosis, ergibt sich durch Multiplikation des Git-
terfaktors mit dem Öffnungsverhältnis, d.h. es ist

$$\eta = f \cdot \Psi.$$

Le <u>"facteur de grille"</u> f représente le facteur par lequel on peutt
multiplier la dose à la surface délivrée avec une grille par rapport
à celle délivrée par un champ simple sans que la tolérance cutanée
soit modifiée. Le facteur augmente lorsque le rapport d'ouverture Ψ
(Ψ = surface ouverte de la grille/surface totale du champ) et la
taille des trous de la grille diminuent.

Le <u>"coefficient d'homogénéité"</u> Q est le rapport de la dose dans les
zônes protegées à la dose dans les zônes irradiées. L'"efficacité"
de la grille η, c'est à dire l'accroissement possible de la dose en
profondeur s'obtient en multipliant le facteur de grille par le rapport d'ouverture:

$$\eta = f \cdot \Psi.$$

El <u>"factor de rejilla"</u> f indica hasta que punto se puede elevar una
dosis superficial suministrada sobre une rejilla, frente a un campo
abierto irradiado, manteniendo la tolerancia de piel. El factor
aumenta cuando la relación de abertura Ψ (Ψ = aberturas/campo
total) y el tamaño de los agujeros de la rejilla disminuye.

El <u>grado de homogeneidad</u> Q es la razón de la dosis bajo la porción
blindada del campo a la dosis bajo las partes expuestas del campo.
Para encontrar la "efectividad" η de la irradiación con rejilla, esto
es el aumento posible en la dosis de profundidad media, se multiplica
el factor de rejilla por la abertura relativa; esto es:

$$\eta = f \cdot \Psi.$$

Lit.: 1. LOEVINGER, R., WOLF, B.S., MINOWITZ, W.: Am.J.Roentgenol.
         <u>64</u>, 999 (1950)
      2. COHEN, O.A., PALAZZO, W.L.: Am.J.Roentgenol. <u>67</u>, 470 (1952)
      3. LOEVINGER, R.: Radiology <u>58</u>, 351 (1952)
      4. JOLLES, B., MITCHELL, R.G.: Brit.J.Radiol. <u>27</u>, 407 (1954)

8.10.2   <u>Practical values for f, η, and Q</u>
         <u>Praktische Werte für f, η und Q</u>
         <u>Valeurs pratiques pour f, η et Q</u>
         <u>Valores prácticos para f, η, y Q</u>

8.10.2.1 <u>Grid factors - Gitterfaktoren - Facteurs de grille -</u>
         <u>Factores de rejilla (f)</u>

Valid for 200 kV= (≈ 1.7 mm Cu HVL); field size ~100 cm^2
and grid holes of about 10 mm diameter - Gültig für
200 kV= (≈ 1,7 mm Cu HWSD), Feldgrößen von ~100 cm^2 und
Gitteröffnungen von 10 mm Durchmesser - Valable pour:
200 kV= (≈ 1,7 mm Cu CHA); champs de 100 cm^2 et diametres
des ouvertures de la grille 10 mm - Válido para: 200 kV=
(≈ 1,7 mm Cu CHR); campos de 100 cm^2 y aberturas de la
rejilla de 10 mm diámetro

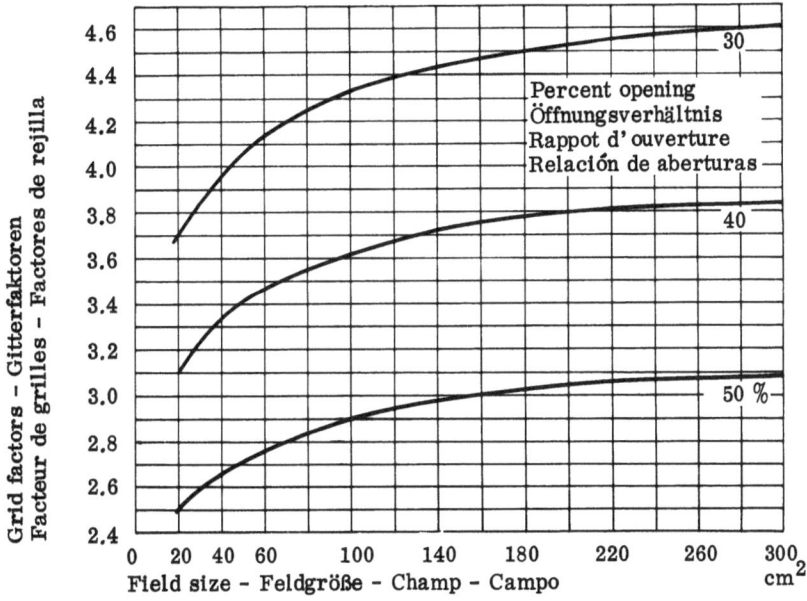

Field Feld Champ Campo cm^2	Grid factors - Gitterfaktoren - Facteurs de grille - Factores de rejilla and - und - et - y					f
	Effectivness - Wirkungsgrad - Efficacité - Efectividad					η
	Percent opening - Öffnungsverhältnis - Rapport d'ouverture - Relación de aberturas					%
	30		40		50	
	f	η	f	η	f	η
20	3.70	1.10	3.10	1.24	2.50	1.25
40	3.95	1.18	3.35	1.34	2.65	1.33
60	4.15	1.24	3.45	1.38	2.75	1.37
80	4.25	1.27	3.55	1.42	3.25	1.43
100	4.35	1.30	3.60	1.44	2.90	1.45
150	4.45	1.34	3.75	1.49	3.00	1.50
200	4.55	1.36	3.80	1.51	3.05	1.53
250	4.60	1.38	3.80	1.53	3.05	1.54
300	4.60	1.39	3.85	1.54	3.10	1.55

Note - Bemerkung - Remarque - Nota:

For fractionated doses the grid factors (f) are optimal (= maximal)
only if the grids are applied in such a way that the same skin areas
are always exposed or protected respectively.

Die Gitterfaktoren (f) sind bei fraktionierter Dosisverabreichung nur
dann optimal (= maximal), wenn die Gitter immer so aufgelegt werden,
daß jedesmal die gleichen Hautstellen offen bzw. abgedeckt sind.

Pour les irradiations fractionnées les facteurs de grille (f) sont
maxima seulement si la grille est mise en place de telle façon que
ce soient les mêmes surfaces de peau qui soient toujours irradiées
ou protegées.

Para dosis fraccionadas los factores de rejilla (f) son optimos (=
maximal) solamente si las rejillas son aplicadas en forma tal, que la
misma área de piel es siempre expuesta o desligada.

8.10.2.2 Degree of homogeneity - Homogenitätsgrad - Degré d'homo-
          généité - Grado de homogeneidad *)

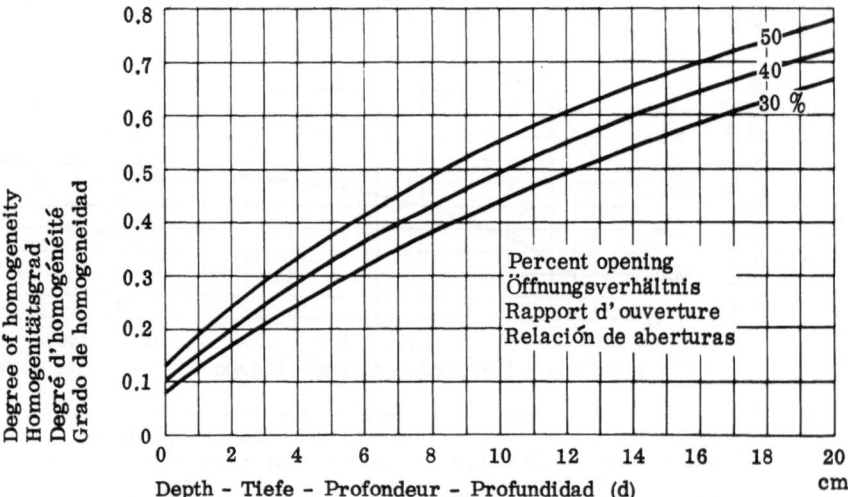

Depth - Tiefe - Profondeur - Profundidad (d)

*) Definition homogeneity see page - Begriff Homogenität siehe
   Seite - Définition d'homogénéité voir page - Definición homo-
   geneidad ver página 208

d cm	Degree of homogeneity - Homogenitätsgrad - Degré d'homo-généité - Grado de homogeneidad			d cm			Q
	ψ				ψ		%
	30	40	50		30	40	50
0	0.08	0.10	0.13	8	0.38	0.43	0.48
1	0.13	0.15	0.18	10	0.44	0.48	0.55
2	0.17	0.20	0.24	12	0.50	0.55	0.60
3	0.21	0.24	0.28	14	0.55	0.60	0.65
4	0.24	0.28	0.33	16	0.60	0.65	0.70
5	0.27	0.33	0.37	18	0.65	0.70	0.75
6	0.32	0.37	0.42	20	0.70	0.75	0.80

Table of contents - Inhaltsverzeichnis
Table des matières - Tabla de materias

9.1 Dose limits for man - Dosisgrenzwerte für Personen
Limites de dose pour les individus - Dosis limites para individuos

Organ Organ Organe Organo	Occupationally exposed persons Beruflich Strahlen-exponierte Travailleurs profes-sionnellement exposés Ocupacionalmente expuesto		Individual member of the public Einzelpersonen der Bevölkerung Individu donné de la population Individuos de la población en general	General population Gesamt-bevölkerung Population Población
	rem/a	rem/1/4 a	rem/a	rem/30 a
Gonads, red bone marrow, whole body Gonaden, rotes Knochenmark, Ganzkörper Gonades, moelle rouge, corps entier Ganados, médula roja, cuerpo total	5	3	0.5	5
Skin, thyroid gland, bone Haut, Schilddrüse, Knochen Peau, thyroïde, os Piel, glándula tiroidea, hueso	30	15	3(1.5)	
Hands, forearms, feet, ankles Hände, Unterarme, Füße, Knöchel Mains, avant-bras, pieds, chevilles Manos, antebrazos, pies, tobillos	75	40	7.5	
All other organs individually Alle anderen Organe einzeln Tout les autres organes individuellement Todos los demás órganos	15	8	1.5	

For a full discussion of dose limits the reader is referred to:
Einzelheiten sind aus folgenden Publikationen zu entnehmen:
Pour une discussion complète sur les limites de dose, le
lecteur est renvoyé à:
Para mayores detalles remitimos al lector a las publicaciones:

ICRP Publ. 9(1966), 2(1967), 10(1968)
22(1973), Oxford: Pergamon Press
IAEA Safety Series No. 9 (1967)
ENEA Radiation Protection Norms 1968
NCRP Report 39, Washington 1971

9.2 Important activities and concentrations (soluble substances)
Wichtige Aktivitäten und Konzentrationen (lösliche Stoffe)
Activités et concentrations notables (matériaux solubles)
Actividades y concentraciones importantes (material solubles)

Nuclide Nuklid Nucléide Nuclido	1 µCi	2 *) µCi	3 *) µCi	4 *) µCi/cm³	5 **) a µCi	5 **) b µCi	6 a rem/µCi	6 b rem/µCi
^{51}Cr	100	800	$2.7 \cdot 10^4$	$4 \cdot 10^{-6}$	$1.3 \cdot 10^3$	$2.7 \cdot 10^3$	$1.2 \cdot 10^{-3}$	$3.3 \cdot 10^{-4}$
^{57}Co	10	200	$8.7 \cdot 10^3$	$5 \cdot 10^{-3}$	$4.3 \cdot 10^2$	$8.7 \cdot 10^2$	$3.6 \cdot 10^{-3}$	$5.5 \cdot 10^{-4}$
^{58}Co	10	30	$2.4 \cdot 10^3$	$3 \cdot 10^{-7}$	$1.0 \cdot 10^2$	$2.4 \cdot 10^2$	$1.5 \cdot 10^{-2}$	$2.4 \cdot 10^{-3}$
^{59}Fe	10	20	$3.7 \cdot 10^2$	$5 \cdot 10^{-8}$	$4.7 \cdot 10^2$	$3.7 \cdot 10$	$3.3 \cdot 10^{-2}$	$4.0 \cdot 10^{-2}$
^{75}Se	10	90	$3.1 \cdot 10^3$	$4 \cdot 10^{-7}$	$2.4 \cdot 10^2$	$3.1 \cdot 10^2$	$6.3 \cdot 10^{-3}$	$5.0 \cdot 10^{-3}$
^{85}Sr	10	60	$5.8 \cdot 10^2$	$8 \cdot 10^{-8}$	$7.6 \cdot 10$	$5.8 \cdot 10$	$1.3 \cdot 10^{-2}$	$3.0 \cdot 10^{-2}$
^{99m}Tc	100	200	$9.5 \cdot 10^4$	10^{-5}	$4.6 \cdot 10^3$	$9.5 \cdot 10^3$	$(3 \cdot 10^{-4})$	$(1.5 \cdot 10^{-4})$
^{113m}In	100	30	$2.1 \cdot 10^4$	$3 \cdot 10^{-6}$	$1.0 \cdot 10^3$	$2.1 \cdot 10^3$	$(5 \cdot 10^{-4})$	$(2.0 \cdot 10^{-4})$
^{125}I	(1)	(1)	$(4 \cdot 10)$	$(5 \cdot 10^{-9})$	(2.4)	(4.0)	(1.2)	(0.75)
^{131}I	1	0.7	$2.1 \cdot 10$	$(3 \cdot 10^{-9})$	1.6	2.1	2.0	1.6
^{132}I	10	0.3	$5.9 \cdot 10^2$	$(8 \cdot 10^{-8})$	4.5	$5.9 \cdot 10$	$6 \cdot 10^{-2}$	$4.5 \cdot 10^{-2}$
^{137}Cs	10	30	$1.6 \cdot 10^2$	$2 \cdot 10^{-8}$	$1.2 \cdot 10$	$1.6 \cdot 10$	$1.1 \cdot 10^{-1}$	$8 \cdot 10^{-2}$
^{197}Hg	100	20	$2.9 \cdot 10^3$	$4 \cdot 10^{-7}$	$2.4 \cdot 10^2$	$2.9 \cdot 10^2$	$5.2 \cdot 10^{-3}$	$4.5 \cdot 10^{-3}$
^{198}Au	10	20	$8 \cdot 10^2$	10^{-7}	$4.1 \cdot 10$	$8 \cdot 10$	$3.4 \cdot 10^{-2}$	$2.6 \cdot 10^{-4}$
^{203}Hg	10	4	$1.8 \cdot 10^2$	$2 \cdot 10^{-8}$	$1.4 \cdot 10$	$1.8 \cdot 10$	$1.0 \cdot 10^{-1}$	$8 \cdot 10^{-2}$

1. Maximum permissible activity for exemption from notification, registration or licensing - Freigrenze - Activité maximale permettant l'exemption de la déclaration où de la demande d'agréement - Limite de libertad

2. Maximum permissible total body burden - Höchstzugelassene Körperaktivität - Activité corporelle maximale permissible - Carga corporal máxima permisible

3. Maximum permissible annual intake by inhalation during working hours - Maximal zulässige Jahresaktivitätszufuhr über die Luft während der Arbeitszeit - Quantité inhalée maximale permissible durant des heures de travail - Aporte de carga anual máximo permisible por inhalación durante las horas de trabajo

4. Maximum permissible concentration in inhaled air; exposure time 168 h/week - Maximal zulässige Konzentration in der Atemluft, Einwirkungsdauer 168 h/Woche - Concentration maximale permissible pour l'air inhalé; temps de référence: 168 h/ semaine - Concentración máxima permisible en el aire inhalado, tiempo de influencia 168 h/semana

5. Limiting value for annual intake by (a) ingestion and (b) inhalation - Grenzwert der Jahresaktivitäszufuhr durch (a) Ingestion und (b) Inhalation - Valeurs limites des quantités annuelles a) ingérée et b) inhalée - Valores límites del aporte de carga anual por a) ingestión b) inhalación

6. Dose commitment (50 a), single intake - Folge-Äquivalentdosis (50 a), einmalige Aufnahme - Dose engagée (50 a), incorporation unique - Dosis sucesiva, equivalente (50 a), toma unica

*) Workers - Arbeiter - Travailleurs - Trabajadores

**) Member of the public - Einzelperson der Bevölkerung - Individu de la population Individuo de la populación

Lit.: See page - Siehe Seite - Voir page - Ver página 212

9.3 Mean doses to the whole body, gonads or organs
     Mittlere Ganzkörper-, Gonaden- oder Organdosen
     Doses moyennes délivrées à l'ensemble de l'organisme, aux
     gonades ou aux différents organes
     Doses medianos a cuerpo entero, gónados or órganos

(Maximal values neglected - Höchstwerte vernachlässigt - Les valeurs
extrêmes n'ont pas été retenues - Valores maximales desuidos)

		min.	mean	max.
1.	Natural sources - Natürliche Strahlenquellen - Sources naturelles - Fuentes naturales		mrad/a	
1.1	Cosmic radiation - Kosmische Strahlung - 0 m	20	30	40
	Rayonnement cosmique - Rayos cósmicos 1000 m	30	40	50
1.2	Terrestrial radiation - Umgebungsstrahlung Rayonnement terrestre - Radiación terrestral	20	45	150
	(Maximum values - Höchstwerte - Valeurs maximales - Valores máximos Kerala/India, Guarapari/Brazil		- ∿1000	>3000)
1.3	Incorporated radionuclides - Inkorporierte Radionuklide - Radionucléides dans le corps humain - Radionúclidos incorporados)	10	20	40
1.4	Additional radiation in houses - Zusätzliche Strahlung in Gebäuden - Irradiations additio- nelles dues aux bâtiments - Radiación adicional en las casas	<0	15	30
	Total - Zusammen - Total - Total	∿60	∿110	∿270
2.	Artificial sources - Künstliche Strahlenquellen Sources d'origine humaine - Fuentes artificiales			
2.1	Medicine - Medizin - Médecine - Medicina Total:	20	50	80
2.1.1	Diagnosis - Diagnostik - Diagnóstic - Diagnóstico	16	48	76
2.1.2	Therapy - Therapie - Thérapie - Terapía	0.5	1	2
2.1.3	Nuclear medicine - Nuklearmedizin - Médecine nucléaire - Medicina nuclear	0.5	1	2
2.2	Occupational exposure - Berufliche Strahlen- belastung - Exposition professionnelle - Exposición ocupacional		<1	
2.3	Radioactivity in consumer goods - Radioakti- vität in Verbrauchsgütern - Radioactivité des biens de consommation - Radiactividad en los productos del consumidor	1	2	4
2.4	Fall-out - Fall out - Retombées - Lluvia radiactiva	3	4	10
2.5	Nuclear power plants - Kernkraftwerke - Centrales nucléaires - Plantas nucleares		< 1	
	Total - Zusammen - Total - Total	∿25	∿60	∿100

9.4 Components of cosmic radiation at various altitudes
Komponenten der kosmischen Strahlung in verschiedenen Höhen
Composants du rayonnement cosmique à diverses altitudes
Componentes de radiación cósmica a diferentes altitudes

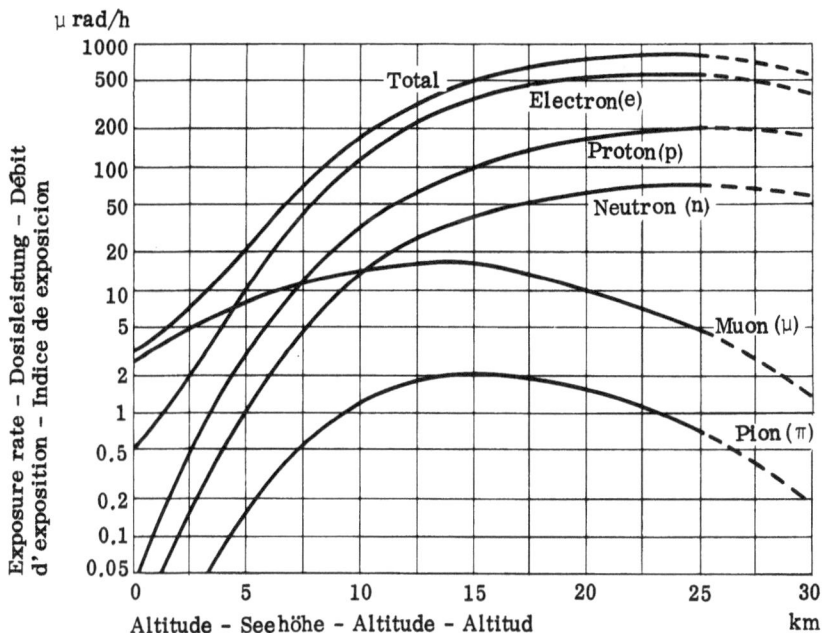

Altitude Seehöhe Altitude Altitud	Exposure rate - Dosisleistung - Débit d'exposition - Indice de exposición μrad/h					
	Particle - Teilchen - Particules - Partículas					
km	π	μ	n	p	e⁻	total
0	(<0.01)	2.7	(0.015)	0.04	0.5	3.2
1	(<0.01)	3.4	0.04	0.12	0.8	4.3
2	(<0.01)	4.2	0.1	0.3	1.4	6.0
3	0.04	5.2	0.25	0.7	2.8	9.0
4	0.08	6.5	0.5	1.5	5.4	14
5	0.15	8.0	1.0	3.0	10	22
7.5	0.35	12	4.4	12	40	69
10	1.2	14	14	34	110	173
12.5	1.8	16	26	60	220	324
15	2.0	15	35	100	360	512
17.5	1.9	13	50	135	450	650
20	1.6	10	62	165	500	740
22.5	1.1	7.0	68	190	550	820
25	0.7	4.5	73	200	550	830
27.5	(0.4)	(2.7)	(65)	(195)	(480)	(750)
30	(0.2)	(1.3)	(58)	(170)	(370)	(600)

Lit.: 1. ICRP Publ. 18, Oxford: Pergamon Press 1972

Average half- and tenth-value layers of shielding materials
Mittlere Halb- und Zehntelwertschichten von Abschirmstoffen
Couches moyennes de demi atténuation et d'atténuation 1/10
pour les matériaux utilisés en radioprotection
Capas hemi y deci reductoras para materiales de blindaje

Broad beams - Breite Felder - Champs larges - Campos anchos

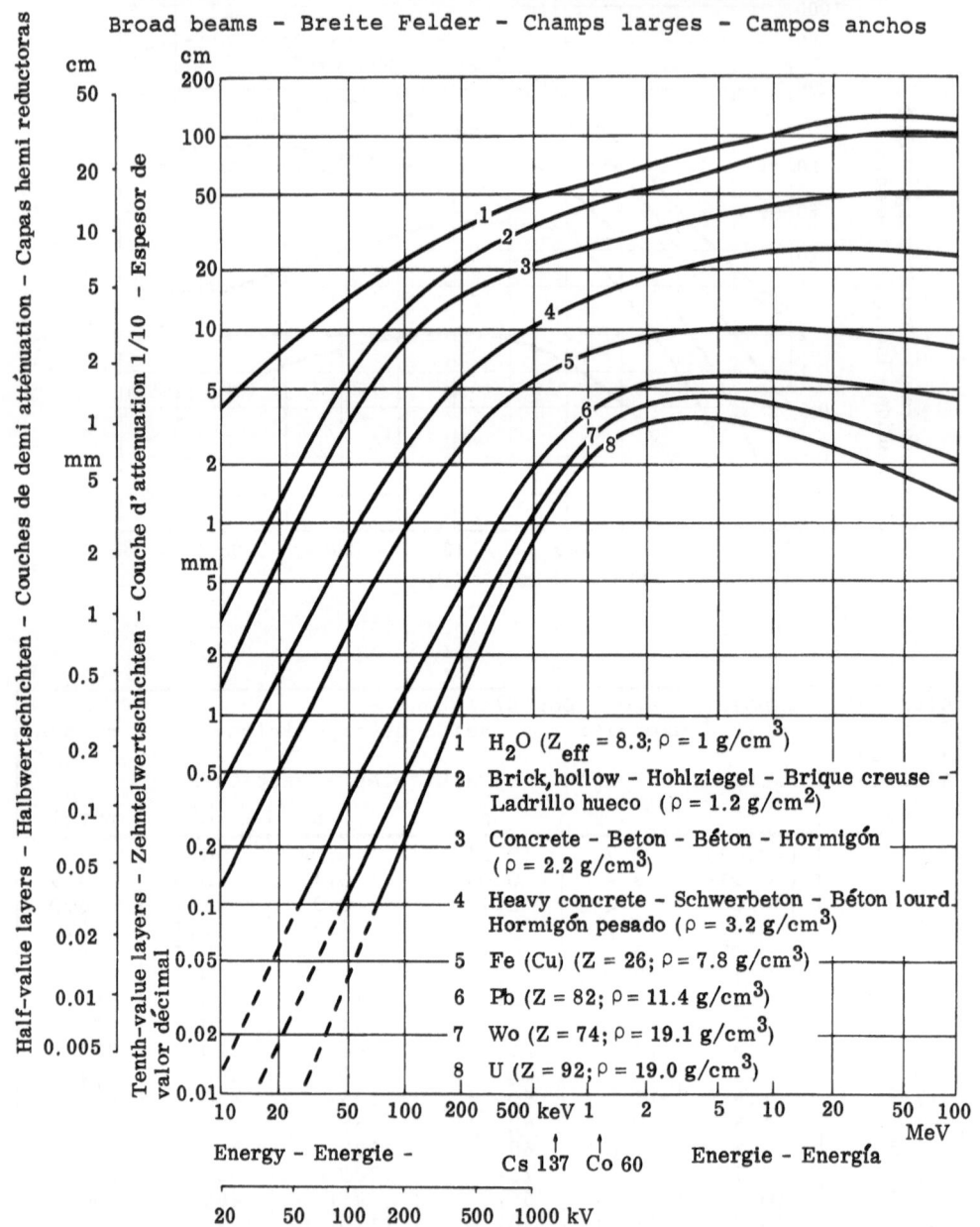

1 H_2O (Z_{eff} = 8.3; ρ = 1 g/cm^3)

2 Brick, hollow - Hohlziegel - Brique creuse - Ladrillo hueco (ρ = 1.2 g/cm^2)

3 Concrete - Beton - Béton - Hormigón (ρ = 2.2 g/cm^3)

4 Heavy concrete - Schwerbeton - Béton lourd, Hormigón pesado (ρ = 3.2 g/cm^3)

5 Fe (Cu) (Z = 26; ρ = 7.8 g/cm^3)

6 Pb (Z = 82; ρ = 11.4 g/cm^3)

7 Wo (Z = 74; ρ = 19.1 g/cm^3)

8 U (Z = 92; ρ = 19.0 g/cm^3)

Energy - Energie -   Cs 137 Co 60   Energie - Energía

20   50   100 200   500 1000 kV

Tube voltage - Röhrenspannung - Tension d'alimentation - Voltaje del tubo

Half-value layers - Halbwertschichten - Couches de demi atténuation - Capas hemi reductoras

Tenth-value layers - Zehntelwertschichten - Couche d'attenuation 1/10 - Espesor de valor décimal

Energy / Energie / Energie / Energía	HVL - HWSD - CDA - CHR (Rounded values - Abgerundete Zahlenwerte - Valeurs arrondies - Valores redondeados) Material - Stoff - Matériau - Material								
E	1 (H$_2$O)	2	3	4	5 (Fe)	6 (Pb)	7 (W)	8 *) (U)	
10 keV	1.2	0.9	0.4	0.12	0.04	(0.004)	-	-	mm
20	2.3	3.9	1.4	0.5	0.16	(0.009)	(0.006)	-	
50	4.2	1.7	1.0	2.3	0.8	0.11	0.035	(0.012)	
100	6.8	3.8	2.5	7.0	2.7	0.38	0.14	0.065	
200	10	6.5	4.4	1.7	7.3	1.35	0.65	0.38	
500	14	10	6.4	3.1	1.6	5.6	3.2	2.3	
Cs 137	15	11	6.8	3.5	1.8	7.0	4.5	3.4	
1 MeV	16	12	7.5	4.2	2.2	1.1	7.8	6.1	cm
Co 60	17	14	8.0	4.5	2.4	1.2	9.0	7.2	
2	20	15'	9.2	5.4	2.7	1.6	1.2	1.0	
5	23	19	11	6.7	3.0	1.7	1.3	1.0	
10	28	22	13	7.2	3.0	1.7	1.2	0.9	
20	35	28	14	7.6	3.0	1.6	1.0	0.7	
50	38	31	15	7.3	2.6	1.4	0.8	0.5	
100	35	30	15	7.0	2.4	1.3	0.63	0.38	
E	1/10 VL - 1/10 WSD - CA 1/10 - C 1/10 R								
10 keV	3.8	3.2	1.4	0.4	0.13	(0.013)	-	-	mm
20	7.6	1.3	6.5	1.7	0.55	(0.06)	(0.018)	-	
50	15	6.0	3.5	8.0	2.7	0.38	0.11	0.04	
100	23	13	9.0	2.4	9.0	1.3	0.45	0.22	
200	34	22	15	5.7	2.6	4.7	2.2	1.3	
500	48	35	22	11	5.5	2.0	1.1	8	
Cs 137	52	39	24	12	6.4	2.8	1.8	1.3	
1 MeV	58	50	26	15	7.6	3.8	2.8	2.2	cm
Co 60	60	51	28	16	7.9	4.0	3.1	2.4	
2	70	54	33	18	9.4	5.5	4.2	3.3	
5	87	66	38	23	10	5.8	4.6	3.5	
10	100	78	44	25	11	5.8	4.2	3.0	
20	120	96	48	26	10	5.5	3.5	2.4	
50	122	104	50	25	8.6	4.9	2.7	1.8	
100	120	103	50	23	8.0	4.4	2.1	1.3	

*) Numbers 1 - 8 see page 216
Zahlen 1 - 8 vergl. Kurven auf Seite 216
Pour les numeros 1 - 8 voir page 216
Cifras 1 - 8 ver página 216

Lit.: 1. GLADYS, WHITE, R.: NBS-Report No. 1003 (1952)
2. LORENTZON, L.: Acta Radiol. 41, 201 (1954)
3. NCRP Report No. 33 (1968)
4. ICRP Report No. 21 (1971)
5. MARUYAMA, R. et al.: Hlth. Phys. 20, 277 (1971)
6. JAEGER, R., HÜBNER, W.: Dosimetrie und Strahlenschutz, Stuttgart: Thieme 1974
7. TROUT, D.E. et al.: Hlth. Phys. 29, 163 (1975)

9.6   Transmission of rays through shielding walls
       Durchlässigkeit von Abschirmwänden für Strahlungen
       Transmission des rayonnements à travers des écrans protecteurs
       Permeabilidad de las radiaciones a través de blindaje

9.6.1   50 - 300 kV X-rays - Röntgenstrahlen - Rayons X - Rayos X

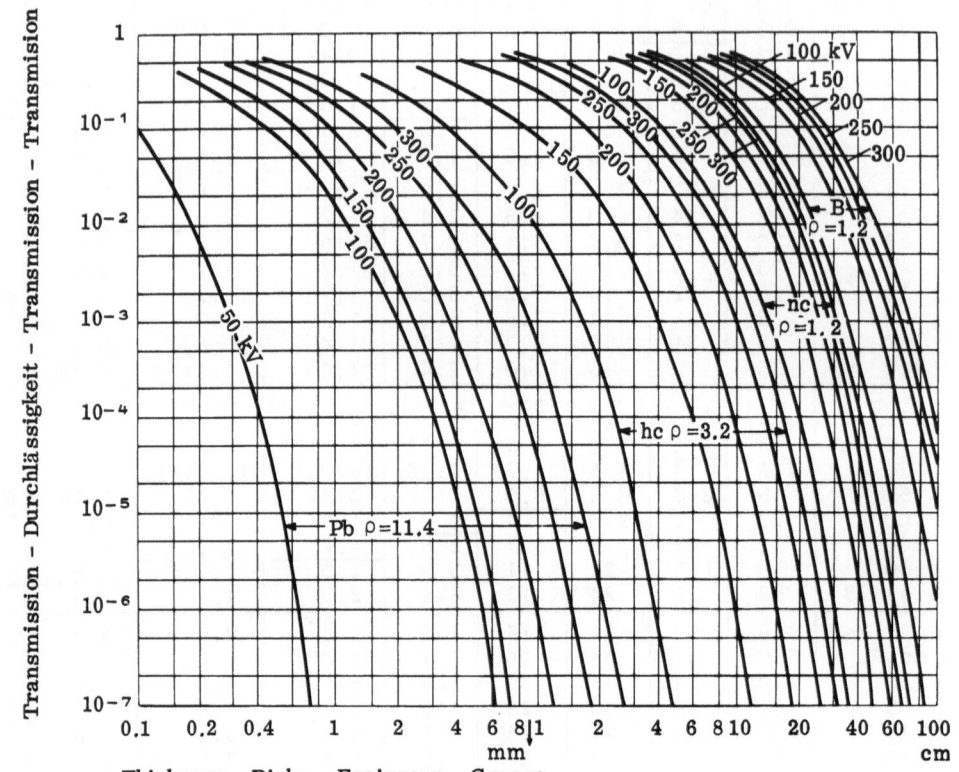

Thickness - Dicke - Epaisseur - Grueso

Pb (ρ = 11.35) = Lead - Blei - Plomb - Plomo

hc (ρ = 3.2) = Heavy concrete - Schwerbeton - Béton lourd - Hormigón
                    pesado

nc (ρ = 2.2) = Normal concrete - Normalbeton - Béton normal -
                    Hormigón normal

B (ρ = 1.2) = Brick - Ziegel - Brique - Ladrillo

kV = Normal radiation - Normalstrahlung - Rayonnement normal -
     Radiación normal

Lit.: 1. ICRP, Suppl. 15, Oxford (1970)
      2. KELLEY, J.P., TROUT, E.D.: Radiology 104, 171 (1972)
      3. DIN 6812, Berlin: Beuth-Verlag, Februar 1974
      4. Authors' measurements - Eigene Messungen - Mesures perso-
         nelles - Medidas propias

Transmission / Durchlässigkeit / Transmission / Transmisión	Required thickness - Erforderliche Abschirmung - Epaisseur nécessaire - Espesor requerido mm, cm											
	With tube voltages - Bei Röhrenspannungen - Tension du tube - Con tensión del tubo kV											
	Lead - Blei / Plomb - Plomo mm						Heavy concrete - Barytbeton / Béton baryté - Hormigón pesado cm					
	kV 50	100	150	200	250	300	kV 50	100	150	200	250	300
10^{-1}	0.10	0.45	0.62	1.0	1.4	2.0	(0.09)	0.35	0.90	1.8	2.9	3.4
$5 \cdot 10^{-2}$	0.12	0.65	0.86	1.3	2.0	3.0	(0.13)	0.5	1.3	2.4	3.5	4.6
10^{-2}	0.17	1.1	1.5	2.2	3.5	5.0	(0.26)	1.0	2.4	4.1	6.1	7.8
$5 \cdot 10^{-3}$	0.20	1.4	1.8	2.7	4.2	6.3	(0.31)	1.2	3.0	5.0	7.2	9.0
10^{-3}	0.27	2.0	2.5	3.6	6.0	9.0	(0.44)	1.7	4.0	6.7	9.8	12
$5 \cdot 10^{-4}$	0.30	2.3	2.8	4.2	6.7	10	(0.49)	1.9	4.6	7.7	11	14
10^{-4}	0.36	3.1	3.5	5.6	8.7	14	(0.65)	2.5	6.0	9.5	14	17
$5 \cdot 10^{-5}$	0.40	3.3	4.0	6.1	9.8	15	(0.70)	2.7	6.4	11	15	18
10^{-5}	0.45	4.3	5.0	7.8	12	17	(0.80)	3.1	7.9	13	18	22
$5 \cdot 10^{-6}$	0.48	4.7	5.4	8.3	13	19	(0.85)	3.3	8.5	14	23	23
10^{-6}	0.54	5.5	6.2	9.9	15	22	(0.98)	3.8	10	16	22	27
$5 \cdot 10^{-7}$	0.57	5.7	6.7	10.5	16	24	(1.04)	4.0	10.5	17	23	28
10^{-7}	0.62	6.0	7.3	12	18	28	(1.14)	4.4	11.5	19	26	31

	Concrete - Beton / Béton - Hormigón cm						Brick - Ziegel / Brique - Ladrillo cm					
	kV 50	100	150	200	250	300	kV 50	100	150	200	250	300
10^{-1}	1.3	4.3	7.3	9.2	10.5	13	3.5	13	18	21	23	25
$5 \cdot 10^{-2}$	1.7	5.6	9.4	12	14	15	4.3	16	22	25	27	30
10^{-2}	2.7	9.0	15	18	20	21	6.2	23	30	35	39	43
$5 \cdot 10^{-3}$	3.2	10.5	17	20	22	22	6.7	25	34	38	44	48
10^{-3}	4.5	15	21	26	29	27	8.5	32	43	49	54	60
$5 \cdot 10^{-4}$	5.1	17	23	29	31	31	9.0	34	46	53	60	64
10^{-4}	6.0	20	28	34	36	36	11	42	53	64	69	75
$5 \cdot 10^{-5}$	6.6	22	30	36	40	37	12	43	56	67	74	(80)
10^{-5}	7.8	26	34	41	46	43	14	50	66	80	-	-
$5 \cdot 10^{-6}$	8.4	28	36	43	50	46	15	54	69	(85)	-	-
10^{-6}	9.3	31	42	50	47	51	17	61	80	-	-	-
$5 \cdot 10^{-7}$	9.5	32	44	52	60	54	17	63	(85)	-	-	-
10^{-7}	10.0	34	48	59	66	60	19	70	-	-	-	-

I 131, Cs 137, Co 60, 5 - 100 MV

X- and gamma rays - Röntgen- und Gammastrahlen - Rayons X et
rayons gamma - Rayos X y gamma

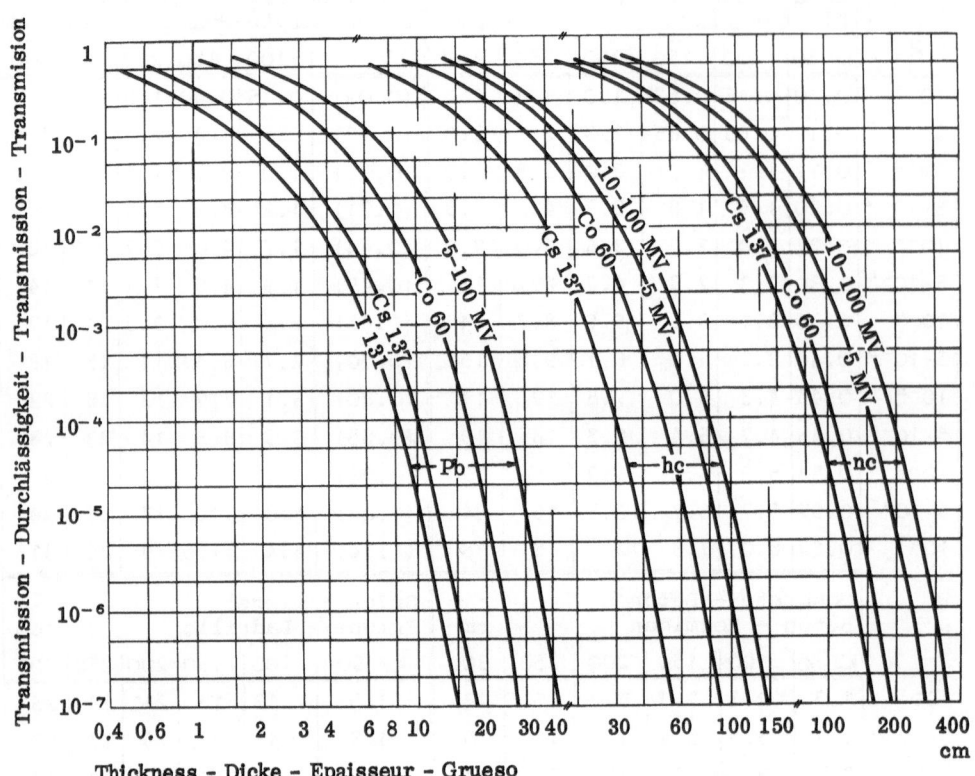

Thickness - Dicke - Epaisseur - Grueso

Pb (ρ = 11.35) = Lead - Blei - Plomb - Plomo

hc (ρ = 3.2) = Heavy concrete - Schwerbeton - Béton lourd - Hormigón
              pesado

nc (ρ = 2.2) = Normal concrete - Normalbeton - Béton normal -
              Hormigón normal

I 131 = γ-radiation of ^{131}I (E = 640 keV) - γ-Strahlung von ^{131}J

        (E = 640 keV) - Radiation γ de ^{131}I (E = 640 keV) - Radiación

        γ de ^{131}I (E = 640 keV)

Lit.: 1. MARUYAMA, T. et al.: Health Phys. 20, 277 (1971)
      2. SAUERMANN, D.F., FRIEDRICH, W., MITLACHER, H.: Tagungsbe-
         richte, Fachverband für Strahlenschutz, 241 (1973)

Transmission / Durchlässigkeit / Transmission / Transmisión	Required thickness - Erforderliche Abschirmung - Epaisseur nécessaire - Espesor requerido mm, cm											
	With γ-radiation of - Bei γ-Strahlungen von - Avec rayonnement γ de - Con radiación γ de kV											
	Lead - Blei Plomb - Plomo mm				Heavy concrete Barytbeton Béton baryte Hormigón pesado cm				Concrete Beton Béton Hormigón cm			
	^{131}I	Cs	Co	5-100 MV	Cs	Co	5 MV	10-100 MV	Cs	Co	5 MV	10-100 MV
$5 \cdot 10^{-1}$	0.46	0.67	1.3	1.9	2.7	4.3	6.6	7.5	7.0	8.5	13	16
$2 \cdot 10^{-1}$	1.0	1.4	2.8	4.5	5.3	8.8	12	14	15	18	26	34
10^{-1}	1.7	2.1	4.2	6.6	7.6	12	17	19	22	26	37	48
$5 \cdot 10^{-2}$	2.1	2.8	5.2	8.0	9.8	17	21	25	28	34	49	63
$2 \cdot 10^{-2}$	3.0	3.9	6.9	11	13	22	28	32	37	46	63	82
10^{-2}	3.7	4.8	8.1	13	15	25	33	39	42	52	74	96
$5 \cdot 10^{-3}$	4.4	5.7	9.4	15	18	28	38	47	50	60	85	110
$2 \cdot 10^{-3}$	5.3	6.8	11	17	21	33	45	52	58	70	104	130
10^{-3}	6.0	7.5	13	19	22	37	50	60	65	80	114	145
$5 \cdot 10^{-4}$	6.7	8.3	14	21	25	41	54	64	71	85	125	160
$2 \cdot 10^{-4}$	7.6	9.4	15	23	28	46	62	72	80	98	140	180
10^{-4}	8.1	10	17	25	30	50	67	80	88	105	150	190
$5 \cdot 10^{-5}$	8.8	11	18	27	32	53	71	85	95	114	160	205
$2 \cdot 10^{-5}$	9.7	12	19	29	36	59	78	94	105	125	180	230
10^{-5}	10.3	12	20	30	38	63	83	103	110	135	190	245
$5 \cdot 10^{-6}$	11	13	22	32	41	67	89	110	115	140	200	260
$2 \cdot 10^{-6}$	12	14	23	34	43	71	96	117	128	155	220	280
10^{-6}	13	15	24	36	46	75	102	123	135	165	240	300
$5 \cdot 10^{-7}$	13	16	25	38	49	79	108	130	140	175	250	315
$2 \cdot 10^{-7}$	14	17	27	40	53	85	112	138	155	180	270	335
10^{-7}	15	18	28	42	55	89	120	145	160	190	275	350

9.7 Quantity and quality of back-scattered X-radiation
Quantität und Qualität rückgestreuter Röntgenstrahlung
Quantité et qualité des rayonnements X rétrodiffusés
Cantidad y calidad de la radiación dispersa de los rayos X

Conditions of measurement - Meßbedingungen - Conditions de mesure - Condiciones de medida

20 x 20 cm^2 Field area - Feldgröße - Champ - Campo

50 cm Distance source/scatterer/radiation detector; thick scattering medium (d > 3 HVL) - Abstand Strahlenquelle/Streukörper/Strahlendetektor; Dicke Streukörper (d > 3 HWSD) - Distance source/milieu diffusant/détecteur; épaisseur de milieu diffusant (d > 3 CDA) - Distancia fuente/cuerpo disperson/detector; espesor del cuerpo dispersor (d > 3 CHR)

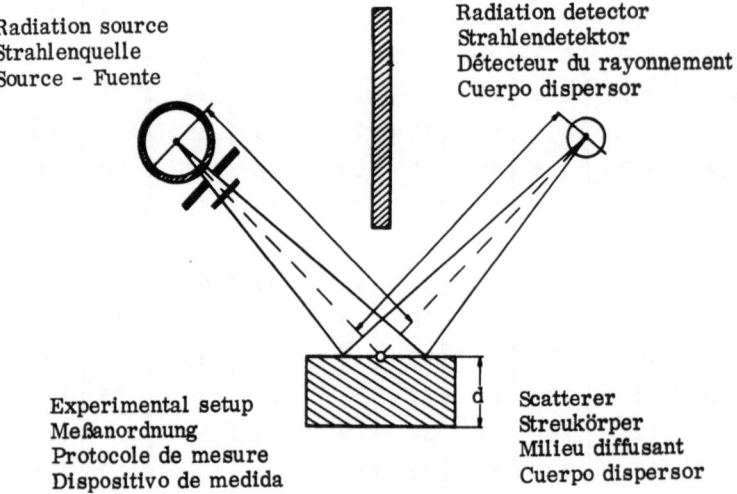

Radiation source
Strahlenquelle
Source - Fuente

Radiation detector
Strahlendetektor
Détecteur du rayonnement
Cuerpo dispersor

Experimental setup
Meßanordnung
Protocole de mesure
Dispositivo de medida

Scatterer
Streukörper
Milieu diffusant
Cuerpo dispersor

The data given in the graphs must be regarded as relative only since they are strongly dependent on the distances and angles between radiation source, scatterer, and detector. Therefore the results are presented only in graphic form.

Die aus den Kurven ablesbaren Daten müssen relativ betrachtet werden, da sie stark von den Abständen und Winkeln Strahlenquelle/Streukörper/Detektor abhängen. Aus diesem Grunde sind die Ergebnisse nur in Kurvenform dargestellt.

Les valeurs figurant sur les courbes sont des données approchées, car elles dépendent beaucoup des distances et des angles entre la source, le diffuseur et le détecteur. C'est pourquoi les résultats sont présentés seulement sous une forme graphique.

Los valores mostrados deben considerarse como relativos ya que - los valores absolutos dependen en gran parte de la distancia y los ángulos de la fuente/cuerpo dispersor/detector y tamaño del campo irradiado.

Lit.: 1. WACHSMANN, F.: Fortschr.Röntgenstr. 101, 308 (1964)
      2. WACHSMANN, F.: Radiologia diagnostica 6, 369 (1965)
      3. ICRP 21, (1971)

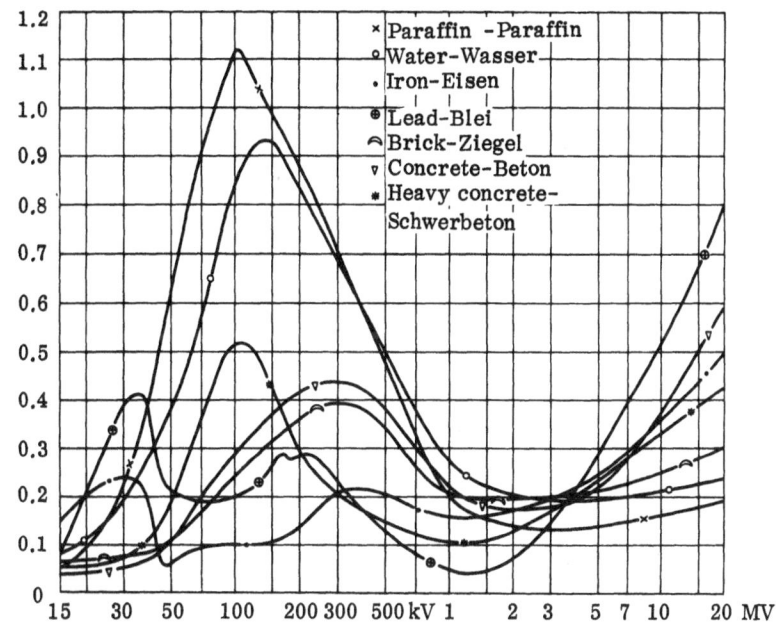

Paraffin - Paraffin
Water - Wasser
Iron - Eisen
Lead - Blei
Brick - Ziegel
Concrete - Beton
Heavy concrete - Schwerbeton

Normal radiation - Normalstrahlung - Rayonnement normal
Radiación normal

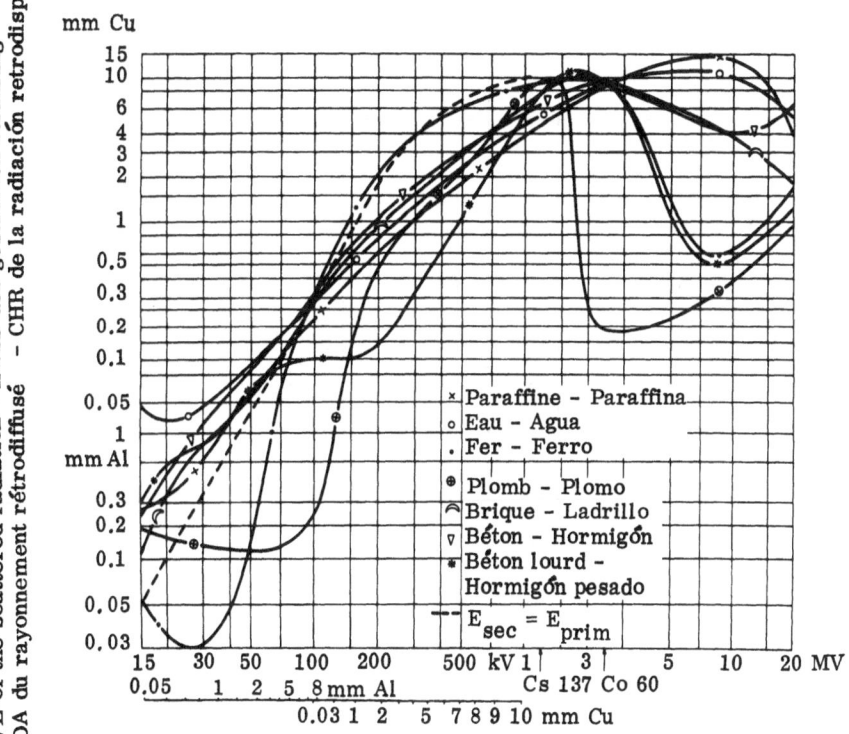

mm Cu

mm Al

Paraffine - Paraffina
Eau - Agua
Fer - Ferro
Plomb - Plomo
Brique - Ladrillo
Béton - Hormigón
Béton lourd - Hormigón pesado
$E_{sec} = E_{prim}$

Cs 137 Co 60

0.05   1   2   5   8 mm Al
0.03 1 2   5   7 8 9 10 mm Cu

Normal radiation - Normalstrahlung - Rayonnement normal
Radiación normal

223

9.8 Radioactivity in building materials
Radioaktivität in Baustoffen
Radioactivité des matériaux de construction
Radioactividad en materiales de construcción

Average values - Richtwerte
Valeurs moyennes - Valores orientativos

Material / Material / Matériaux / Material	Activity - Aktivität - Activité - Actividad nCi/kg ^{40}K			^{226}Ra			^{232}Th		
	min.	med.	max.	min.	med.	max.	min.	med.	max.
Sand and gravel / Sand und Kies / Sable et gravier / Arena y grava	0.2	7	18	0.1	<0.4	0.8	0.1	<0.4	1
Other natural stone / Andere Natursteine / Autres pierres natur. / Otras piedras naturales	1	<13	25	0.5	0.7	1.2	0.5	<0.8	1.4
Lava, basalt / Tuffstein, Basalt / Lave, basalte / Toba, basalto	11	38	55	0.4	1.1	2.3	0.2	<0.5	1.4
Slate, granite / Schiefer, Granit / Ardoise, granit / Pizarra, granito	24	40	96	0.8	1.5	3.6	1.1	2.2	5.2
Brick - Ziegel / Brique - Ladrillo	4	17	69	0.6	2.2	6.7	0.5	2.6	10
" with 30 % red mud / " mit 30 % Rotschlamm / " avec 30 % boue rouge / " con 30 % de barro rojo		13			5			5	
Pumice - Bimsstein / Pierre ponce / Piedra pomez	13	24	30	0.7	2.2	3.6	1.1	2.3	4.6
Slag-stone / Schlackensteine / Scories / Piedra de escorias	3	9	16	1.2	2.2	3.2	0.6	2.8	5.6
Cement - Zement / Ciment - Cemento	0.5	<4	7	0.3	<1.4	5.3	0.3	<1.4	5.2
Gypsum, nat.-Naturgips / Gypse naturel / Yeso natural	0.7	2.4	5		<0.7			<0.5	
Gypsum, techn. / Technischer Gips / Gypse techn. / Yeso artificial técnico	0.8	<2	6	7	14	28		<0.5	
Flagstone-Fliesen / Carrelage - Baldosas	5	13	31	0.6	1.7	2.7	0.7	1.9	4.9

Lit.: 1. Schmier, H.: Jahresbericht Bundesgesundheitsamt, Berlin
Bundesministerium des Innern 1973

9.9 Typical dose values in radiation protection
    Typische Dosiswerte im Strahlenschutz
    Valeurs des doses typiques en radioprotection
    Valores típicos de dosis en protección

1. Dose limits for the total population and for professionally exposed persons, in whole-body and partial irradiation - Dosisgrenzwerte für die Gesamtbevölkerung und die beruflich Strahlenexpo-
   nierten bei Ganz- und Teilkörperbestrahlungen - Limites de dose
   pour l'ensemble de la population et pour les travailleurs profes-
   sionnellement exposés lors d'irradiations totales ou partielles -
   Dosis límites para la población total y para personas afectadas
   de exposición por razones profesionales, radiación corporal total
   y parcial

       See page - Siehe Seite - Voir page - Ver página 212

2. Symptoms following a single total-body exposure
   Symptome bei einmaliger Ganzkörperbestrahlung
   Symptômes suivant une irradiation totale unique
   Síntomas a consecuencia de una exposición unica
   del cuerpo total

       Initial symptoms - Erste Symptome - Symptômes
       initiaux - Primeros síntomas   >50 rad

       Life-threatening radiation sickness - Lebensbedrohliche
       Strahlenkrankheit - Maladie des irradiations menaçant
       la vie - Enfermedad radioactiva con peligro mortal   >200 rad

       50 % lethal dose for man - 50 % Letaldosis/Mensch
       Dose létale 50 % chez l'homme - 50 % dosis letal
       para el hombre (LD_{50}) 350 rad

       Gastrointestinal death, which cannot be
       arrested even by bone marrow transplantation
       Gastrointestinaler Strahlentod, der auch durch
       Knochenmarktransplantation nicht aufzuhalten ist
       Mort intestinal ne pouvant être évitée même avec
       une greffe de moelle
       Muerte radioactiva gastrointestinal que no se puede
       detener incluso con trasplante de médula ósea   >10000 rad

3. Natural background radiation - Höhe der natürlichen
   Strahlenbelastung - Irradiation naturelle - Nivel de
   carga radioactiva ambiental

       Cosmic radiation at sea level - Höhenstrahlung in
       Meereshöhe - Rayonnement cosmique au niveau de la
       mer - Radiación cósmica al nivel del mar   2 µR/h

       Environmental radiation above sedimentary rocks,
       limestone and sand - Umgebungsstrahlung über Sediment-
       oder Kalkstein und Sand - Irradiation d'ambiance au
       dessus d'un terrain sédimentaire, de calcaire, et
       de sable - Radiación ambiental sobre piedra sedimen-
       taria o calcárea y arena   2-5 µR/h

       Same above volcanic rock - Desgl. über vulkanischem
       Gestein - Idem au-dessus de roches volcaniques -
       Idem sobre roca volcánica   10-25 µR/h

Zones with exceptionally high background radioactivity
Zonen mit besonders hohem Strahlenuntergrund
Zônes ayant une radioactivité specialement élevée
Zonas con radiación de fondo especialmente elevada 1)
(Neendakara/Kerala - Guarapari-Brasil) $<300~\mu R/h$
(Yearly doses - Jahresdosen - Doses annuelles -
Dosis anuales mR/a $\approx \mu$R/h x 10)

4. Incorporated natural radionuclides - Inkorporierte
   natürliche Radionuklide - Radionucléides naturels
   incoporés - Radionúclidos naturales incoporados 1)

   ^{14}C (Whole body - Ganzkörper - Corps entier -
       Totalidad del cuerpo)   1.6 mrem/a

   ^{40}K (Whole body - Ganzkörper - Corps entier -
       Totalidad del cuerpo)   10-20 mrem/a

   ^{210}Po (Bone - Knochen - Os - Huesos)   14 mrem/a

   ^{222}Rn (Whole body - Ganzkörper - Corps entier -
       Totalidad del cuerpo)   2 mrem/a

   ^{222}Rn (Lungs - Lungen - Poumons - Pulmones)   150 mrem/a

   ^{226}Ra (Whole body - Ganzkörper - Corps entier -
       (Totalidad del cuerpo)   3-5 mrem/a

   ^{226}Ra (Bone - Knochen - Os - Huesos)   35 mrem/a

5. Levels of genetically significant doses from man made
   exposures - Genetisch signifikante Dosen aus künst-
   lichen Strahlenquellen - Dose génétique importante
   provenant des sources de rayonnement artificielles -
   Dosis geneticamente significantes a partir de fuentes
   des radiación artificiales 1)

   Fall out 1975   2-4 mrem/a

   Medicine - Medizin - Médecine - Medicina
   (Developed countries - Industrialisierte Länder -
   Pays développés - Paises desarrollados)

   Diagnostic radionuclides   30-50 mrad/a

   Radiation therapy   2-3 mrad/a

   Diagnostic isotopes   0.3-1 mrad/a

   Radioactivity in consumer goods - Radioaktivität
   in Verbrauchsgütern - Radioactivité dans les biens
   de consommation - Radioactividad en productos de
   consumo $<$ 1-2 mrad/a

   Nuclear power - Kernkraft - Centrales nucléaires -
   Potencia nuclear (1975) $<$ 1 mrad/a

   Idem expected - Erwartet - Idem, attendu -
   Predicción (2000)   1-3 mrad/a

   Average exposure of X-ray diagnosticians in Germany
   Mittlere Exposition von Röntgendiagnostikern in
   Deutschland - Irradiation moyenne des radiologistes
   en Allemagne - Exposición media de rayos X por médicos
   diagnósticos en Alemania   160 mrad/a

6. Radiation risk after whole-body irradiation with 1 rem
   Strahlenrisiko nach Ganzkörperbestrahlung mit 1 rem
   Risque dûe à l'irradiation du corps entier avec 1 rem
   Riesgo por exposición del cuerpo total de 1 rem

Leukaemia	1:100 000
Carcinogenesis	1: 10 000

7. Blackening of photographic emulsions - Schwärzung von
   fotografischen Emulsionen - Noircissement des émulsiones
   photographiques - Ennegrecimiento de emulsiones
   fotográficas

   See page - Siehe Seite - Voir page - Ver página 184

8. Dosis which can be detected by solid-state dosimeters
   Dosen, die mit Festkörperdosimetern festgestellt
   werden können - Doses pouvant être mesurées par des
   détecteurs à l'état solide - Dosis detectables con
   dosímetros sólidos 2)

Change of color - Verfärbung - Modification de la couleur - Cambio de color	1 kR-100 MR
Photoluminescence (PLD)	10 mR-10 kR
Thermoluminescence (TLD)	50 µR-1 MR
Exo electron emission (EED)	10 µR-100 R

9. Polimerisation of plastics - Polimerisation von
   Kunststoffen - Polimérisation des plastiques -
   Polimerización de plásticos   100-1000 krad

10. Radiation resistance of building materials
    Strahlenfestigkeit von Baustoffen - Résistance
    à l'irradiation des matériaux de construction -
    Resistencia a la radiación de materiales

Plastics - Kunststoffe - Plastiques - Plásticos	10^7-10^{10} rad
Ceramics - Keramische Stoffe - Céramiques - Materiales cerámicos	$10^{10}-10^{14}$ rad
Metals - Metalle - Métaux - Metales	$10^{15}-10^{20}$ rad

Lit.: 1. UNSCEAR: Report of the United Nations, Scientific Committee
         on the Effects of Atomic Radiation, Off. Rec. XXVII Session
         Suppl. No. 25 (A/8725), New York 1972
      2. UNSCEAR: Ionizing Radiation: Levels and Effects, Vol. I
         Levels, New York 1972
      3. BEIR-Report: The Effects on Populations of Exposure to Low
         Levels of Ionizing Radiation, Nat. Acad. of Sciences
      4. GROSSE-SCHULTE, M. in E. SCHRÜFER: Strahlung und Strahlen-
         meßtechnik in Kernkraftwerken, Berlin: Elitera 1974
      5. BECKER, K., SCHARMANN, A.: Einführung in die Festkörper-
         dosimetrie, 56, Thiemig: München 1975

10. Subject index

10. Sachverzeichnis

233

10. Index

10. Indice

Related Titles

J. Gershon-Cohen: **Atlas of Mammography**

W. Wenz: **Abdominal Angiography**

S. Wende, E. Zieler, N. Nakayama: **Celebral Magnification Angiography.**
Physical Basis and Clinical Results

S. Takahashi, S. Sakuma: **Magnification Radiography**

T. Nomura: **Atlas of Cerebral Angiography**

Angiography/Scintigraphy. Symposium of the European Association
of Radiology, Mainz, 1–3 October. 1970, Editor: L. Diethelm

Advances in Cerebral Angiography. Anatomy – Stereotaxy – Embolization –
Computerized Axial Tomography. INSERM-Symposium, Marseille,
May 13–16, 1975. Editor: G. Salamon

Encyclopedia of Medical Radiology/Handbuch der medizinischen Radiologie
In 19 volumes (approx. 52 subvolumes) with contributions in German and
English. Further information upon request

N. Hassani: **Ultrasonography of the Upper Abdomen**

W. A. McAlpine: **Heart and Coronary Arteries.** An Anatomical Atlas for Clinical
Diagnosis, Radiological Investigation, and Surgical Treatment

Radiological Exploration of the Ventricles and Subarachnoid Space.
By G. Ruggiero et al.

G. Salamon, Y. P. Huang: **Radiologic Anatomy of the Brain**

A. Wackenheim: **Roentgen Diagnosis of the Craniovertebral Region**

Biological Aspects of Radiation Protection. Proceedings of the International
Symposium, Kyoto, October 1969. Editors: T. Sugahara, O. Hug

Springer-Verlag Berlin Heidelberg New York

Related Titles

H. Dertinger, H. Jung: **Molecular Radiation Biology.** The Action of Ionizing Radiation on Elementary Biological Objects (Heidelberg Science Library, Vol. 12)

Frontiers of Nuclear Medicine/Aktuelle Nuklearmedizin. Editor: W. Horst

W. A. Fuchs, J. W. Davidson, H. W. Fischer: **Lymphography in Cancer** (Recent Results in Cancer Research, Vol. 23)

K. Kawai, H. Tanaka: **Differential Diagnosis of Gastric Diseases**

A. S. Takahashi: **An Atlas of Axial Transverse Tomography and its Clinical Application**

A. Wackenheim, J. P. Braun: **Angiography of the Mesencephalon.** Normal and Pathological Findings

Journals

Neuroradiology
Organ of the European Society of Neuroradiology

Pediatric Radiology

Radiation and Environmental Biophysics
Fundamentals and Applications

Biophysics of Structure and Mechanism

Medical Progress through Technology

Springer-Verlag Berlin Heidelberg New York